MEDICAL RADIOLOGY

Diagnostic Imaging

Editors:
A. L. Baert, Leuven
M. Knauth, Göttingen
K. Sartor, Heidelberg

S. Peer · G. Bodner (Eds.)

High-Resolution Sonography of the Peripheral Nervous System

2nd Revised Edition

With Contributions by

G. Bodner · H. Gruber · S. Kiechl · P. Kovacs · S. Peer · H. Piza-Katzer

Foreword by

A. L. Baert

With 207 Figures in 402 Separate Illustrations, 76 in Color and 6 Tables

Springer

Siegfried Peer, MD
Professor, Department of Radiology
Section for Diagnostic and
Interventional Sonography
Innsbruck Medical University
Anichstrasse 35
6020 Innsbruck
Austria

Gerd Bodner, MD
Professor, Department of Radiology
St. Bernards Hospital
Europort 1–4
Gibraltar

Medical Radiology · Diagnostic Imaging and Radiation Oncology
Series Editors:
A. L. Baert · L. W. Brady · H.-P. Heilmann · M. Knauth · M. Molls · C. Nieder · K. Sartor

Continuation of Handbuch der medizinischen Radiologie
Encyclopedia of Medical Radiology

ISBN 978-3-642-08036-4 eISBN 978-3-540-49084-5
DOI 10.1007/49084-5

Medical Radiology · Diagnostic Imaging and Radiation Oncology ISSN 0942-5373

Cover design and Layout: Verlagsservice Teichmann, 69256 Mauer

Printed on acid-free paper

9 8 7 6 5 4 3 2 1 0

springer.com

Foreword

Technological progress in hard- and software of ultrasound equipment for clinical use has been tremendous in recent years.

Exquisite morphological visualisation of soft tissues and related pathology is now possible in clinical daily routine work. Periarticular anatomy and pathology of ligaments, bursae or tendons can now be depicted with unprecedented precision by sonography. This technique provides important support for better management of patients affected by trauma or diseases of the locomotor system.

The important role of high resolution sonography in the visualisation and management of traumatic or tumoral conditions of the peripheral nervous system is less well known.

This volume provides an excellent and comprehensive overview of our current knowledge in this emerging field of radiological imaging. It is the result of considerable original sonographic research by the authors in close collaboration with colleagues from several other disciplines including anatomists, neurologists and surgeons.

Dr. S. Peer and Dr. G. Bodner are internationally renowned pioneers in the new area of peripheral nerve sonography and their book is based on extensive personal experience and exhaustive study of the existing literature on the topic. I would like to congratulate them on this outstanding work.

I am confident that this superbly illustrated volume is a very timely and well needed work and that it will find great interest among radiologists, neurologists and specialists in reconstructive and plastic surgery, as well as among trauma surgeons and all those involved in rehabilitation medicine. I sincerely hope that it will meet with the same success among readers as the previous volumes published in this series.

Leuven

Albert L. Baert

Preface

Contrary to our initial expectations, the first edition of this book was a huge success and very quickly sold out. This was somewhat surprising, since it covers only a very narrow segment of radiology in general and sonography in particular.

We received a lot of feedback on the first edition - mostly positive - from various medical professionals and we realized that there is a growing interest in peripheral nerve sonography, not only among radiologists, but more so among neurologists, orthopedic and plastic surgeons and traumatologists. Many of these people told us that they feel sonography fills a gap in their daily diagnostic regime by providing a quick and reliable diagnosis for a variety of peripheral nerve diseases. For many of these, other imaging methods yield only dismal results and/or are expensive, time consuming and uncomfortable for the patient.

Much of the feedback we received, together with new insights into various aspects of nerve sonography – gained either from in-house research or from the growing international scientific community dedicated to this method – went into this second edition. In addition to scientific progress, scanner and especially transducer technology has evolved further, prompting us to replace all anatomical, and as many as possible of the clinical sonograms for state of the art high resolution images in this second edition.

It would not have been possible to achieve this without the help of several people, none of whom may go unmentioned: Special thanks go to the series editor, Prof. Albert Baert, for his trust and confidence in our work, and who immediately agreed when asked about a possible second edition. Also, we would like to express our thanks to the editorial staff of Springer Verlag (especially Mrs. Ursula Davis) for their contribution to the editing and production of this volume.

Innsbruck — Siegfried Peer
Gibraltar — Gerd Bogner

Contents

High Resolution Sonography of the Peripheral Nervous System: General Considerations and Technical Concept

Siegfried Peer

CONTENTS

S. Peer, MD
Professor, Department of Radiology, Section for Diagnostic and Interventional Sonography, Innsbruck Medical University, Anichstrasse 35, 6020 Innsbruck, Austria

1.1 Introduction to High Resolution Sonography of the Peripheral Nervous System

In 1988 Radiology published Bruno Fornage's report on the feasibility of sonographic imaging of peripheral nerves (Fornage 1988). At that time he used an ALOKA 210-DX scanner (which is meanwhile hardly found in museums) with a 5–7.5 MHz linear array transducer and with his report opened up a new field of sonographic imaging. In the first edition of our book we mentioned the technical developments in sonography, which were achieved since this event and until now only 4 years have passed. Nevertheless the technical success story of sonography has continued and will certainly do so in the future. Meanwhile, high resolution transducers of up to 17 MHz are a must for imaging of superficial nerves and dedicated artifact reduction software is a standard tool in almost every modern ultrasound scanner. This has changed the role of sonography in musculoskeletal diagnosis in general, and for inspection of the peripheral nerve sonography may meanwhile really be regarded as the number one imaging modality. The spectrum of peripheral nerve disease entities accessible to sonography has since the first edition of this book also broadened, but still there are white spots on the map, which warrant further research.

Besides being cheap and commonly available, sonography spares the patient from ionizing radiation and is an interactive and non-discomforting method, which makes it first choice from a patient's viewpoint. In this paragraph a short overview of the historical development of sonography of the peripheral nervous system, the rationale for the widespread use of sonography in the work-up of patients with peripheral nerve disease, the technical requisites for performance of nerve sonography and the basic image features of peripheral nerves on sonography will be given.

1.1.1 Historical Development of Peripheral Nerve Sonography

As already mentioned, the first report on the feasibility of peripheral nerve sonography was presented by Fornage (1988). This report also demonstrated the typical tubular structure of peripheral nerves with a speckled internal appearance for the first time. Fornage also stated that the identification of a nerve is facilitated by identification of surrounding anatomic landmarks. Besides this, Fornage focused more on the identification and differential diagnosis of peripheral nerve tumors. How technical aspects hampered the more widespread introduction of this newly presented method into clinical routine may be realized if we imagine that it took 3 more years for the first report to appear in the literature concerned with direct evaluation of a single peripheral nerve (the sciatic nerve, which is the largest peripheral nerve in the body), for an attempt on sonographic diagnosis of various disease entities such as nerve compression and trauma as well as for a first report on the appearance of a surgically reconstructed nerve (Graif et al. 1991). One of the first evaluations of special disease entities in the peripheral nervous system with sonography was published shortly thereafter and concentrated on the diagnosis of carpal tunnel disease (Buchberger et al. 1991). While Buchberger and coworkers were able to show the potential of sonography for the differential diagnosis of this common disease entity, sonography did not gain wide acceptance. In their work they correlated the presence of carpal tunnel disease with flattening of the median nerve on sonography (Fig. 1.1a,b), but to go deeper into the ultrastructure of the impaired nerve was beyond the abilities of their equipment.

Silvestri et al. (1995) presented a basic report on the ultrastructural sonographic/histological correlation of peripheral nerves and for the first time reported the meanwhile commonly known criteria which aid in the differentiation of nerves and tendons. While nerves consist of multiple hypoechoic nodular (transverse scan plane) or continuous longitudinal structures (sagittal scan plane) with a thin echoic stroma (Fig. 1.2a,b), small discontinuous hyperechoic speckles interspersed with hypoechoic elements represent the typical appearance of tendons (Fig. 1.2a). With angulation of the scanhead a tendon changes markedly from hyperechoic to a more hypoechoic appearance, while the echotexture of a peripheral nerve is influenced to a much lesser extent (Fig. 1.3a,b).

Since then, various reports in the literature underlined the high potential of sonography for imaging of peripheral nerve diseases (Martinoli et al. 1996; Chiou et al. 1998; Bodner et al. 1999; Peer et al. 2001, 2002; Gruber et al. 2003, 2005, 2007). We already stated this in the first edition of this book, but what has happened since? We realized some interesting developments: if you perform a literature research on papers related with peripheral nerve sonography you find about 10 articles concerned with ultrasound guided anesthesia or nerve stimulation for every article concerned with the clinical application of nerve sonography. Nevertheless among the latter are some interesting new developments, such as the application of diagnostic sonography on the diagnosis of vasculitic neuropathy (Takao et al. 2007), multifocal motor neuropathy (Beekmann et al. 2005), functional studies (Altinok et al. 2004) or the ultrastructural definition of nerve tumors (Gruber et al. 2007). Like we stated in the first edition, the application of sonography to the diagnosis

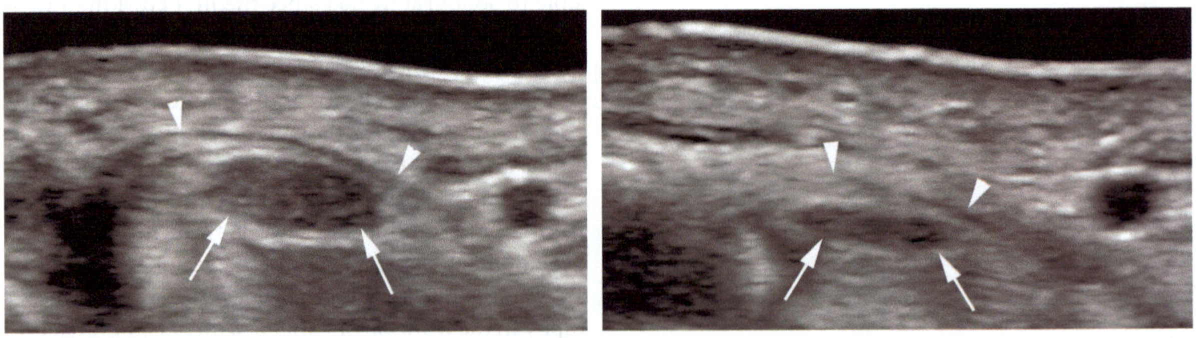

Fig. 1.1a,b. Transverse sonograms through proximal (**a**) (*arrowheads* = flexor retinaculum) and distal (**b**) carpal tunnel in a patient with carpal tunnel disease. In the proximal carpal tunnel the median nerve (*small arrows*) is enlarged because of edema with loss of fascicular echotexture. There is marked flattening of the nerve in the distal carpal tunnel

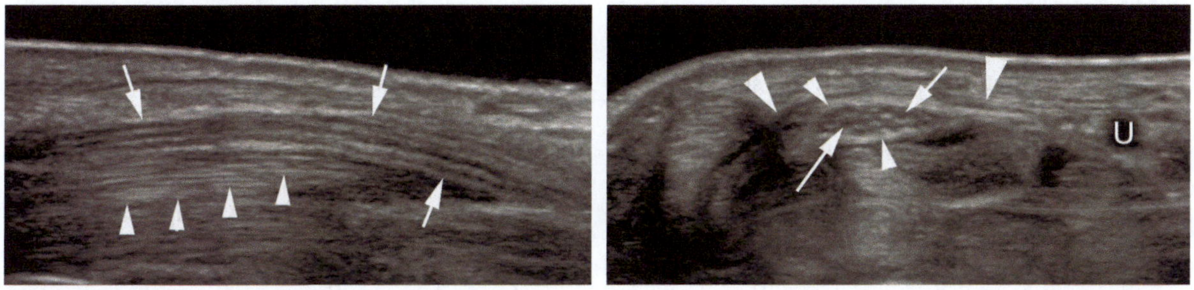

Fig. 1.2. a Longitudinal sonogram of the wrist in a healthy volunteer demonstrating typical appearance of peripheral nerve (*arrows* = median nerve) with continuous hypoechoic longitudinal elements (fascicle groups) interspersed with echoic peri- and epineurium and tendons (discontinuous hyperechoic speckles = *arrowheads*). **b** Transverse sonogram showing dotted appearance of normal nerve with multiple rounded hypoechoic fascicle groups (*arrows*) surrounded by hyperechoic peri- and epineurium (*small arrowheads*). *U* = ulnar artery, large arrowheads = flexor retinaculum

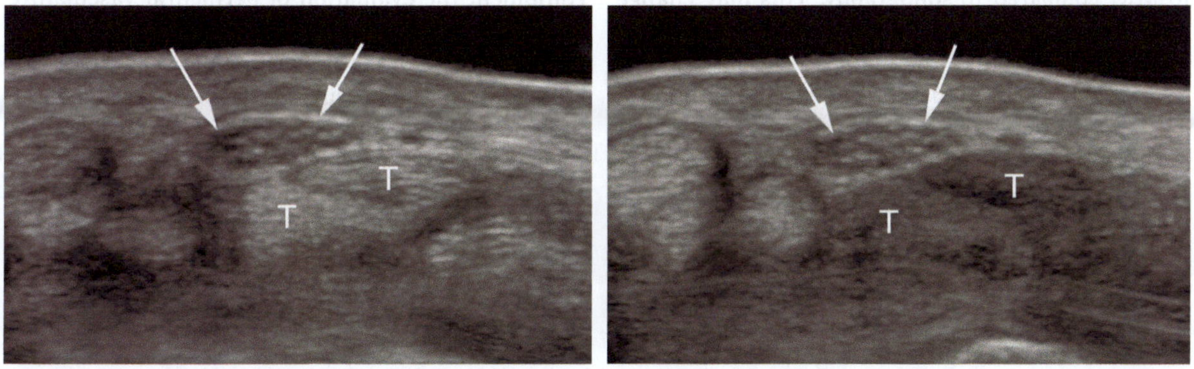

Fig. 1.3a,b. Transverse sonogram through median nerve at level of the wrist with different angulation of scanhead in images **a** and **b** Note markedly changing echotexture of tendons (*T*) with rather consistent echotexture of nerve (*arrows*)

of peripheral nerve diseases is still limited to a few centers around the world but interest in this method is constantly rising, mainly in non-radiologists, i.e., in neurologists, anesthetists, orthopedic and plastic surgeons, traumatologists and other professionals involved in the diagnosis and treatment of peripheral nerve diseases. Walker et al. (2004) presents a review of the current status of nerve and muscle ultrasound and states "ultrasound is an ideal tool for the clinical and research investigation of normal and diseased nerve and muscle" and "it will likely assume a more significant role in these areas, as those most able to exploit its potential, clinical neurophysiologists and neuromuscular physicians, incorporate its use at the bedside". I think we are not far from this becoming reality.

1.1.2 Why Sonography of the Peripheral Nervous System?

Sonography is user dependent, difficult to perform (imagine the complex regional anatomy) and not widely accepted – so why should we use it?

From an imaging point of view this question is, in our opinion, easily answered. There is no real alternative! The only thing we might possibly think of is MRI, but the reader who has already been involved with magnetic resonance imaging of peripheral nerve disease will agree that MRI of peripheral nerves – despite MRI's high soft tissue contrast and multiplanar capabilities – is often less than satisfying. The basic problem with MRI lies in the only subtle contrast differences of nerves and surrounding tissues (Fig. 1.4a,b) and besides this the resolution of MRI is still far below that of sonography. We stated this in the first edition and so far – despite ongoing progress in MRI techniques – this statement is still valid.

While with bigger nerves surrounded by fat the nerve and its ultrastructure may be accessible to MRI (Filler et al. 1996), the visualization of small nerves is limited. Only with small high resolution surface coils and special imaging sequences may the fascicular pattern of a small peripheral nerve be visualized with MRI (Fig. 1.5), although at the expense of a small field of view and only for nerves lying close to the skin surface.

Therefore, besides the lower resolution which limits MRI to imaging of bigger nerves only, above all the ultrastructure of nerves is not as easily accessible to MRI compared to sonography. This may change with the advent of new ultra-high field 3.0-Tesla clinical MR-scanners and this may be proven with correlative studies, but today MRI is second in line regarding anatomic and pathophysiologic analysis of peripheral nerves. Another reason for the low impact of MRI for diagnosis of peripheral nerve disease is the oblique course of nerves in the extremities – while it is easy to follow a nerve with a sonographic scan, this is difficult to accomplish with MRI. The use of 3-D sequences and advanced postprocessing may be a choice with MRI, but this is highly time consuming. In this regard the only region where MRI may challenge sonography is the examination of the brachial or sacral plexus (Hayes et al. 1997; Gierada and Erikson 1993; Gierada et al. 1993; Blake et al. 1996), and if we look at the MRI literature concerned with imaging of peripheral nerves, this is the main topic of interest (besides the differential diagnosis of peripheral nerve tumors), but despite limitations in the diagnosis of radicular avulsions the peripheral parts of the plexus are much more easily assessed with sonography compared to MRI. An important asset of MRI in the evaluation of peripheral nerves is the possibility to acquire images after intravenous administration of gadolinium contrast agents, which may add some information regarding nerve inflammation or hyperperfusion and inflammatory edema in neuritis or chronic nerve compression. The same information will probably be gained with color Doppler and power Doppler sonography of peripheral nerves, but there are no data in the literature on the value of Doppler techniques for diagnosis. Nevertheless, with modern equipment the evaluation of perineural vasculature is certainly within reach. In this regard some promise may also lie in the application of sonographic microbubble contrast agents for the investigation of the peripheral nerve, but to date there are no literature reports on this technique.

Besides the problems with MRI, there are other reasons which advocate sonography of peripheral nerves and one lies in the limitations of electrodiagnostic methods, which will be discussed in more detail later in this book. While electrodiagnosis is able to confirm definitely and in many cases localize a nerve lesion, to define the nature of the underlying pathology is often beyond its reach. The latter however is important information for planning of treatment and may in many cases be gained from careful sonographic evaluation.

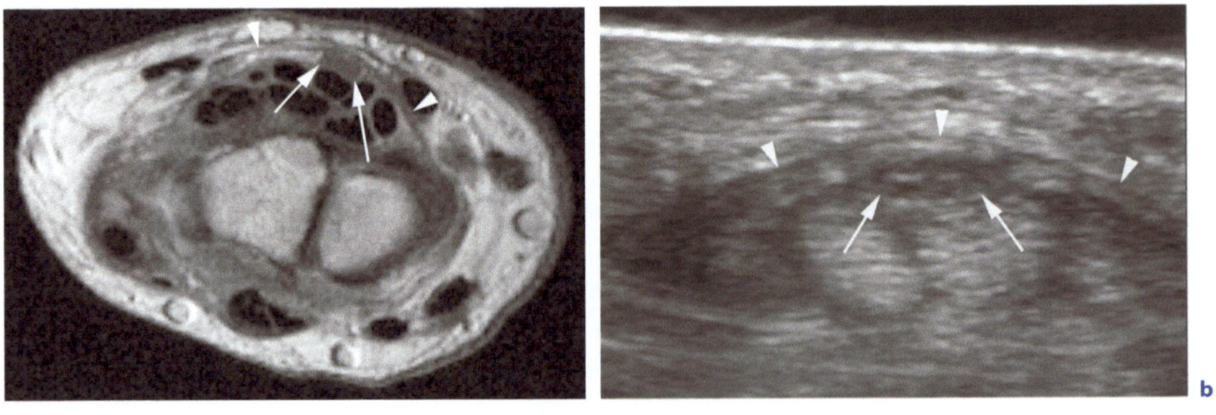

Fig. 1.4a,b. Transverse T1 weighted MR-image (**a**) and sonogram (**b**) through median nerve (*arrows*) at level of the carpal tunnel. Note slight flattening of median nerve (*arrows*) underneath the flexor retinaculum (*arrowheads*). While the median nerve is only faintly visible in the MR-image acquired with a normal surface coil, the outer margin of the nerve and its inner structure is readily visualized in the sonogram – thickening of flexor retinaculum (*arrowheads*) is easily assessed in the sonogram, while hardly identified in the MR-image

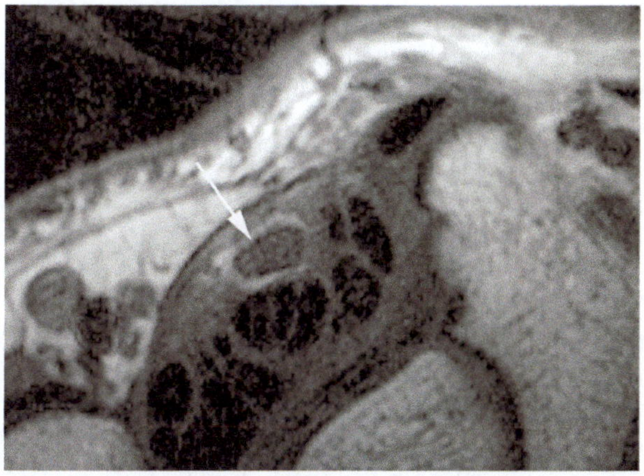

Fig. 1.5. Transverse high resolution MR-image of median nerve at wrist level (*arrow*) with small loop type surface coil. Note visibility of nerve fascicles inside median nerve but at the expense of increased noise

Another favorable aspect of sonography lies in the interactive nature of the procedure. The examination is easily tailored to the exact location of a patients pain sensations, areas of hypersensitivity (such as a Tinel-Sign) or areas of possible coexisting trauma. It is quick and lacks the discomfort caused by pricking with needles during electrodiagnostic studies or by positioning in MRI. The possible interaction between examiner and patient with the ability to react on clues in a patients history is a further important asset and so is the possibility to perform a functional ultrasound examination tailored to the investigation of reduced nerve mobility (an important sign in compression neuropathies or postoperative patients with scar formation) or nerve dislocation (in snapping triceps syndrome for example).

1.2 Ultrasound Scanner Hard- and Software Requirements

The results which may be obtained in the diagnosis of peripheral nerve disease with sonography are to a large extent influenced by the availability of state of the art equipment. We will not touch on the basic physical principals of sonographic imaging but only on some of the aspects which are especially critical for nerve examinations. In addition, some of the newer developments which are likely to influence clinical practice will be discussed in the next paragraphs.

1.2.1 Hardware Requirements

Imaging with ultrasound depends on both contrast and resolution. With current clinically available transducers imaging of superficial structures is possible at frequencies of up to 17 MHz, which results in an axial resolution of 250–500 microns. Spatial detail in a sonogram, however, is not only dependent on axial resolution but also on resolution within the scan plane (lateral resolution) and the slice thickness (elevation). High frequency broad band linear array transducers are state of the art for small parts sonography and "sine qua non" as far as imaging of peripheral nerves is concerned. Future transducer development will supply us with multidimensional arrays, which will further enhance resolution in the elevation plane with reduction of clutter (Wildes et al. 1997). For peripheral nerve sonography the choice of transducer depends on the anatomical region to be examined, but generally speaking a high frequency scanhead is preferred wherever possible. For superficially lying nerves, therefore, a 15–17-MHz transducer is highly recommended, while for deep lying nerves such as the sciatic nerve a 12- or even 9-MHz linear array transducer may be more feasible.

Until recently peripheral nerve sonography asked for a high end state of the art ultrasound scanner, which meant a quite bulky machine stuffed with several kilos of fancy electronics. This may change in the near future, as several ultrasound companies provide us with portable systems that almost reach the image quality of their bigger counterparts. In particular the concept of zone-sonography is very promising in this regard – we were unable to apply it to a bigger sample of routine patients, but first impressions of nerve examinations we performed on a Zonare-Z.One portable ultrasound system (Zonare Medical Systems, CA, USA) were very impressive. Thus the "sonographic stethoscope", with the potential to perform bedside nerve sonography easily, seems not far away.

1.2.2 Software Requirements

1.2.2.1 Compound Imaging

While real time compound imaging is common in modalities such as CT and MR, ultrasound systems have traditionally lacked the power needed for acquisition and processing of such images in real time. New developments in the processing speed of ultrasound scanners made this technique available. The computed beam steering software is used to steer the ultrasound beam "off axis", which results in several lines of sight to a sonographic target within a single scan. With powerful signal processing software the single image frames are accurately rendered according to the visualized geometry and updated in real time. A schematic illustration of compound imaging technology is given in Figure 1.6.

The clinical value of compound imaging lies in the reduction of sonographic artifacts (Piccoli et al. 2000). By scanning from different view angles, different artifact patterns are produced in the single views. By averaging these single frames into a compound image, artifacts such as speckle, noise, dropout or refractive shadowing are suppressed. This results in a sharper delineation of tissue interfaces and better discrimination of lesions against their background, as well as improvement of image contrast and detail resolution (Fig. 1.7a–h).

In addition the mode of compound technology applied can be changed by the examiner to either target the beam to enhanced resolution of regions of interest or to a quicker overview mode.

1.2.2.2 Tissue Harmonic Imaging

Tissue harmonic imaging is another sonographic technology which improves image quality of sonograms in state of the art scanners (Burns et al. 1996). The fundamental ultrasound signal transmitted to the tissue consists of a broad band of low frequencies. The transmitted signal resonates off tissue in the body at a frequency twice the transmitted signal and only these high frequency resonant signals are detected by the scan head. In a normal scan the signal travels into the body and back to the transducer again, which means the ultrasound beam passes tissue interfaces twice and therefore artifacts increase. With tissue harmonic imaging the detected signal (which is produced by resonance inside the tissue) travels only one way towards the transducer, which means it is not at-

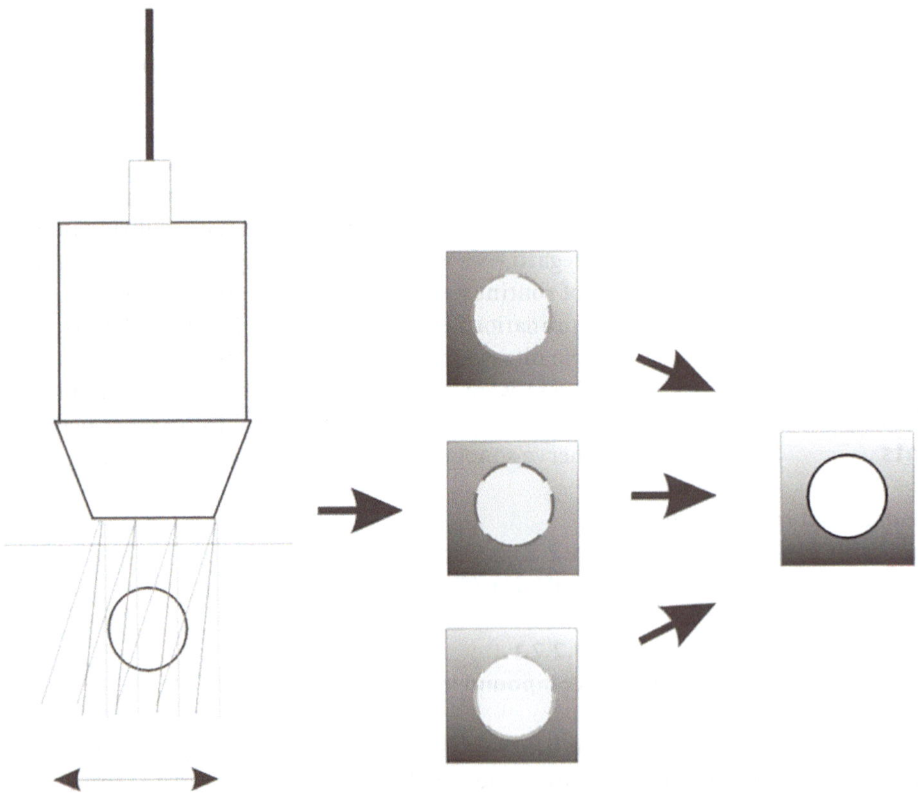

Fig. 1.6. Schematic drawing of compound imaging technology. A structure is scanned from different view angles by use of beam steering, which results in single images with somewhat different representation of the structure and different artifact pattern. The latter are added in real time format and a "compound image" is reconstructed

tenuated by round-trip travel through tissue and therefore we experience a reduction of artifacts. In addition, resonance at object margins (the main source of artifacts in a normal scan) is of very low energy and therefore does not contribute to the image to the same extent compared to conventional imaging. Despite good results in other areas of small part sonography, the value of tissue harmonic imaging for ultrasound of the peripheral nerve is limited by adding only little improvement to the image quality (Fig. 1.7a–h).

We might add that somehow the value of this technology for B-mode imaging has in our opinion been surpassed by compound imaging and other artifact reduction techniques, which are certainly the better choice for imaging of peripheral nerves.

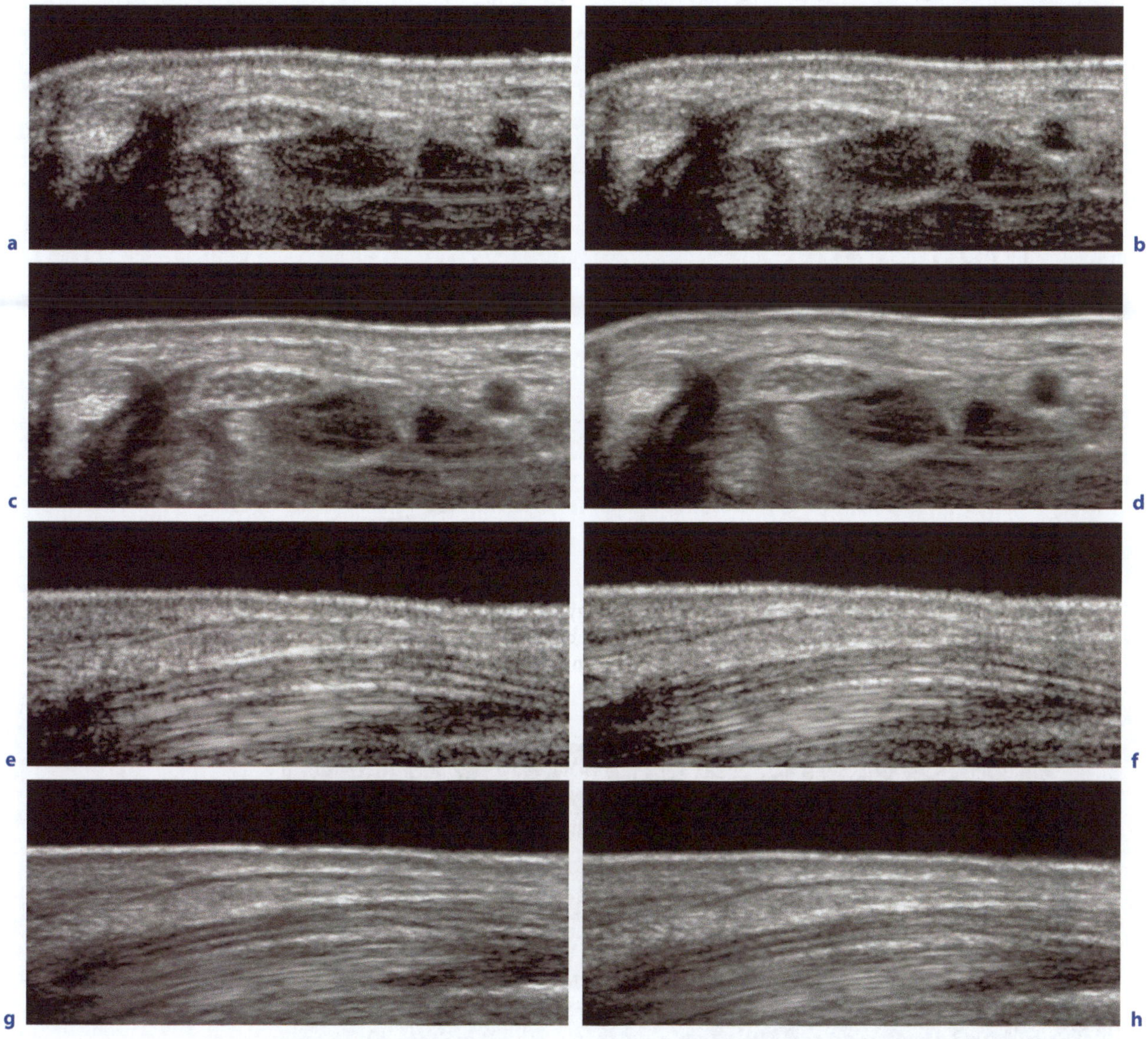

Fig. 1.7a–h. Transverse and longitudinal sonograms through median nerve at wrist level in normal B-mode (**a,e**), with addition of tissue harmonic imaging (**b,f**), image compounding (**c,g**) and compound imaging + artifact reduction software (XRES[W]) (**d,h**). Addition of tissue harmonic imaging adds only little improvement of image quality; nevertheless the interfaces between individual fascicular bundles inside the median nerve as well as between the nerve and its surroundings are sharper (**b,f**). Note marked improvement of image sharpness, with better definition of tissue borders and an overall reduction of image noise in images acquired in compound mode (**c,g**) and the additional effect of artifact reduction software (**d,h**) especially on image homogeneity

1.2.2.3 Extended Field of View Imaging

With extended field of view imaging (also called panoramic imaging by some manufacturers) the possibility of sonography to display longitudinal structures is enhanced. With this technique the transducer is swept longitudinally along a structure of interest and dedicated software reconstructs an image out of single scans along the course of the sweep (Fig. 1.8).

Newer technology not only uses pixel information at the edge of the scan for reconstruction of the panoramic image but, by application of a pattern recognition algorithm, extracts information of every entire single scan and adds it to the final panoramic view. This technique not only yields better image quality in panoramic scans but also enables the user to redirect his sweep easily by moving back and forth with continuous update of the panoramic view and without having to restart his sweep. Once the panoramic image has been acquired, dedicated software allows one to refine the image further by application of various postprocessing tools such as magnification, rotation, etc.! With high end ultrasound scanners, panoramic imaging is also possible in compound mode, which adds the benefit of improved resolution (Fig. 1.9).

From a clinical point of view, panoramic imaging is mainly a tool for documentation or presentation of results, which – as far as the peripheral nerve is concerned – may add valuable information for the planning of surgical interventions.

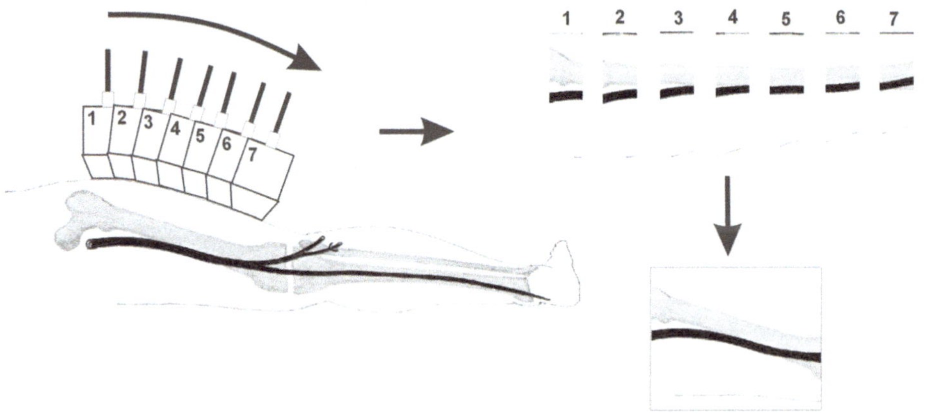

Fig. 1.8. Schematic drawing of panoramic imaging technology. Continuous single images (as wide as the width of the scanhead allows) acquired at a fixed distance during a longitudinal sweep along an anatomic structure are summed up and reconstructed to a "panoramic view" of the structures along the whole sweep

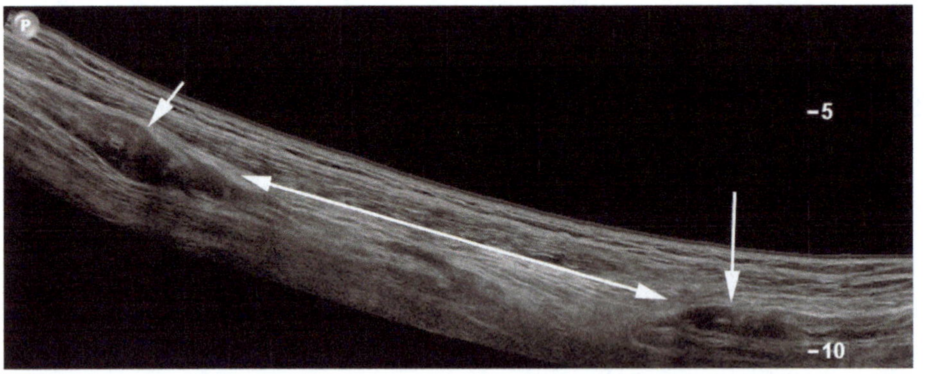

Fig. 1.9. Panoramic image in compound mode along the dorsal aspect of the thigh in a patient with traumatic rupture of the sciatic nerve. The proximal (*short arrow*) and distal (*long arrow*) nerve stump is demonstrated with marked swelling and disorganized blind ending neural elements in the proximal stump due to neuroma formation. The panoramic image nicely demonstrates the huge gap in between the nerve stumps measuring almost 20 cm (*double headed arrow*)

1.2.2.4 High Resolution Imaging

Within the last few years, different ultrasound companies have tried to enhance the quality of sonographic images with the introduction of various image processing tools. One of these tools, which was recently introduced into clinical practice, is XRES™ by ATL/Philips. This pattern analysis tool takes place at the pixel level. It looks at the predominate patterns within groups of pixels and brings them into order. By emphasizing patterns and de-emphasizing speckle, noise and clutter, XRES™ imaging enhances diagnostic features by reducing artifacts, improving visibility of existing tissue texture patterns and bringing margins and borders into greater definition. One of the special aspects of XRES™ imaging is the ability to combine this tool with image compounding, thus adding further to image improvement by significantly improving the visibility of the tissue patterns that are detected in SonoCT mode, so that the patterns are more vivid and clearly evident. Images take on a significant depth they did not have before. There is also an overall sharpening of margins, borders and tissue interfaces. A comparison of XRES™ imaging with simple compound imaging is given in Figure 1.7a–h.

1.3 General Technique of Sonographic Nerve Examination

In this section we will focus briefly on some general recommendations for examination of peripheral nerves and documentation of results.

1.3.1 Anatomic Considerations

Nerves are round or ovoid structures with a complex internal architecture resembling a cable. The single nerve fibers are composed of axons, myelin sheaths and Schwann cells. Several of these fibers form a single fascicle and a variable number of such fascicles combine into an individual nerve. The size of a single fascicle and the numbers of fascicles included in a nerve depend on the size of the nerve, its location (distance from its origin, type and tightness of surrounding tissue) and its type (amount of motor or sensory elements). The single nerve fascicles and the nerve as a whole are interwoven and surrounded by supportive tissue, the interfascicular and superficial epineurium. The latter two may be identified to a certain extent with sonography, while the connective tissue comprising the endoneurium, which surrounds a single nerve fiber and the perineurium surrounding a fascicle are very thin membranes and below sonographic resolution. Sonographic histological correlations first presented by Silvestri et al. (1995) confirmed the ability of sonography to identify the fascicular architecture of a peripheral nerve: On transverse sonograms a normal nerve shows an echotexture of tiny hypoechoic dots – the fascicles (or fascicle groups) – embedded in a hyperechoic meshwork of connective tissue – the interfascicular and superficial epineurium (Fig. 1.10).

However, we must note that the overall number of fascicles visualized on sonograms does not correspond exactly with the real number of fascicles in a nerve, probably due to coalescence of some adjacent fascicles in a single image. Another reason for this lies in the somewhat interwoven course of nerve fascicles, and this is also why the analysis of the continuity of single fascicles in traumatic lesions or after nerve repair has to be done with caution. We must also be aware that a reduction of transducer frequency leads to a diminishing number of individual fascicles, which may be visualized in the image.

In contrast to tendons, nerves are highly vascularized structures, with small vessels running along the perineurium and supplying a tight microvascular plexus. With newer high resolution transducers and improved color Doppler sensitivity these vessels may quite frequently be visualized with color or power Doppler (Fig. 1.11). To date we do not know the amount of vasculature or which Doppler-waveforms are characteristic for an individual normal nerve, as studies with sonoanatomic correlation of a nerve's vascular state are lacking. Thus, if vessels are visible inside a nerve with color Doppler, we have to keep in mind that this may be a normal finding, and not immediately think of pathologic hypervascularization – although we do know that an altered vascular state is an important aspect of the pathophysiology of nerve entrapment and compression injuries (Dahlin 1991). In our experience a detected increase of vessels inside and along the surface of a nerve, when compared with the normal, clinically unsuspicious contralateral nerve, may be a sign of a hypervascular state in a postoperative nerve (Fig. 1.12), in perineuritis or in a nerve proximal to a compression. However, this is still preliminary experience with lack of confirmation in larger statistically controlled clinical trials.

Variations of the course or shape of peripheral nerves are known and may be studied with sonography. Not uncommonly, variations of the median nerve may be found in the carpal tunnel, for example, which should be known to the examiner as they may be important in a preoperative setting. In 20% of asymptomatic volunteers a unilateral persistent median artery and in 6% a bilateral persistent median artery is detectable with sonography (GASSNER et al. 2002), which may associated with a high division or a bifid median nerve (Fig. 1.13a,b).

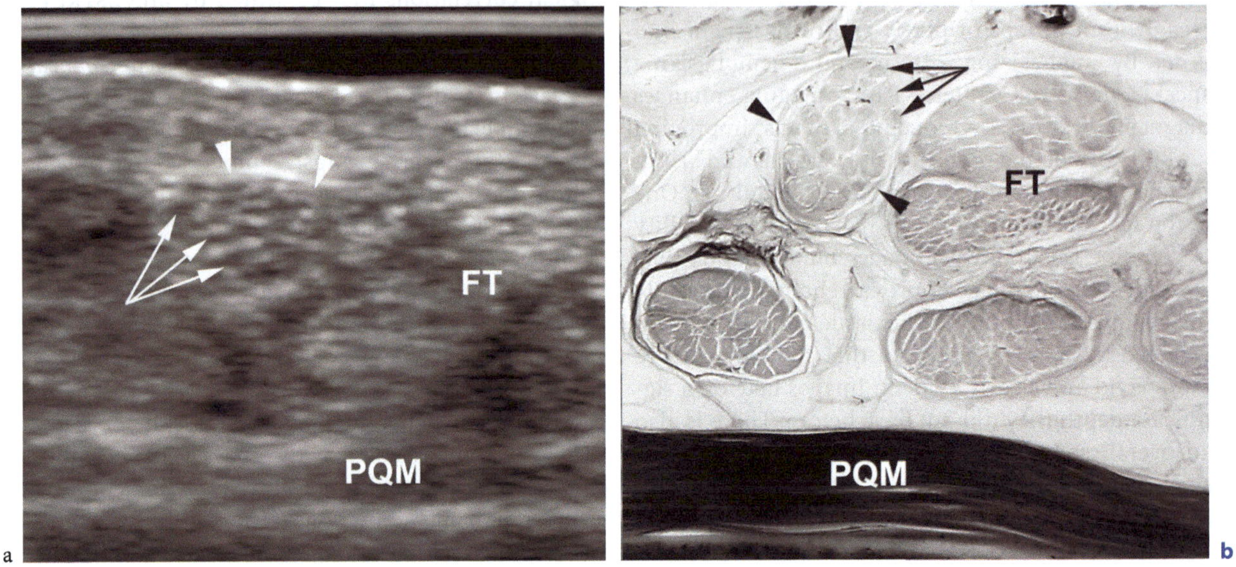

Fig. 1.10a,b. Corresponding transverse sonogram (**a**) and plastinated anatomic section (**b**) of cadaver specimen acquired at distal forearm. The median nerve fascicles (*arrows*) are clearly visualized as hypoechoic nodular structures in the sonogram. Note also visualization of superficial epineurium (*arrowheads*) with tiny extensions between the nerve fascicles. *PQM* = pronator quadratus muscle, *FT* = flexor tendons

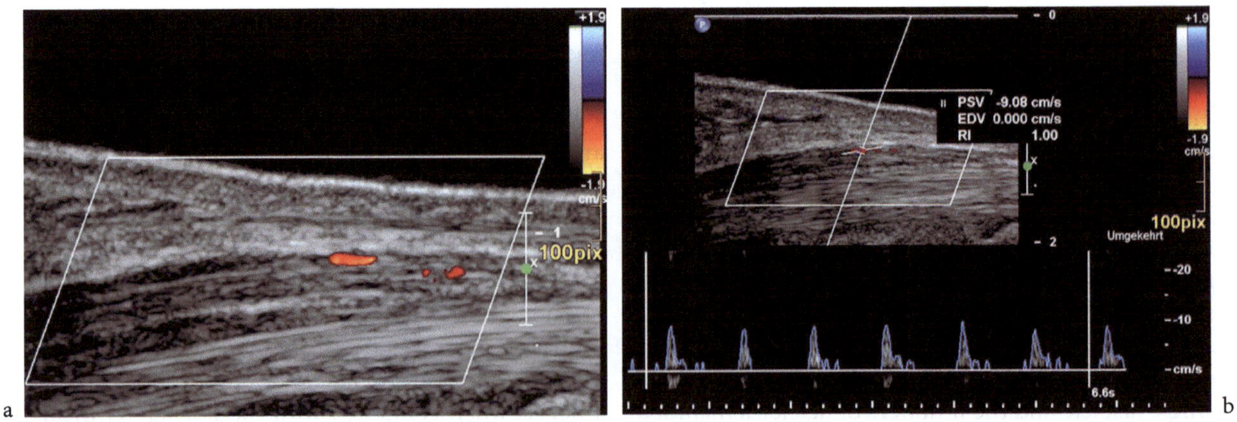

Fig. 1.11a,b. Longitudinal color Doppler sonogram (**a**) along median nerve (*arrowheads*) in a healthy volunteer. A small vessel is identified along the surface (but inside the outer epineurium) of this normal nerve. Spectral wave analysis (**b**) shows a monomorphic high resistance waveform

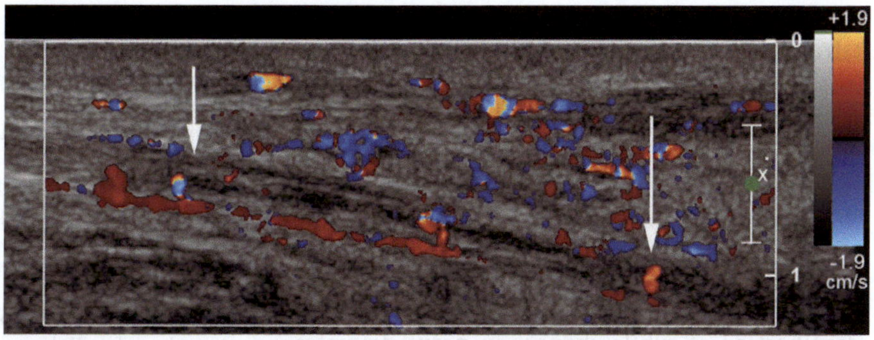

Fig. 1.12. Longitudinal color Doppler sonogram through peroneal nerve in a patient with a compression fracture of the tibial condyle and coexistent peroneal palsy. The peroneal nerve (*arrows*) is continuous surrounded by edema and hematoma and shows marked hypervascularization especially along its surface due to unspecific reactive neuritis

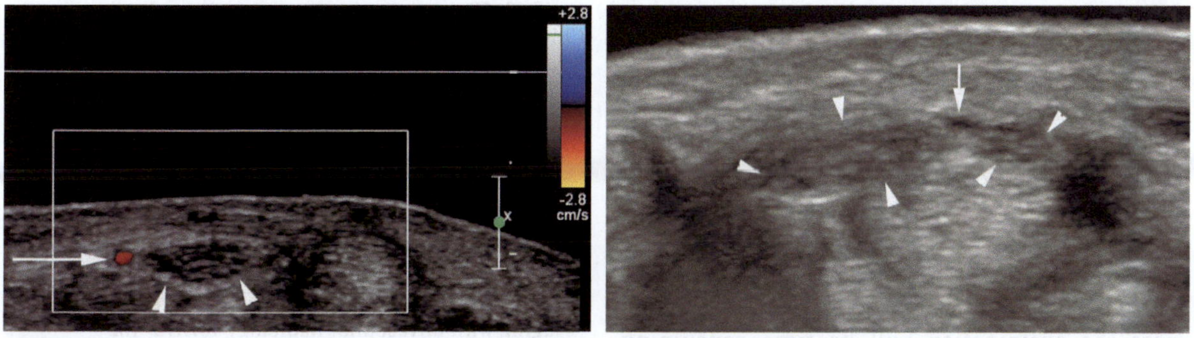

a b

Fig. 1.13. a Transverse color Doppler sonogram through carpal tunnel in a patient with suspected carpal tunnel disease. Single median nerve stem with normal configuration and fascicular texture (*small arrowheads*) is accompanied by a small eccentrically positioned median artery (*arrow*). **b** Transverse sonogram through carpal tunnel in another patient with suspected carpal tunnel disease shows bifid median nerve with a larger radial and a smaller ulnar portion (*arrowheads*) and a interposed median artery (*arrow*)

1.3.2 Nerve Examination

The examination of a peripheral nerve should include transverse and longitudinal scanning. For superficially lying nerves (median nerve) or nerves coursing along bony ridges we generally recommend the use of a stand off gel pad, which improves the contact of the transducer with the skin surface and results in substantial improvement of image quality. The identification of a nerve inside an image scan is easily accomplished if common anatomical landmarks are observed (i.e., the peroneal nerve at the fibular neck, or the tibialis nerve following the course of the posterior tibial artery and veins, etc.) and Chapter 2 will focus extensively on these relationships. For the evaluation of nerve compression syndromes the recommendation is straightforward, as they typically occur in distinct locations along the course of a nerve, i.e., the carpal tunnel, the ulnar sulcus etc.! If a patient's history and/or clinical examination is typical for one of these compressive lesions, the sonographic exam will be tailored to evaluation of the site where the nerve lies close to ligaments, bony ridges or spurs or tight to a bony surface and is followed for 5–10 cm proximal and distal to this area. While transverse scanning is better suited to identifying edematous swelling of nerve fascicles proximal to a compressive lesion, longitudinal scans or panoramic views are better suited to revealing a sudden change in the diameter of a nerve traversing underneath a ligament for example. In cases of unclear or atypical symptoms an attempt to scan the whole course of a nerve, searching for pathology, is to be taken and sometimes it will be necessary to scan even the brachial plexus of the affected side. In these cases we often prefer to identify the nerve at a site where it lies close to the surface or near distinct anatomical landmarks and follow it from there to the level of suspected pathology. This type of examination is highly recommended in cases where the nerve lies inside scar tissue or close to hematomas, as the nerve itself is often rather difficult to distinguish at the level of the lesion in such situations.

Another general recommendation concerns the examination of the nerve at the unaffected side. The diagnosis of nerve pathology is often achieved with identification of subtle changes in nerve diameter or echotexture, which is why we always confirm our local findings in comparison with the contralateral unaffected side. The latter is of utmost importance if measurements of nerve diameters or cross sectional area are used for the identification of a compression syndrome. High inter-individual variations in these measurements exist and a reliable diagnosis of pathology is only possible in correlation with the measurement of the normal contralateral nerve. We will comment on this in other chapters of this book and want to remind the reader that evaluation of the ultrastructure is key for the diagnosis of a peripheral nerve lesion.

Positioning of the patient is another important aspect in sonographic nerve examinations. In some cases the examination will be time consuming, which is why a position that is comfortable to sustain for the patient and at the same time allows for easy access to the region of interest for the sonographer should be sought. In many cases we use supportive cushions or pillows to put a patients extremity in a position which allows easier access to a nerve.

While peripheral nerves may be scanned with normal B-mode sonography, we always use compound imaging and additional artifact reduction software available on the scanner, because of the resulting gain in soft tissue resolution (see above). We further use color or power Doppler in general nerve examinations because of our interest in the vascular situation of a nerve. We highly recommend this for all cases with inflammatory lesions, tumors or postoperative nerves, as the demonstration of increased vascular supply to a nerve (correlation with contralateral nerve!) may have important implications on diagnosis and treatment. For the examination of nerve tumors, color Doppler sonography is absolutely mandatory. In contrast to neurofibromas, schwannomas for example are generally hypervascular lesions, which helps in the differential diagnosis of neurogenic tumors (Gruber et al. 2007).

References

Altinok MT, Baysal O, Karakas HM, Firat AK (2004) Sonographic examination of the carpal tunnel after provocative exercises. J Ultrasound Med 23:1301–1306

Beekman R, van den Berg LH, Franssen H et al. (2005) Ultrasonography shows extensive nerve enlargements in multifocal motor neuropathy. Neurology 65:305–307

Blake LC, Robertson, WD, Hayes CE (1996) Sacral plexus: optimal imaging planes for MR assessment. Radiology 199:767–772

Bodner G, Huber B, Schwabegger A et al. (1999) Sonographic detection of radial nerve entrapment within a humerus fracture. J Ultrasound Med 18:703–706

Buchberger W, Schoen G, Strasser et al. (1991) High resolution ultrasonography of the carpal tunnel. J Ultrasound Med 101:531–537

Burns PN, Powers JE, Hpe SD et al. (1996) Harmonic imaging: principles and preliminary results. Angiology 47:63–69

Chiou HJ, Chou YH, Cheng SP et al. (1998) Cubital tunnel syndrome: diagnosis by high resolution ultrasonography. J Ultrasound Med 17:643–648

Dahlin LB (1991) Aspects on pathophysiology of nerve entrapments and nerve compression injuries. Neurosurg Clin N Am 2:21–29

Filler AG, Kliot M, Howe FA et al. (1996) Application of magnetic resonance neurography in the evaluation of patients with peripheral nerve pathology. J Neurosurg 85:299–309

Fornage BD (1988) Peripheral nerves of the extremities: imaging with ultrasound. Radiology 167:179–182

Gassner E, Schocke M, Peer S, Schwabegger A, Jaschke W, Bodner G (2002) Persistent median artery in the carpal tunnel – color Doppler ultrasonographic findings. J Ultrasound Med 21:455–461

Gierada DS, Erickson SJ (1993) MR imaging of the sacral plexus: abnormal findings. AJR Am J Roentgenol 160:1067–1071

Gierada DS, Erickson SJ, Haughton WM et al. (1993) MR imaging of the sacral plexus: normal findings. AJR Am J Roentgenol 160:1059–1065

Graif M, Seton A, Nerubali J et al. (1991) Sciatic nerve: sonographic evaluation and anatomic pathologic considerations. Radiology 181:405–408

Gruber H, Kovacs P, Peer S, Marth R, Bodner G (2003) The ultrasonographic appearance of the femoral nerve and cases of iatrogenic impairment. J Ultrasound Med 22:163–172

Gruber H, Peer S, Meirer R, Bodner G (2005) Peroneal nerve palsy associated with knee luxation: evaluation by sonography-initial experiences. AJR Am J Roentgenol 185:1119–1125

Gruber H, Glodny B, Bendix N, Tzamkov A, Peer S (2007) High resolution ultrasound of peripheral neurogenic tumors. Eur Radiol (Epub ahead of print)

Hayes CE, Tsuruda JS, Mathis CM, Maravilla KR, Kliot M, Filler AG (1997) Brachial plexus: MR imaging with a dedicated phased array of surface coils. Radiology 203:286–289

Martinoli C, Serafini G, Bianchi S et al. (1996) Ultrasonography of peripheral nerves. J Periph Nerv Syst 1:169–174

Peer S, Bodner G, Meirer R et al. (2001) Evaluation of postoperative peripheral nerve lesions with high resolution ultrasound. AJR Am J Roentgenol 177:415–419

Peer S, Kovacs P, Harpf C et al. (2002) High resolution sonography of lower extremity peripheral nerves: anatomic correlation and spectrum of pathology. J Ultrasound Med 21:315–322

Piccoli C, Merrit CRB, Forsberg F et al. (2000) Real-time compound imaging of the breast. Presented at the Annual meeting of the American Institute of Ultrasound in Medicine, San Francisco CA, April 2000

Silvestri E, Martinoli C, Derchi LE et al. (1995) Echotexture of peripheral nerves: correlation bewteen US and histologic findings and criteria to differentiate tendons. Radiology 197:291–296

Takao I, Masanori K, Takashi W et al. (2007) Ultrasonography of the tibial nerve in vasculitic neuropathy. Muscle Nerve 35:379–382

Walker FO, Cartwright MS, Wiesler ER, Caress J (2004) Ultrasound of nerve and muscle. Clin Neurophysiol 115:495–507

Wildes DG, Chiao RY, Daft CMW et al. (1997) Elevation performance of 1.25D and 1.5D transducer arrays. IEEE Trans Ultrasonics Fer Freq Control 44:1027–1031

Sonographic Anatomy of the Peripheral Nervous System

2

HANNES GRUBER and PETER KOVACS

CONTENTS

One of the major advantages of sonography compared to other modalities for imaging of the soft tissues, such as MRI and CT, is its ability to acquire images in virtually every orientation along the course of a peripheral nerve. This however results in a very complex regional topographic anatomy. Therefore a well-founded knowledge of regional anatomy and topography is an indispensable prerequisite for the sonographic assessment of peripheral nerves. The typical sonographic appearance of nerves must be distinguished from other soft tissue structures and may change substantially depending on the type of surrounding tissue elements. Usually nerves present as longitudinal bands with a mixture of hyperechoic (peri- and epineurium) and hypoechoic elements (fascicle groups) in longitudinal sonograms. In the transverse plane a variable number of hypoechoic dots (fascicle groups) is surrounded by hyperechoic epineurium with hyperechoic septa between the fascicles (SILVESTRI et al. 1995). Even low-flow feeding vessels, called vasa nervorum, can be depicted using color Doppler sonography Figure 2.1a. Usually one small vessel can be found showing arterial flow in pulsed wave Doppler (Fig. 2.1b). In case of inflammation, nerve entrapment or after nerve repair the detectable vessels increase in number and size and show a higher blood flow.

In the following chapter the regional anatomy of nerves, which may be assessed with state of the art sonographic equipment, is demonstrated by correlation of representative sonograms with anatomic cryosections of fresh cadaver specimens. Transverse and longitudinal sonograms in typical locations for peripheral nerve disease were acquired. The sonographic scan planes were marked on the cadaver surface and correlative anatomic cryosections were produced along the skin markings with a fine needle tooth band saw. In this way an exact correlation of paired sonograms and cross-sections was achieved in order to recapitulate topographic relations and to present the normal topographic anatomy of the peripheral nerves. The figures represent typical sonographic scan planes, that are routinely used for clear visualization of peripheral nerves. Special emphasis was laid on the presentation of useful anatomic landmarks that allow for easier recognition of the individual nerves. That is why cutaneous nerves and terminal nerve branches were excluded from the presentation as their detection is very tricky and sometimes only possible in pathological states.

H. GRUBER, MD
Associate Professor, Department of Radiology, Innsbruck Medical University, Anichstrasse 35, 6020 Innsbruck, Austria
P. KOVACS, MD
Department of Radiology, Innsbruck Medical University, Anichstrasse 35, 6020 Innsbruck, Austria

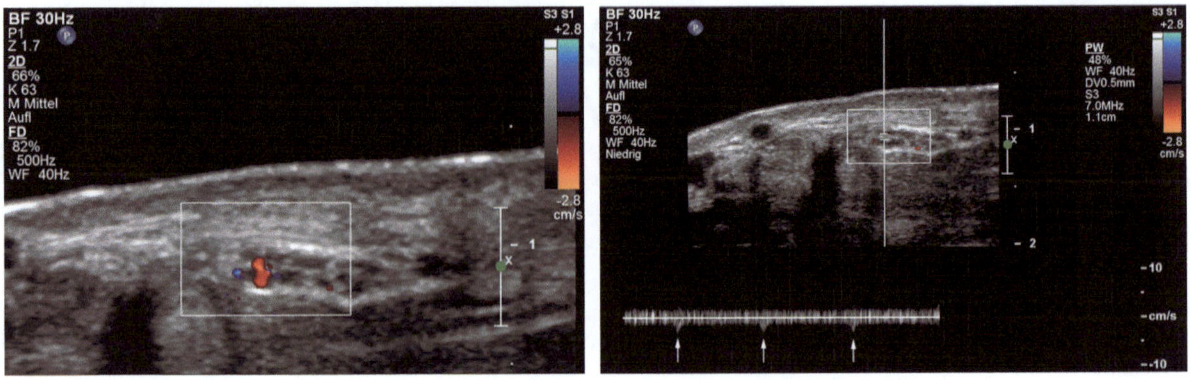

a b

Fig. 2.1a,b. Transverse US scan of the median nerve at the wrist using Color Doppler US (**a**) to depict feeding vessels (vasa nervorum), which are small in size and show low, arterial flow in pulsed wave Doppler (*arrows*) (**b**)

2.1 Sonographic Anatomic Correlation in the Head and Neck Region

2.1.1 Cranial Nerves

The 12 cranial nerve-pairs originate from the brainstem to the mesencephalon and course mainly in small channels inside the bony parts of the neuro- and/or viscerocranium, which is why they are only poorly accessible to sonography. The facial, the accessory and the vagal nerve however may be visualized to a certain extent along their extracranial course. Sonographic imaging, however, is limited by the caliber of the nerves and by influences of surrounding soft tissues, which sometimes impair direct visualization.

The facial nerve (cranial nerve number 7) enters the facial soft tissues at its emission through the stylomastoid foramen of the temporal bone. Consisting completely of motor fibers for viscerocranial muscles (mimic muscles and parts of the chew musculature) it enters directly into the parotid gland, where it usually spreads into two or three main branches. The latter are interconnected by thin nerve fibers forming the so-called parotid plexus. From here the nerve distributes into five nerve-branch-groups (each with one to four branches): the temporal, the zygomatic, the buccal and the marginal mandibular branches as well as one cervical branch (usually anastomosing with branches of the cervical plexus in the superficial cervical ansa).

Sonographic identification of the facial nerve is easiest after its emission from the temporal bone posterior to the perpendicular mandibular branch. Its visualization gets difficult after it enters the parotid gland, where the two or three main branches may only occasionally be visualized with very high-frequency transducers (more than 15 MHz). Within the more ventral parts of the parotid gland nerve branches must be distinguished clearly from the equally hypoechoic minor and major exocrine parotid duct (Fig. 2.2). The latter are always oriented towards the mouth, where they usually end in the region of the premolar teeth of the upper jaw. The terminal peripheral branches of the facial nerve inside the mimic musculature cannot be discerned sufficiently even with state of the art sonographic equipment.

The vagal nerve (cranial nerve number 10) represents the strongest parasympathetic nerve and exits from the jugular foramen where it forms its two ganglia: the superior ganglion (Ganglion jugulare) and the bigger inferior ganglion (Ganglion nodosum). Releasing several branches with several different neuronal qualities, it descends inside a common soft tissue sheath together with the internal jugular vein, the internal carotid artery and more caudal with the common carotid artery.

The vagal nerve is best assessed at the level of the carotid sinus (division of the common carotid artery), where it lies in the posterior triangular space between the slightly offset venous and arterial lumen (Fig. 2.3). The superior cervical sections of the vessels and the nerve lie directly ventral of the sloping anterior scalene muscle. More inferior the vagal nerve directly abuts the cervical prevertebral fascia. Its main stem can be followed with sonography from inframandibular (along a short individual stretch cranial to the hyoid bone) down to the division of the brachiocephalic trunk on the right side and to the origin of the common carotid artery from the aortic arch on the left side. Within the inferior cervical space the detection of the nerve becomes difficult because of interposed fat impairing sonographic contrast.

The two major branches of the vagal nerve (the superior laryngeal and the recurrent laryngeal nerve) may not be clearly visualized with sonography due to their complex course and limited sonographic depth resolution.

The accessory nerve (cranial nerve number 11) being a mere motor nerve also exits from the jugular foramen and hands its internal branch over to the neighboring vagal nerve. The residual external branch (forming the proper accessory nerve) is responsible for the innervation of the sternocleidomastoid and trapezius muscle (Fig. 2.4). In its superior part it lies ventral to the cervical splenius muscle turning onto the lateral surface of the internal jugular vein, usually perforating the superior third of the sternocleidomastoid muscle at a variable height. Its further course follows the medial part of the superior margin of the trapezius muscle, where it may be detected easiest with sonography, before its entrance into the muscle. However, the loose fatty and connective tissue in the lateral cervical region may result in artifacts, which sometimes impair the investigation of the nerve (Bodner et al. 2002).

2.1.2 Cervical and Brachial Plexus

In the fetal period the upper extremity forms paddle-like, being supplied by the according neural segments of the rump wall (metameric segmentation of the vertebrate rump). In later life this ontological specialty finds its expression in the distribution of the sensory dermatomes in relation to the spinal nerves. The annular organization of the dermatomes on the rump wall is continued in a longish fashion in the extremities (segments C3–Th1 for the upper extremity). The order of the axons of the according spinal segments passes through rather complicated combinations and reorganizations compared to the simple distribution of the nerves in the rump wall. This redistribution of the segmental axons mainly takes place at the level of the cervical and brachial plexus, where the individual peripheral nerves of the extremity are formed (Kahle 1991).

The cervical plexus forms out of the ventral roots of the first four spinal nerves (C1–C4). The recombination of the involved axons takes place in the intermuscular soft-tissue resulting in several sensible cutaneous nerves, which are all perforating the lateral superficial cervical fascia at the posterior margin of the sternocleidomastoid muscle to run onward subcutaneously.

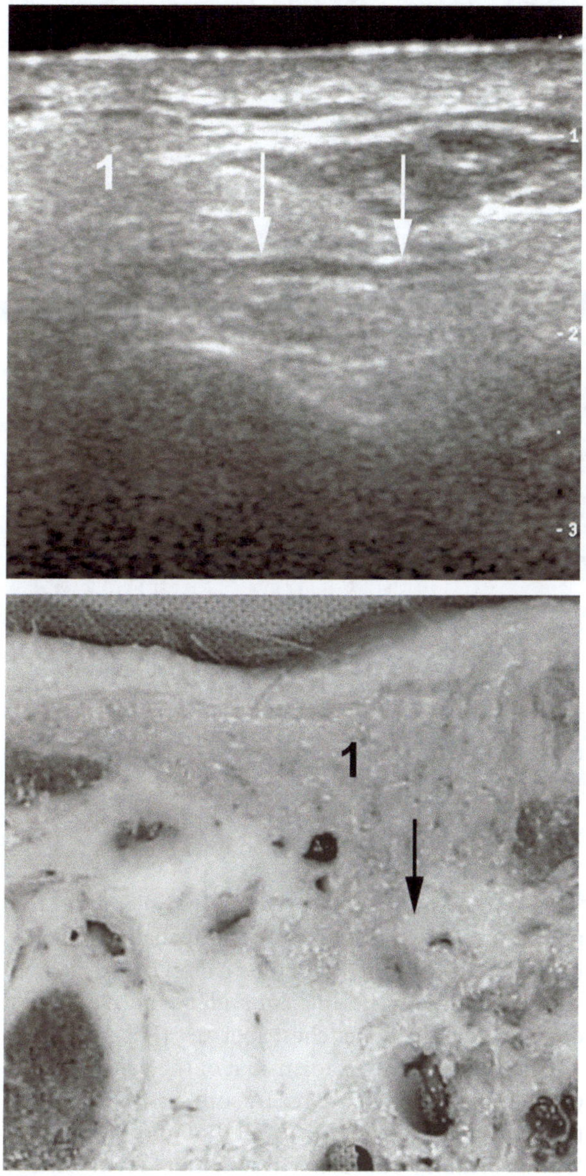

a

b

Fig. 2.2a,b. Longitudinal US scan with corresponding cryosection of facial nerve (*arrows*) in its course within the parotid gland (*1*) with high contrast of the fascicular parts of the nerve to the surrounding glandular tissue

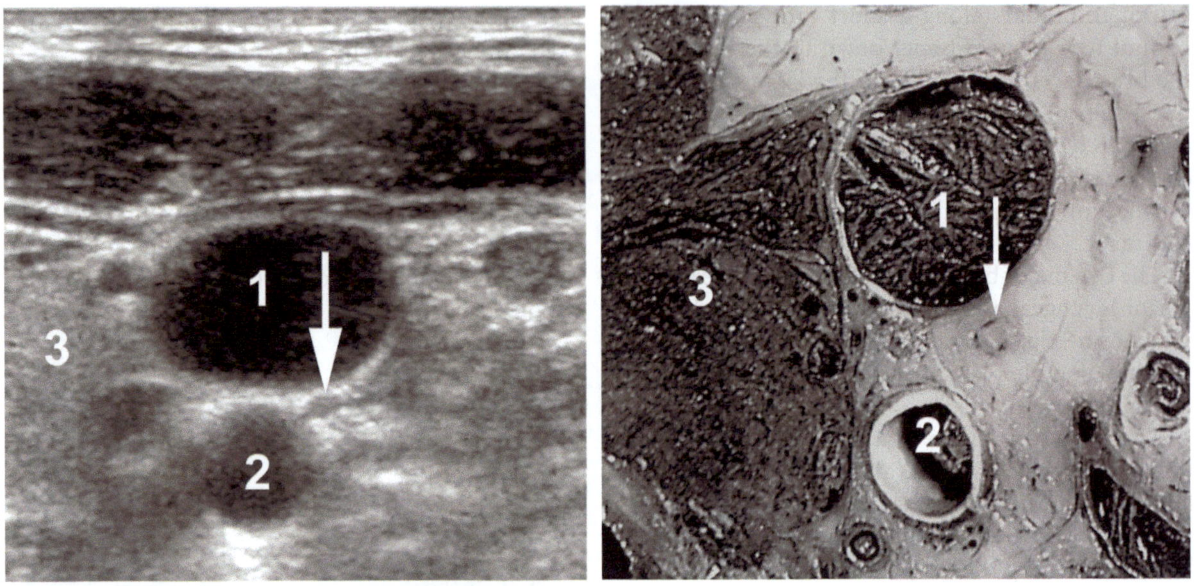

a b

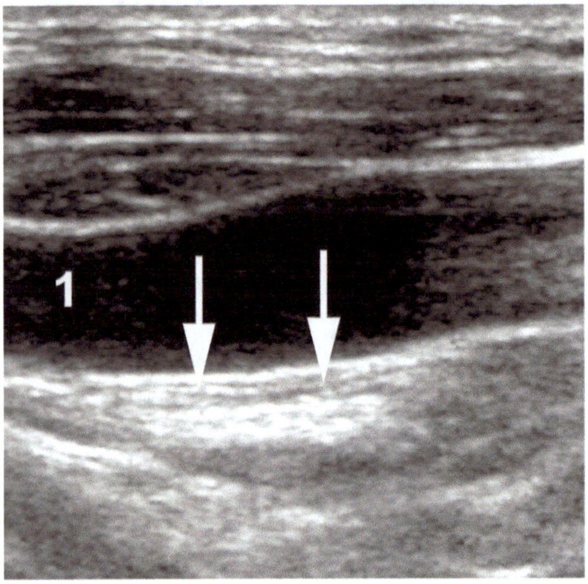

c

Fig. 2.3a–c. Transverse US scan (**a**) with the corresponding cryosection (**b**) showing the vagal nerve (*arrow*) in typical position between the internal jugular vein (*1*) and the common carotid artery (*2*) (thyroid gland *3*). **c** Longitudinal US scan of the vagal nerve (*arrow*) lying adjacent to the internal jugular vein (*1*)

The most important nerve of this plexus is the phrenic nerve, which innervates the ipsilateral hemidiaphragm. It is formed by axons from C3 and C4 and – lying ventral on the anterior scalene muscle – runs downward to the upper chest aperture (Fig. 2.5).

The brachial plexus forms out of the ventral roots of the spinal nerves C5–Th1. Its supra-clavicular section consists of a superior, a medial and an inferior trunk (primary chords). These trunks form within or somewhat lateral to the gap between the anterior and medial scalene muscle (inter-scalene gap). Inferior to the clavicle the three plexus fascicles (medial, lateral and posterior or dorsal) are formed by interchange of axons between the different trunks and they are named according to their relation to the axillary artery (secondary chords). Out of these fascicles the three main nerves of the upper extremity (median, ulnar and radial nerve) as well as the axillary, the musculocutaneous and several cutaneous nerves are formed.

The sonographic identification of the plexus trunks is best achieved in a transverse plane through the interscalene gap, with a slight cranial tilt of the transducer (Fig. 2.6). The three trunks present as hypoechoic nodules positioned on a virtual line from dorso-cranial to ventro-caudal. They are embedded in loose connective and fatty soft tissue and must not be mixed up with small regional lymph nodes on transverse sonograms. Orientation of the probe in a longitudinal plane along the course of the trunks reveals the typical fascicular pattern of peripheral nerves (Yang et al. 1998).

Two distinct nerves leave the plexus trunks at this level: the long thoracic nerve with fibers from the superior and medial trunk and the thoracodorsal nerve with fibers from the medial and inferior trunk. These two nerves are responsible for the lateral, superficial rump muscles (serratus anterior muscle and dorsal latissimus muscle) and run downwards almost perpendicular to each other. The thoracodorsal nerve is in its distal course usually accompanied by a branch of the axillary artery (thoracodorsal artery). Due to only minimal difference in echotexture against the surrounding tissue a clear visualization of these nerves is only achieved in selected cases.

The plexus fascicles in proximity of the axillary artery can be visualized best with an abducted or elevated arm and with the transducer oriented along the course of the axillary artery. The posterior fascicle continues into the axillary and radial nerve, the lateral fascicle together with axons of the medial fascicle (median loop) – after releasing the musculocutaneous nerve directly underneath the clavicle – into the median nerve. The medial fascicle forms the ulnar nerve and the nerves responsible for the sensibility of the medial arm.

a b

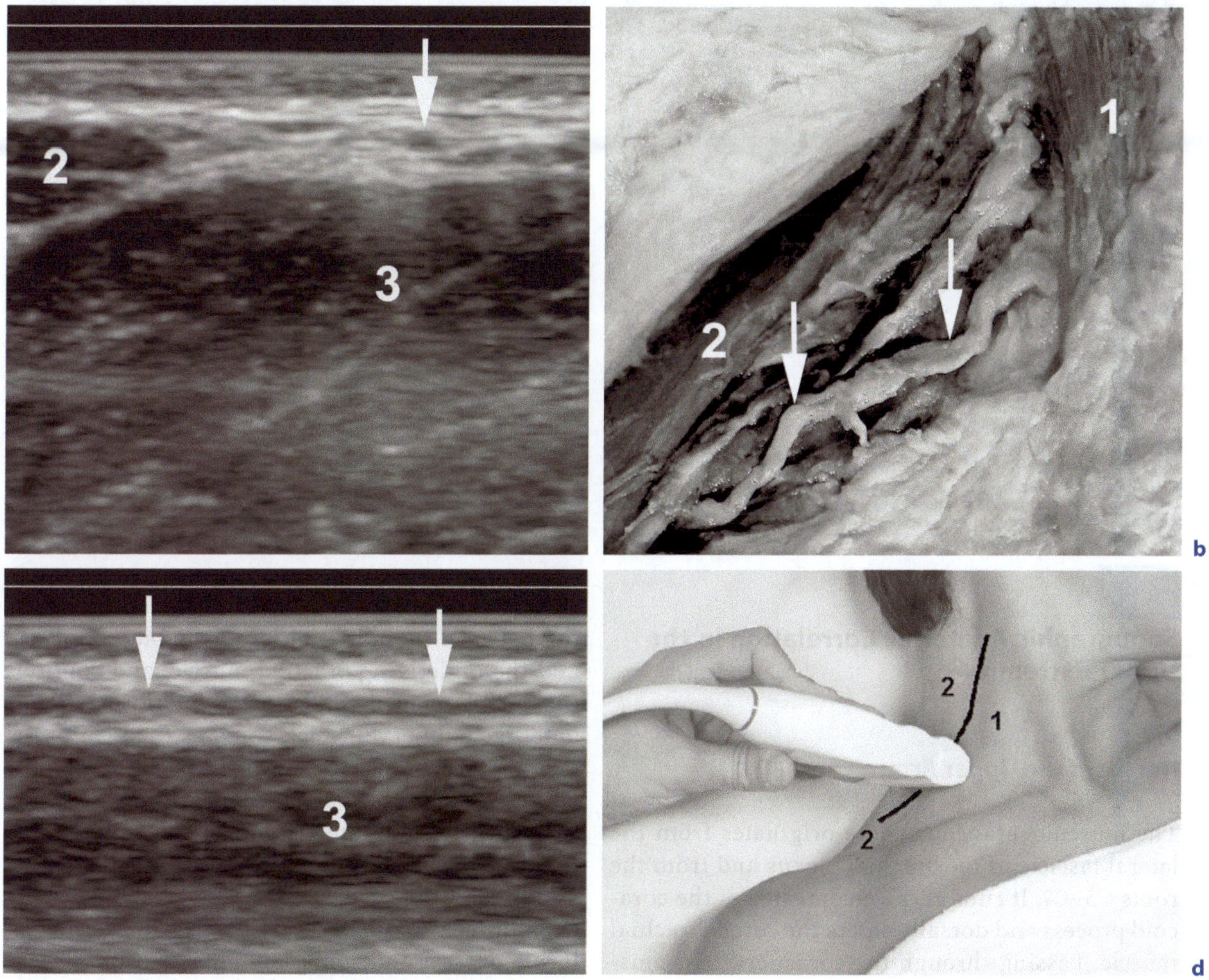

c d

Fig. 2.4a–d. Transverse US scan (**a**) with according anatomical cryosection (**b**) showing the accessory nerve (*arrows*) in its typical topographic situation lying on the scalene muscles (*3*) ventral to the anterior border of the trapezius muscle (*2*) (sternocleidomastoid muscle *1*). **c** Longitudinal US scan according to the course of the accessory nerve (*arrows*) lying on a scalene muscle (*3*). **d** Scheme with the projection of the accessory nerve (*line*) onto the skin surface. Landmarks for identification of scanhead position are the sternocleidomastoid muscle (*1*) and the trapezius muscle (*2*)

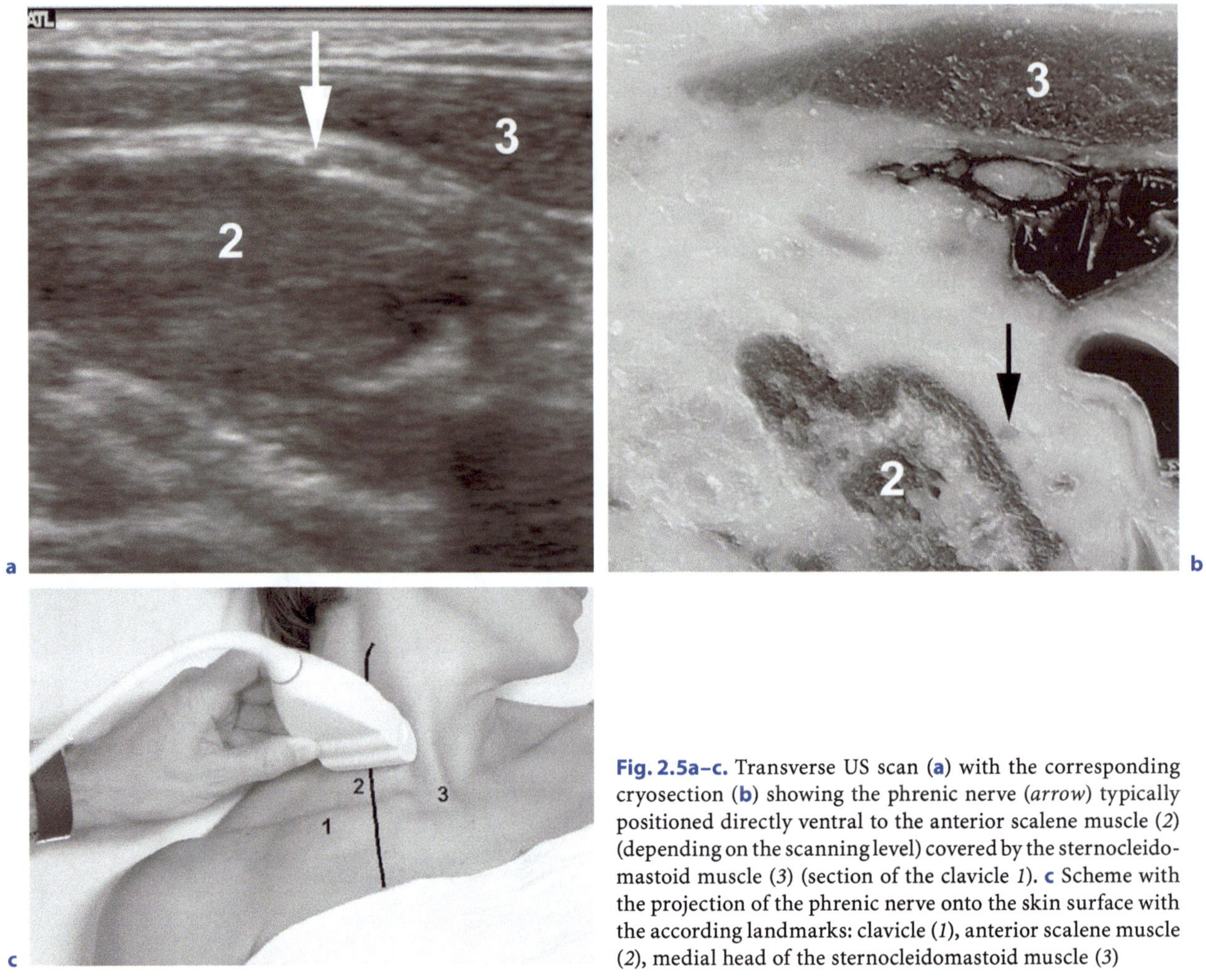

Fig. 2.5a–c. Transverse US scan (**a**) with the corresponding cryosection (**b**) showing the phrenic nerve (*arrow*) typically positioned directly ventral to the anterior scalene muscle (*2*) (depending on the scanning level) covered by the sternocleidomastoid muscle (*3*) (section of the clavicle *1*). **c** Scheme with the projection of the phrenic nerve onto the skin surface with the according landmarks: clavicle (*1*), anterior scalene muscle (*2*), medial head of the sternocleidomastoid muscle (*3*)

2.2 Sonographic Anatomic Correlation in the Upper Extremity

2.2.1 Nerves of the Upper Arm

The musculocutaneous nerve originates from the lateral fascicle of the brachial plexus and from the roots C5–C7. It runs at the medial side of the coracoid process and dorsally enters the coracobrachial muscle. Passing through the coracobrachial muscle the nerve reaches the fascial space between the brachial biceps and the brachial muscle. Usually covered by the muscle belly of the short head of the brachial biceps muscle it heads for the region of the radial epicondyle of the humerus (Fig. 2.7). In this region it comes closer to the surface exiting between the radial onset of the biceps muscle and the underlying brachial muscle, and continuing subcutaneously ends in the lateral cutaneous antebrachial nerve, which supplies the skin of the lateral forearm (sensory branches). The musculocutaneous nerve is a very small nerve and identified easiest with sonography along its course medial to the coracoid process or between the brachial biceps and brachial muscle. From here it may invariably be followed proximally and distally – depending on local contrast and sonographic resolution. It usually is well contrasted by the embedding muscles along a fair distance.

The median nerve is formed out of parts of the lateral and medial fascicle of the brachial plexus (median loop). It runs ventral to the brachial ar-

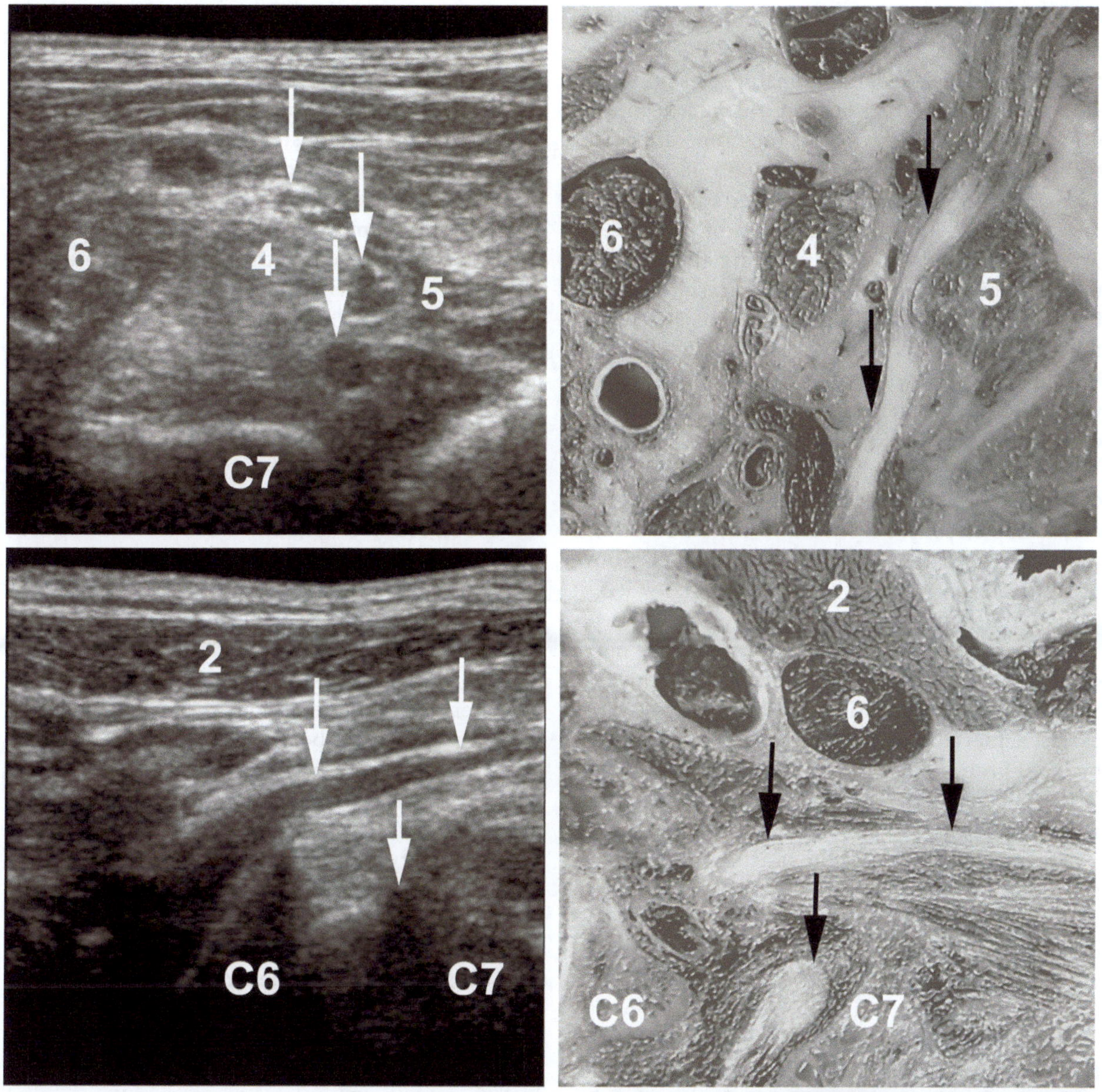

a b c d

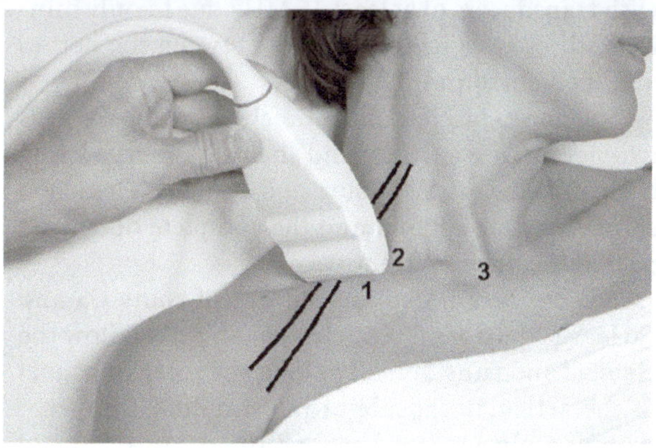

e

Fig. 2.6a–e. Transverse US scan (**a**) with the corresponding cryosection (**b**) showing the roots and trunks of the brachial plexus (*arrows*) between the anterior (*4*) and middle (*5*) scalene muscle in typical topographic relation to the internal jugular vein (*6*) (body of the seventh cervical vertebra *C7*). US scan (**c**) and corresponding cryosection (**d**) according to the course of the roots and the proximal trunks of the brachial plexus (*arrows*) (sternocleidomastoid muscle *2*, internal jugular vein *6* and bodies of the sixth and seventh vertebra *C6*, *C7*). **e** Scheme with the projection of the trunks of the brachial plexus onto the skin surface with the according landmarks: lateral (*2*) and medial (*3*) part of the sternocleidomastoid muscle, clavicle (*1*) tery in the medial bicipital groove directly heading downward to the elbow, where it usually lies in between the two heads of the pronator teres muscle in 95%, between the ulnar head of the muscle and the ulna in 3%, or even perforates the humeral head of the muscle in 2% of cases. The pronator teres muscle is the most proximal muscle supplied by the median nerve. Very seldom the perforation of parts of the pronator teres muscle by the median nerve may lead to a kind of entrapment-syndrome, resulting in an impairment of the ventral forearm muscles. Being the biggest nerve of the upper arm the median nerve is easily identified with sonography along its course within the medial bicipital groove ventral to the brachial artery (Fig. 2.8).

The ulnar nerve as the main branch of the medial fascicle of the brachial plexus (roots C8–Th1) also heads directly downward to the elbow within the medial bicipital groove, and reaches the "groove of the ulnar nerve" (sulcus nervi ulnaris) where it bends around the lower margin of the medial epicondyle of the humerus. In the upper arm the nerve does not release any motor or sensory branches. Sonographic identification of the ulnar nerve is easiest achieved along its course within the medial bicipital groove posterior to the brachial artery, or as the single structure within the groove of the ulnar nerve (Fig. 2.9).

The medial fascicle of the brachial plexus is responsible for two additional sensory nerves supplying the medial skin of the upper extremity: the medial brachial cutaneous and the medial antebrachial cutaneous nerve – both originating from roots from C8 and Th1 and both running downwards epi-fascially and subcutaneously. Sonographic identification of these nerves is only possible in selected cases with transducers of at least 15 MHz due to only minimal differences in echotexture between the nerves and their surroundings.

The dorsal fascicle of the brachial plexus releases two nerves: the axillary and the radial nerve being both mixed nerves (motor and sensory elements) supplying the shoulder and the complete dorsal aspect of the upper extremity.

The axillary nerve formed out of roots C5 and C6 leaves the dorsal fascicle at or slightly below the clavicle and runs dorsally along the inferior aspect of the articular capsule of the shoulder (humeroscapular joint) to bend around the surgical neck of the humerus (collum chirurgicum humeri). It exits the lateral axillary hiatus (foramen axillare laterale, defined laterally by the humerus, proximally by the minor teres muscle, distally by the minor teres muscle and medially by the long head of the triceps muscle) where motor branches take off for the teres muscles. The axillary nerve reaches the deltoid muscle from posterior with several branches for the muscle and additionally provides sensory branches for the skin of the shoulder. A short way after its exit from the dorsal fascicle the axillary nerve is accompanied by the posterior circumflexing artery and veins of the humerus, which supply the deltoid muscle and the muscles at the border of the lateral axillary hiatus. The axillary nerve may sonographically be detected with elevation of the arm in the posterior axillary fold (lateral axillary hiatus). Here it represents a rounded, tubular structure entering the deltoid muscle accompanied by two vessels. From here it may be followed upward to its reunion with the radial nerve in the dorsal fascicle (Fig. 2.10).

The radial nerve (roots of C5–C8) supplies the extensor muscles of the whole upper extremity plus the dorsal skin. It pursues the course of the dorsal fascicle in relation to the axillary and brachial artery. Ventral to the tendinous origin of the dorsal latissimus muscle it bends to the posterior surface of the humerus and continues to the proximal end of the osseous "groove of the radial nerve" (sulcus nervi radialis). It is accompanied by the profound brachial artery and vein. In its spiral course directly at the surface of the humerus between the proximal lateral and distal medial head of the brachial triceps muscle, it reaches the region of the lateral epicondyle where it finally lies at the flexor side of the elbow (cubita) between the brachial and brachioradial muscle. Along its whole course the radial nerve releases motor and sensory branches to the extensor muscles and dorsal skin. The nerve is most easily assessed with sonography in its course within the musculo-osseous channel formed by the bellies of the brachial triceps muscle and the humerus (Fig. 2.11). From this region it may be followed proximally and distally with adherence to the anatomic landmarks mentioned above (axillary/brachial artery, muscular interposition).

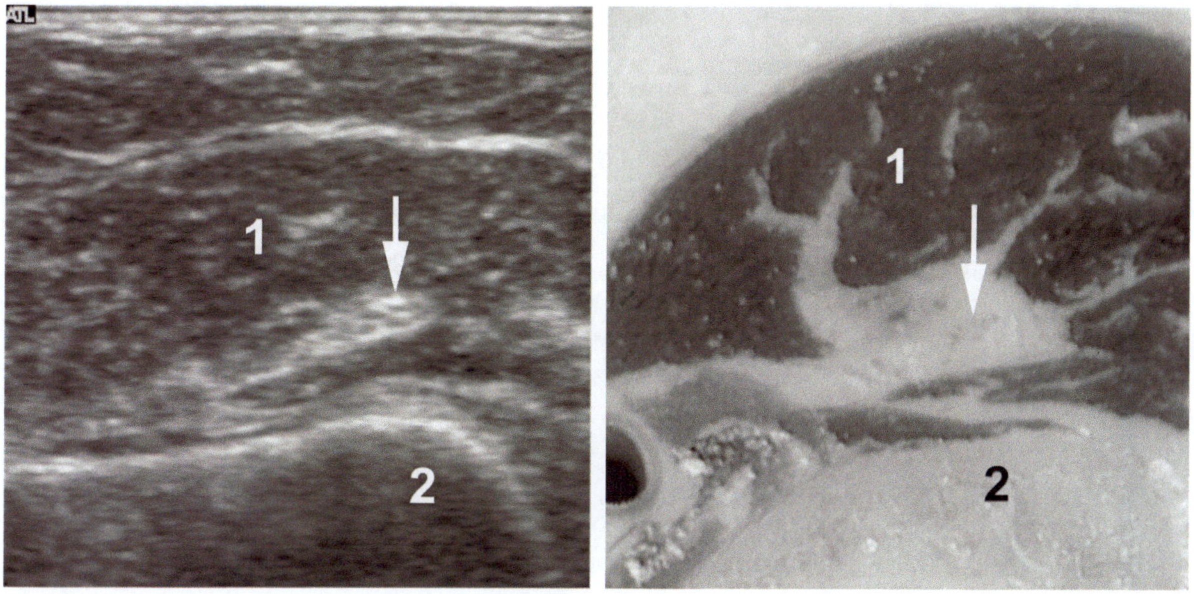

Fig. 2.7a,b. Transverse US scan (**a**) with the corresponding cryosection (**b**) showing the musculocutaneous nerve (*arrow*) lying within the brachial biceps muscle (*1*) ventral to the humerus (*2*)

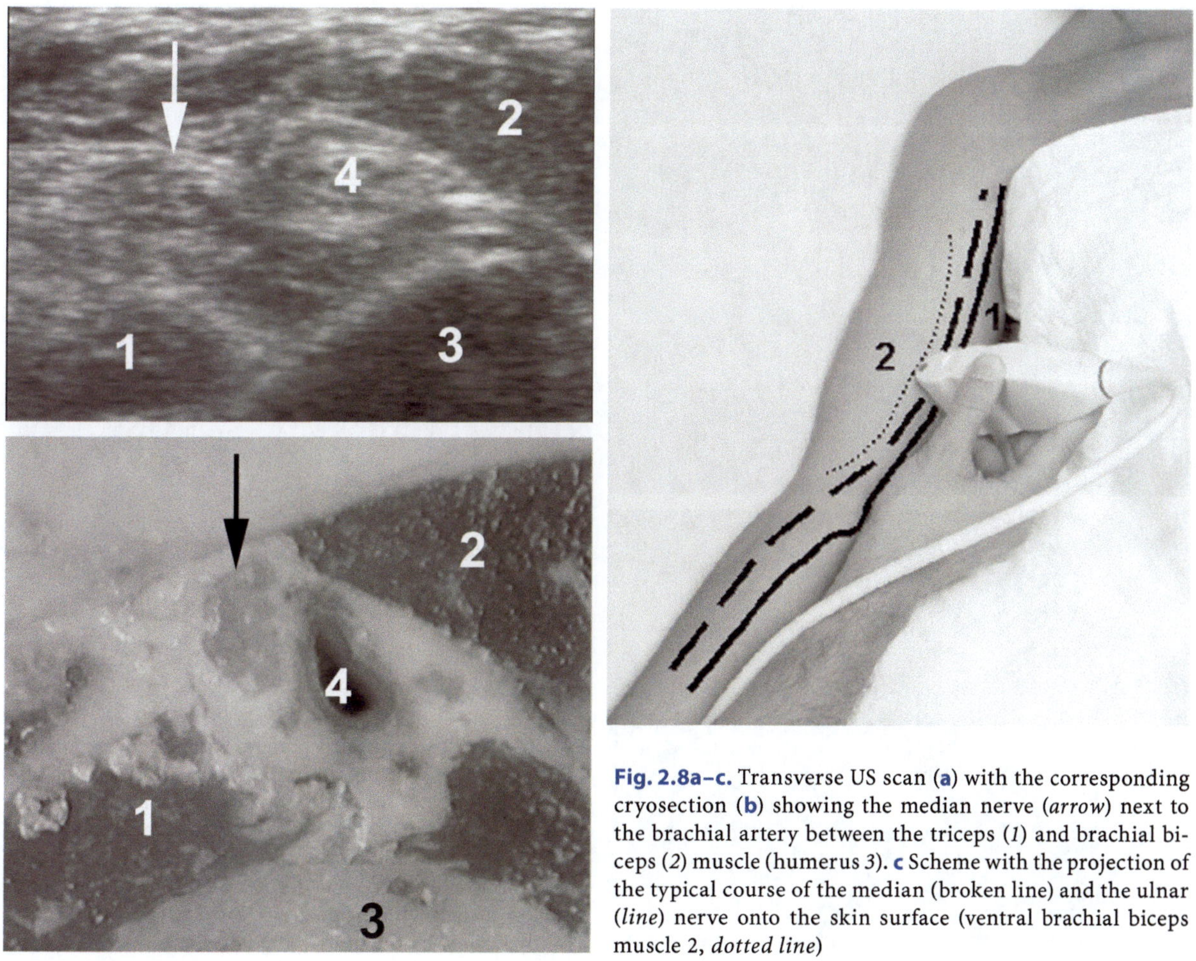

Fig. 2.8a–c. Transverse US scan (**a**) with the corresponding cryosection (**b**) showing the median nerve (*arrow*) next to the brachial artery between the triceps (*1*) and brachial biceps (*2*) muscle (humerus *3*). **c** Scheme with the projection of the typical course of the median (broken line) and the ulnar (*line*) nerve onto the skin surface (ventral brachial biceps muscle 2, *dotted line*)

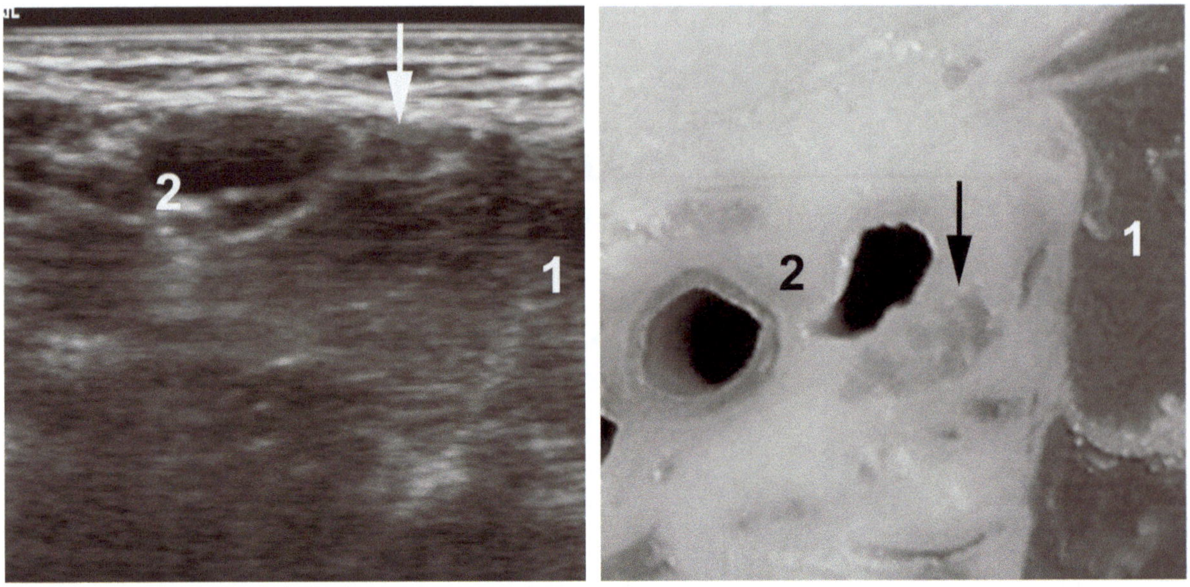

a b

Fig. 2.9a,b. Transverse US scan (**a**) with the corresponding cryosection (**b**) showing the ulnar nerve (*arrow*) in its typical position close to the brachial vascular bundle (brachial artery and vein *2*) ventral to the triceps muscle (*1*)

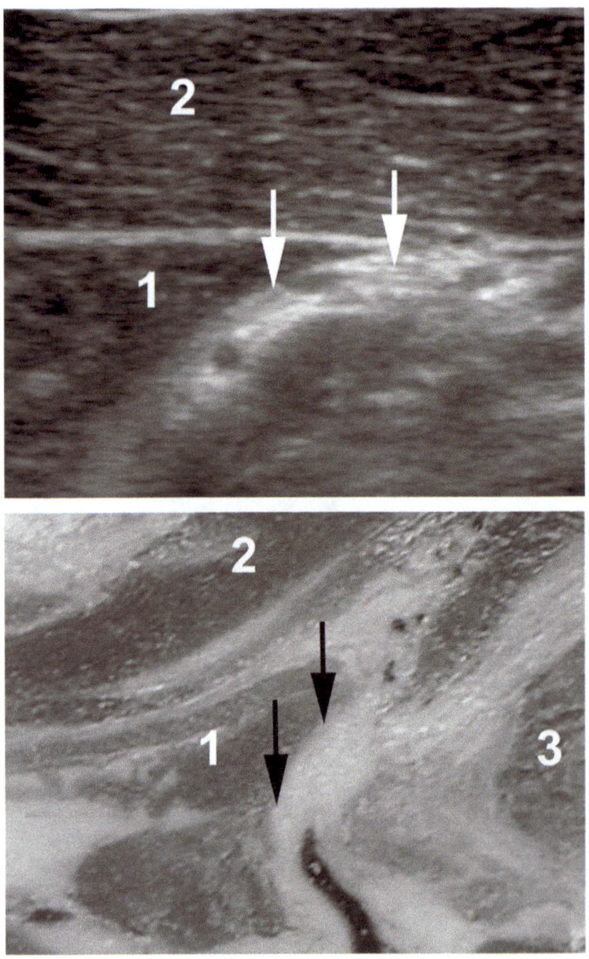

a b

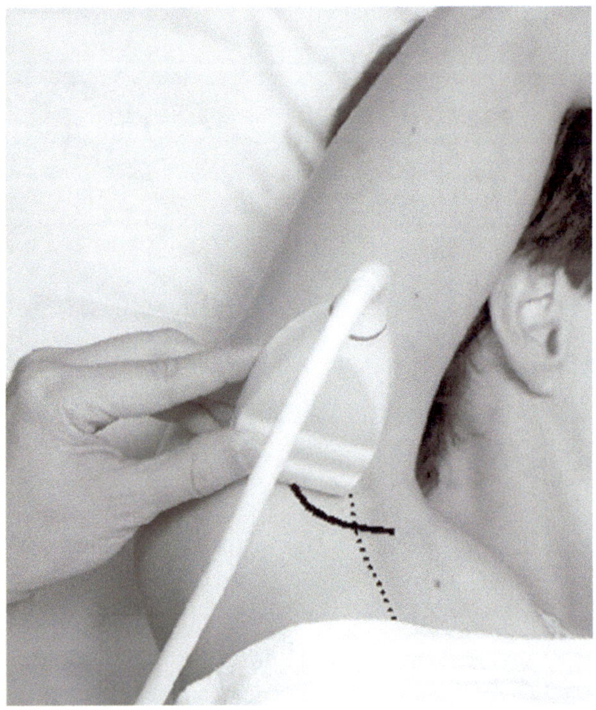

c

Fig. 2.10a–c. Transverse US scan (**a**) with the corresponding cryosection (**b**) showing the axillary nerve and accompanying vessels (*arrows*) ventrally covered by the lateral parts of the latissimus dorsi muscle (*1*) and the pectoral muscle (*2*) inferior to the glenoid part of the scapula (*3*). **c** Scheme with the projection of the course of the axillary nerve (*line*) onto the skin surface with the posterior axillary fold (*dotted line*) mainly formed by the underlying latissimus muscle

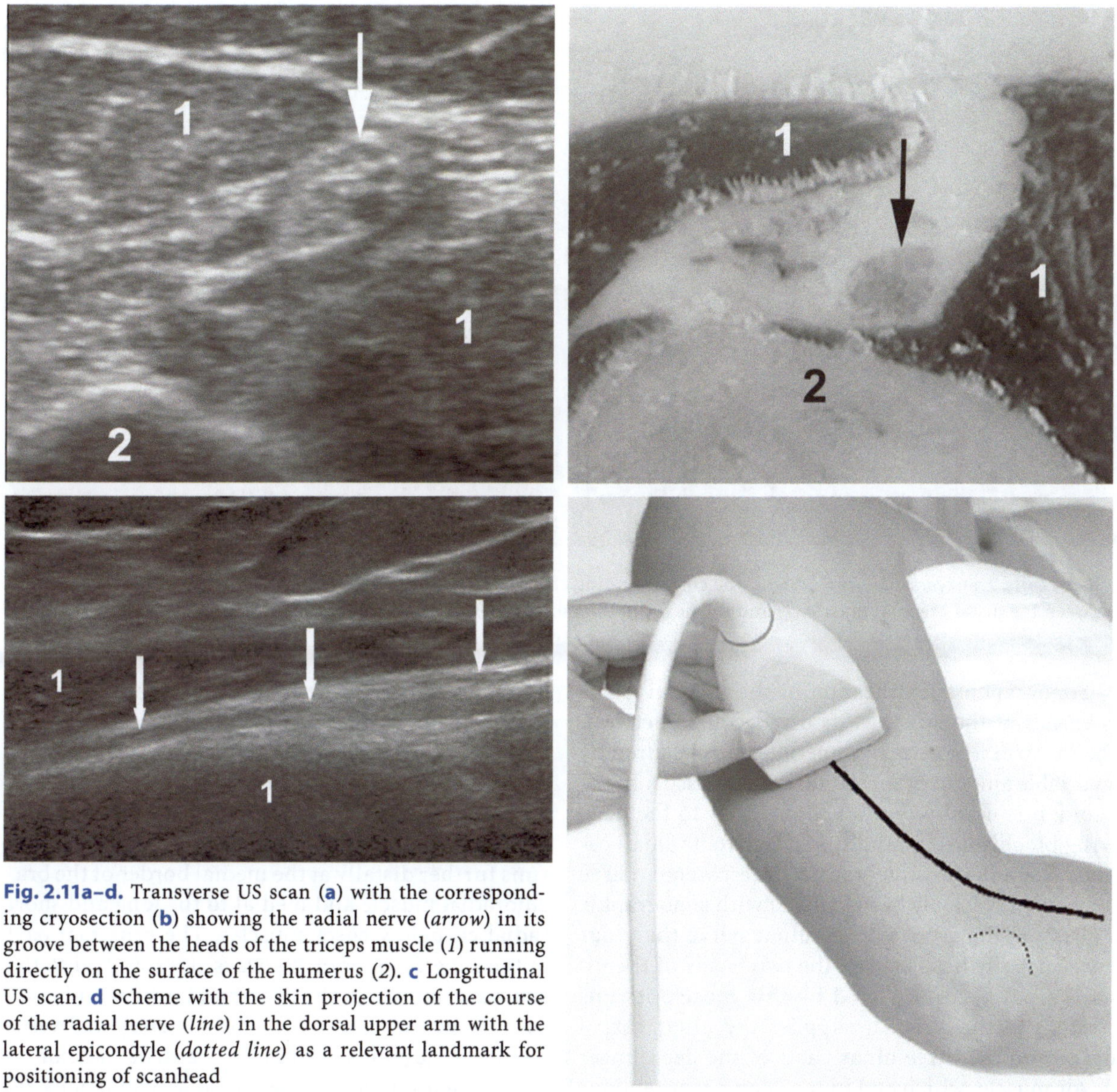

Fig. 2.11a–d. Transverse US scan (**a**) with the corresponding cryosection (**b**) showing the radial nerve (*arrow*) in its groove between the heads of the triceps muscle (*1*) running directly on the surface of the humerus (*2*). **c** Longitudinal US scan. **d** Scheme with the skin projection of the course of the radial nerve (*line*) in the dorsal upper arm with the lateral epicondyle (*dotted line*) as a relevant landmark for positioning of scanhead

2.2.2
Nerves of the Forearm

In the forearm the median nerve, after passing the pronator teres muscle, enters the fascial space between the main flexor groups of the upper extremity: it runs downward to the wrist between the superficial and the profound finger flexors. In its course many muscular branches supply different ventral muscle groups of the forearm. Several ulnar flexors of the forearm however are omitted by this nerve and their supply will be mentioned later. One remarkable branch of the median nerve is the anterior antebrachial interosseous nerve being released in the cubita-region and running downward to the carpus lying directly on the interosseous membrane. This branch finally reaches the square pronator muscle, and along its course supplies the long flexor of the thumb and the radial parts of the deep finger flexors.

In the region of the wrist the median nerve lies directly under the tendon of the long palmar muscle, interposed between the flexor tendons and covered by a thin layer of the forearm fascia (Fig. 2.12). In this region the median nerve may already have split into two parts (common digital nerve trunks), in which case an interposed median artery may coexist as an anatomic variant (Gassner et al. 2002).

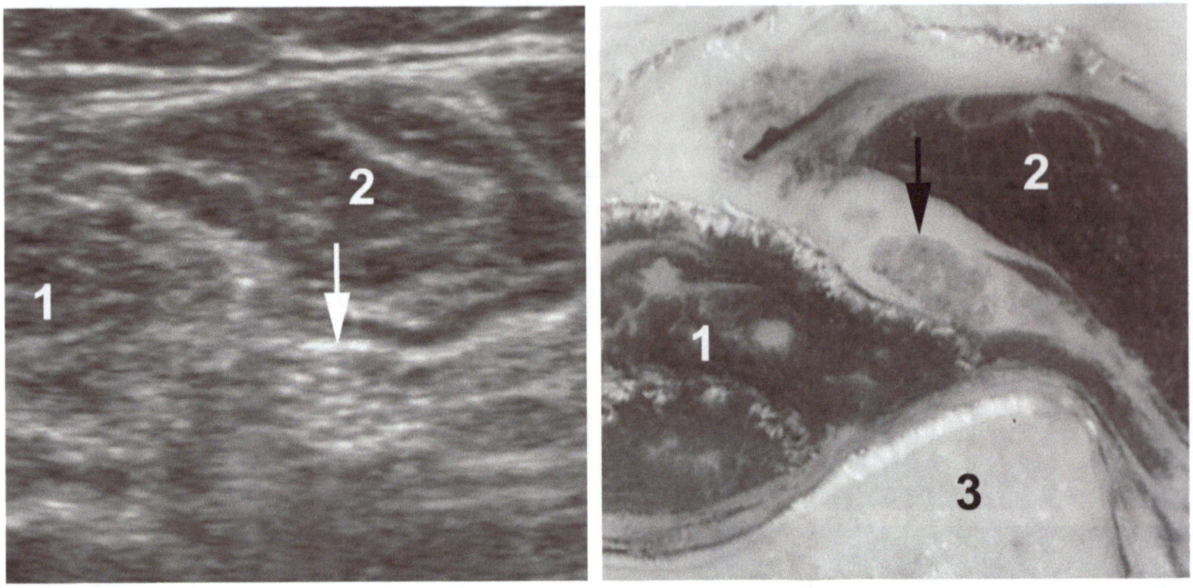

a b

Fig. 2.12a,b. Transverse US scan (**a**) with the corresponding cryosection (**b**) showing the median nerve (*arrow*) interposed between the distal brachial muscle (*1*) and the flexor of the radial carpus (*2*) muscle (trochlea of the humerus *3*)

Sonographic identification of the median nerve is easiest at the wrist, as its distal course between the forearm flexors may sometimes be obscured by a variable amount of surrounding fatty tissue. In the cubita it is usually positioned medially to the deep lying brachial artery and veins. Due to its small caliber the anterior antebrachial interosseous nerve may only invariably be visualized with sonography.

Passing the groove of the ulnar nerve the ulnar nerve usually lies between the two heads of the ulnar carpal flexor. Covered by this muscle it runs straight to the wrist. It supplies the ulnar carpal flexor and the three ulnar parts of the deep finger flexor muscle, which end in the deep flexor tendons of the three ulnar fingers. In the distal part of the forearm the ulnar nerve lies medially between the tendon of the ulnar carpal flexor muscle and lateral of the ulnar artery and veins. The ulnar artery and the ulnar nerve both lie superficially to the thin layer of the forearm fascia, only covered by loose subcutaneous fat and connective tissue. Sonographic visualization of the ulnar nerve is easiest before its entrance into the ulnar carpal flexor muscle at the elbow and in the distal third of the forearm in its typical position between the tendon of the ulnar carpal flexor muscle and the ulnar artery (Fig. 2.13). As it is embedded in inhomogeneous echogenic tissue in the wrist region and is smaller than the neighboring median nerve its identification at this site may sometimes be difficult.

On its course in the cubita and the forearm the radial nerve runs at the ventral side between the brachial and the brachioradial muscle. At the level of the radial head (caput radii) bifurcates in its both terminal branches: the superficial and the profound branch. The superficial branch of the radial nerve runs further distally at the medial border of the brachioradial muscle and medial to the long and short radial carpal extensor muscles. The proximal part of the superficial branch always stays ventral to the supinator muscle in the proximal forearm and is accompanied medially by the radial artery and veins along an individual distance. The distal section of this branch returns to the dorsal subcutaneous region of the extremity through the distal part of the brachioradial muscle and crosses the extensor retinaculum dorsally. The profound branch of the radial nerve enters the supinator muscle at an individual distance from the radial-nerve-bifurcation passing through a small, tendinous arch (the arch of Frohse). In most asymptomatic subjects the profound branch of the radial nerve shows a relative change in caliber at its entry into the supinator muscle through the arch of Frohse (Riffaud et al. 1999). If this arch is too small the profound branch of the radial nerve may be compressed – especially during hand extension and pronation, which further reduces the width of the supinator arch (Thomas et al. 2000). On its course through the supinator muscle the profound branch releases several muscular branches and finally enters the space between the superficial and profound hand extensors. It ends as the posterior antebrachial interosseous nerve lying on the posterior surface of the interosseous membrane.

Sonographic identification of the radial nerve and its branches in the forearm, is easiest at their course between the brachial and brachioradial muscle, where they show a high contrast difference compared with the surrounding muscular tissue. The superficial branch is best assessed medially to the brachioradial muscle. The terminal branches of the superficial radial nerve branch can only be visualized with the use of transducers with a frequency of at least 15 MHz. The profound branch of the radial nerve is easily visualized inside the supinator muscle due to the high sonographic contrast difference between the nerve and the surrounding muscle (Fig. 2.14). The posterior antebrachial interosseous nerve is only detectable with present sonographic equipment in rare cases due to its small size and insufficient contrast.

2.2.3
Nerves of the Wrist and Hand

In some subjects the division of the median nerve begins in the region of the distal forearm, at latest in the region of the carpal tunnel. Usually the first common digital palmar nerve (for the thenar and the thumb) is the first branch leaving the nerve. The infrequently found median artery, which is a variable branch of the proximal section of the ulnar artery and leads into the also variable superficial palmar arterial arch (Hafferl 1969; Von Lanz and Wachsmuth 1972; Platzer 1982), may be found inside the carpal tunnel interposed between the first common digital palmar nerve and the median nerve remnant. The bifurcation of the residual median nerve into the second (second finger and radial part of third finger motor and sensory supply) and third (ulnar third and radial fourth finger motor and sensory supply) common digital palmar nerve usually takes place inside or directly

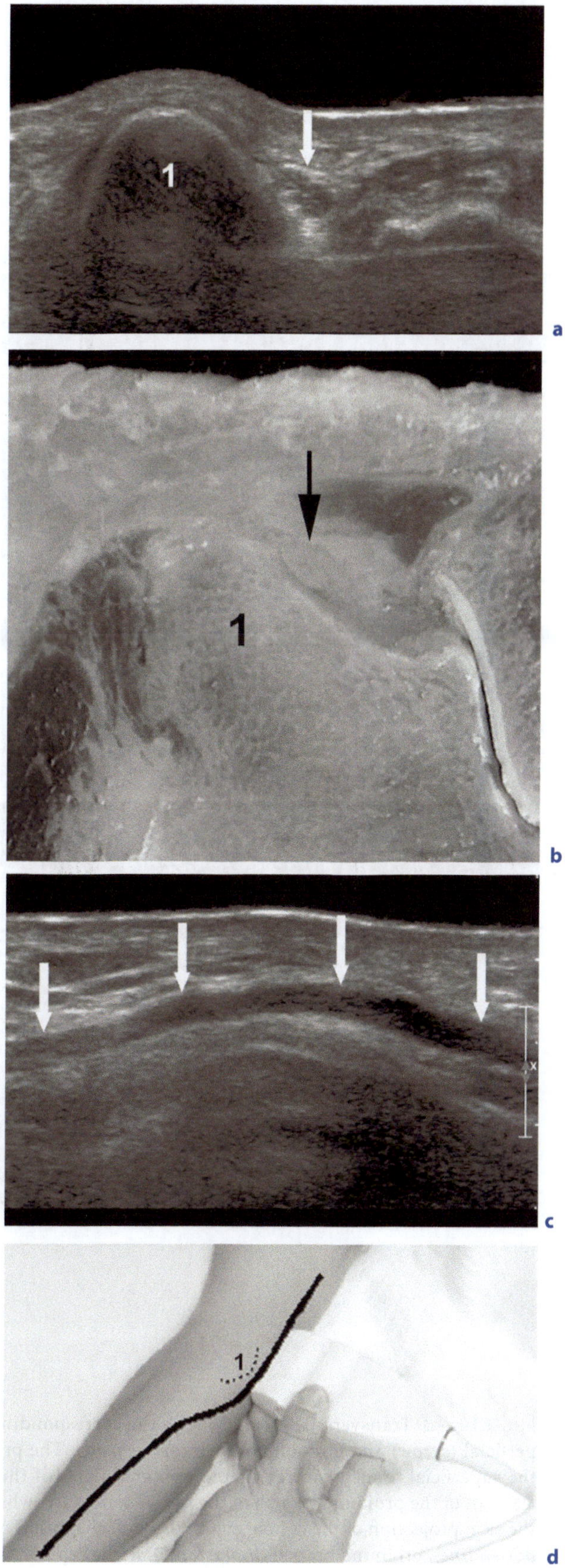

Fig. 2.13a–d. Transverse US scan (**a**) with the corresponding cryosection (**b**) showing the ulnar nerve (*arrow*) in its course within the "sulcus nervi ulnaris" formed by connective tissue and the distal humerus (*1*). **c** Longitudinal US scan of the ulnar nerve (*arrows*) within the "sulcus nervi ulnaris". **d** Scheme with skin projection of the ulnar nerve (*line*) in the cubita relative to the ulnar epicondyle of the humerus (*dotted line*)

distal to the carpal tunnel. The median nerve or its terminal branches always appear more or less oval or flattened, with considerable individual variation in healthy subjects. (Sarria et al. 2000; Duncan et al. 1999) (Fig. 2.15).

The terminal peripheral branches of the median nerve – the paired proper palmar finger nerves (palmar supply of finger 1–3 and the radial palmar side of finger 4) – are sensory branches emerging of the common digital palmar nerves, which are directly positioned on the tendons or tendon sheaths of the long flexor muscles (Fig. 2.16). They may only be visualized with transducers of at least 15 MHz using a stand-off pad. Each of them is accompanied by a proper palmar finger artery, usually lying more superficially (Fig. 2.17).

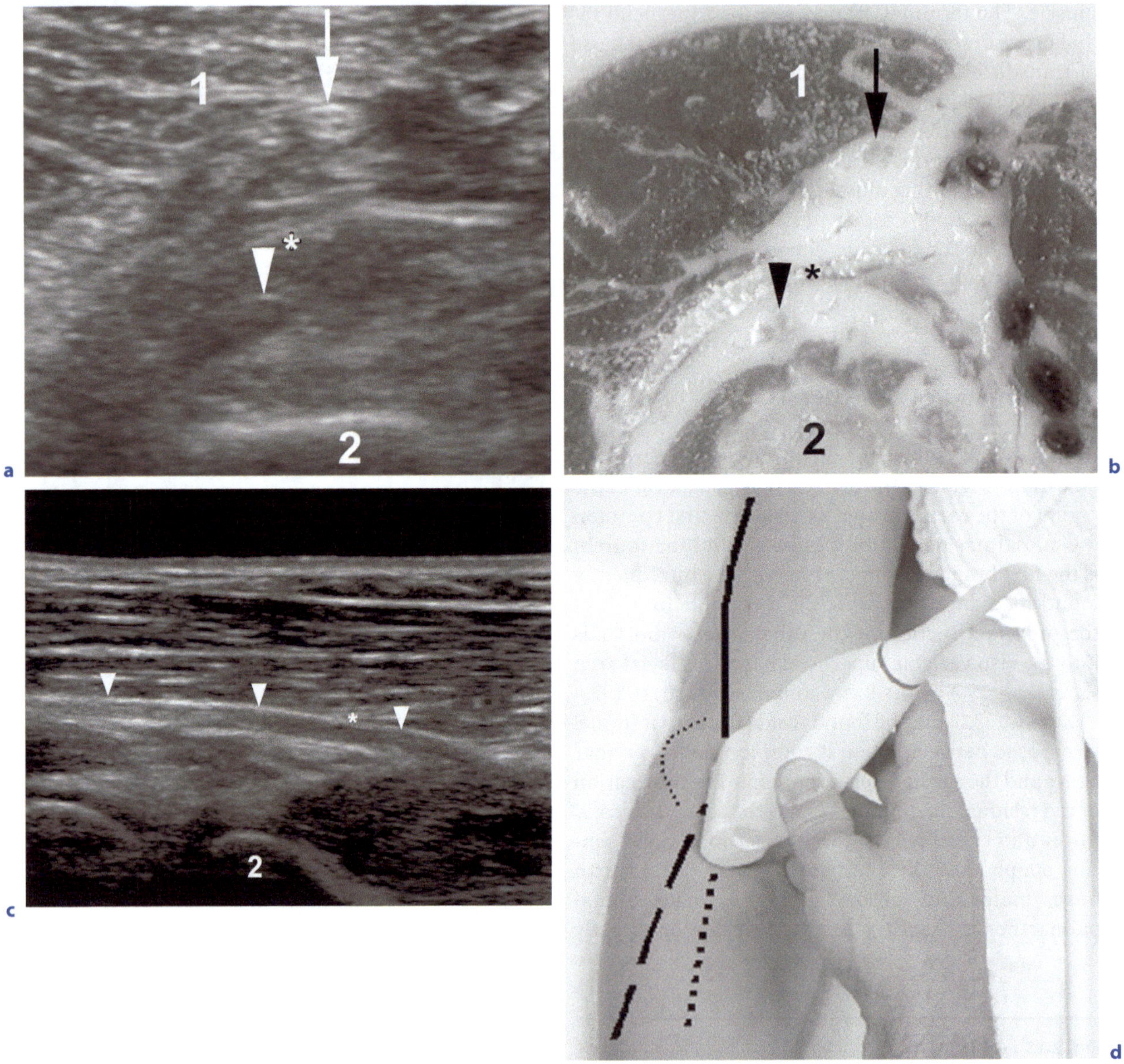

Fig. 2.14a–d. Transverse US scan (**a**) with the corresponding cryosection (**b**) showing the division of the radial nerve: superficial (*arrow*) and profound branch (*arrowhead*). The profound branch typically covered by the arch of Frohse (*) and the superficial branch covered by the proximal parts of the brachioradial muscle (*1*) (proximal radius *2*). **c** Longitudinal US scan of the profound branch of the radial nerve (arrowheads) with the arch of Frohse (*) (radial head *2*). **d** Scheme with the skin projection of the course and division of the radial nerve in the cubita: radial nerve (*line*), superficial branch (thick *dotted line*), profound branch (*broken line*). Radial epicondyle of the humerus (thin *dotted line*) as landmark

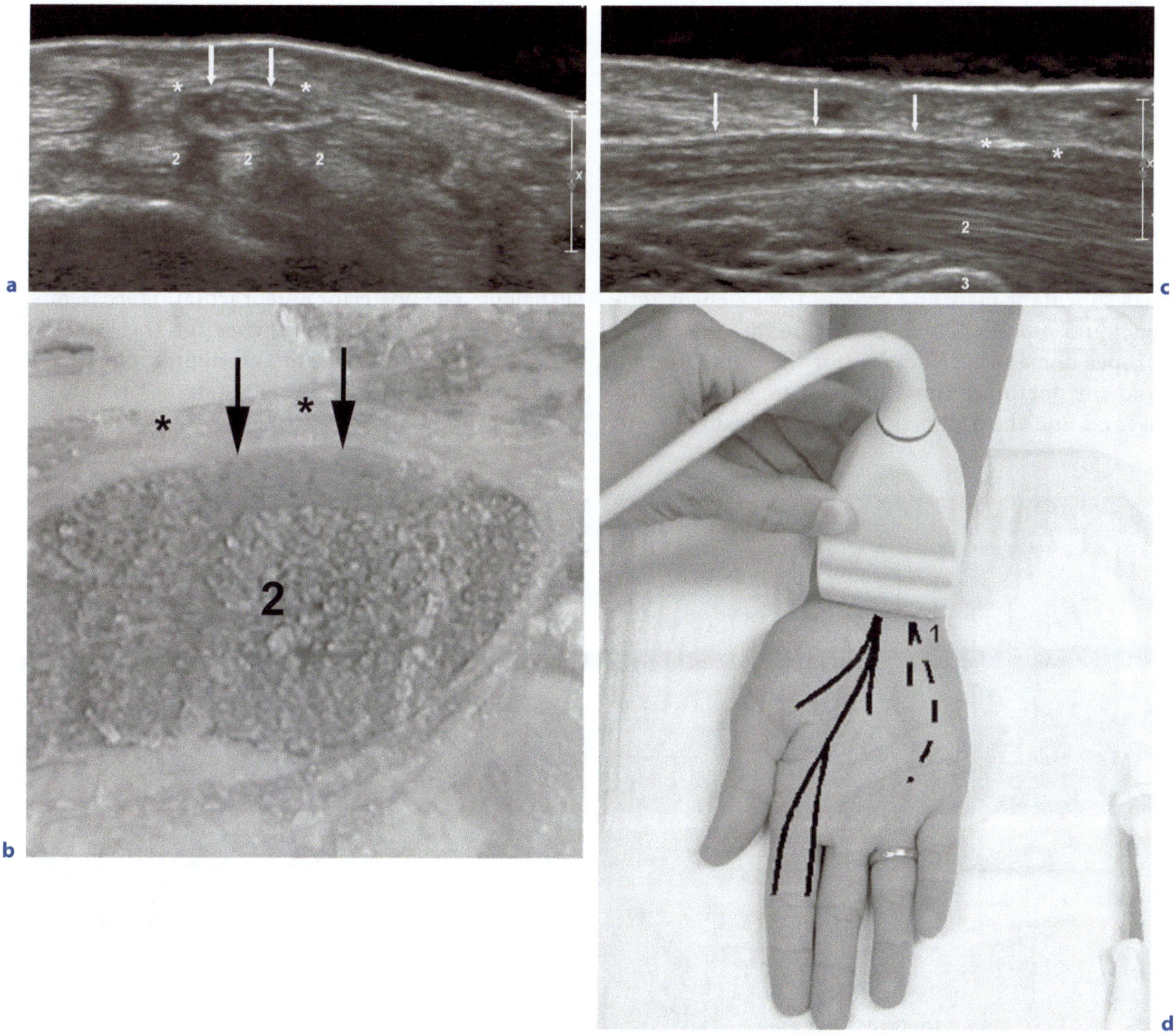

Fig. 2.15a–d. Transverse US scan (**a**) with the corresponding cryosection (**b**) showing the median nerve in the wrist (*arrows*) together with the cross sections of the finger flexor tendons within the carpal tunnel (*2*) covered by the transverse ligament of the carpus (*). **c** Longitudinal US scan of the distal median nerve (*arrows*) with the underlying finger flexor tendons (*2*) (distal radius *3*). **d** Scheme with skin projection of representative branches of the median nerve (*lines*) and the ulnar nerve (*broken lines*) in the wrist and hand. Pisiform bone (*1*) as landmark

The ulnar nerve reaches the hand running superficially to the flexor retinaculum and accompanied laterally by the ulnar artery. Here it bifurcates releasing the profound branch, which forms a neural arch supplying the muscles of the hypothenar, the interosseous muscles and finally even part of the thenar muscles, between the proximal parts of the small flexor and the abductor of the small finger. The residual ulnar nerve (fourth common digital palmar nerve ends in the paired proper palmar finger nerves (supplying the radio-palmar aspect of the fourth and the palmar aspect of the fifth finger). Just like the terminal median nerve-branches the terminal ulnar branches are accompanied by the proper palmar finger arteries (the terminal arterial branches of the superficial palmar arch). A very small side-branch of the ulnar nerve – the dorsal branch of the ulnar nerve – which exits the ulnar nerve in the middle of the forearm, reaches the hand subcutaneously and dorso-medially to the styloid process of the ulna (Fig. 2.18). It ends in the sensory proper finger nerves for the dorsal aspect of the fourth and fifth finger being accompanied by subcutaneous veins. The sonographic visualization of the terminal branches (proper palmar finger nerves) and their proximal nerve stems only succeeds with high frequency transducers of at least 15 MHz using a stand-off pad.

The radial nerve ends in three common dorsal finger nerves, having already formed in the region of the distal forearm. Each of these neural branches lies subcutaneously and crosses the extensor retinaculum superficially. The division into the paired proper dorsal finger nerves (for the dorsal thumb and the dorso-proximal parts of finger 2–4 – the second and third dorsal finger – are usually supplied by the median nerve) takes place at variable locations. The terminal dorsal branches are accompanied by the barely visible terminal arterial branches of the dorsal carpal branch of the radial artery. The visualization of these flimsy branches of the radial nerve is achieved best in the region of the lateral extensor retinaculum. The branches are embedded in subcutaneous fat and connective tissue, which is why their presentation may be insufficient. The posterior antebrachial interosseous nerve and its terminal branches for the sensory supply of the dorsal carpal and digital joints may not be visualized with present state of the art ultrasonography.

a c

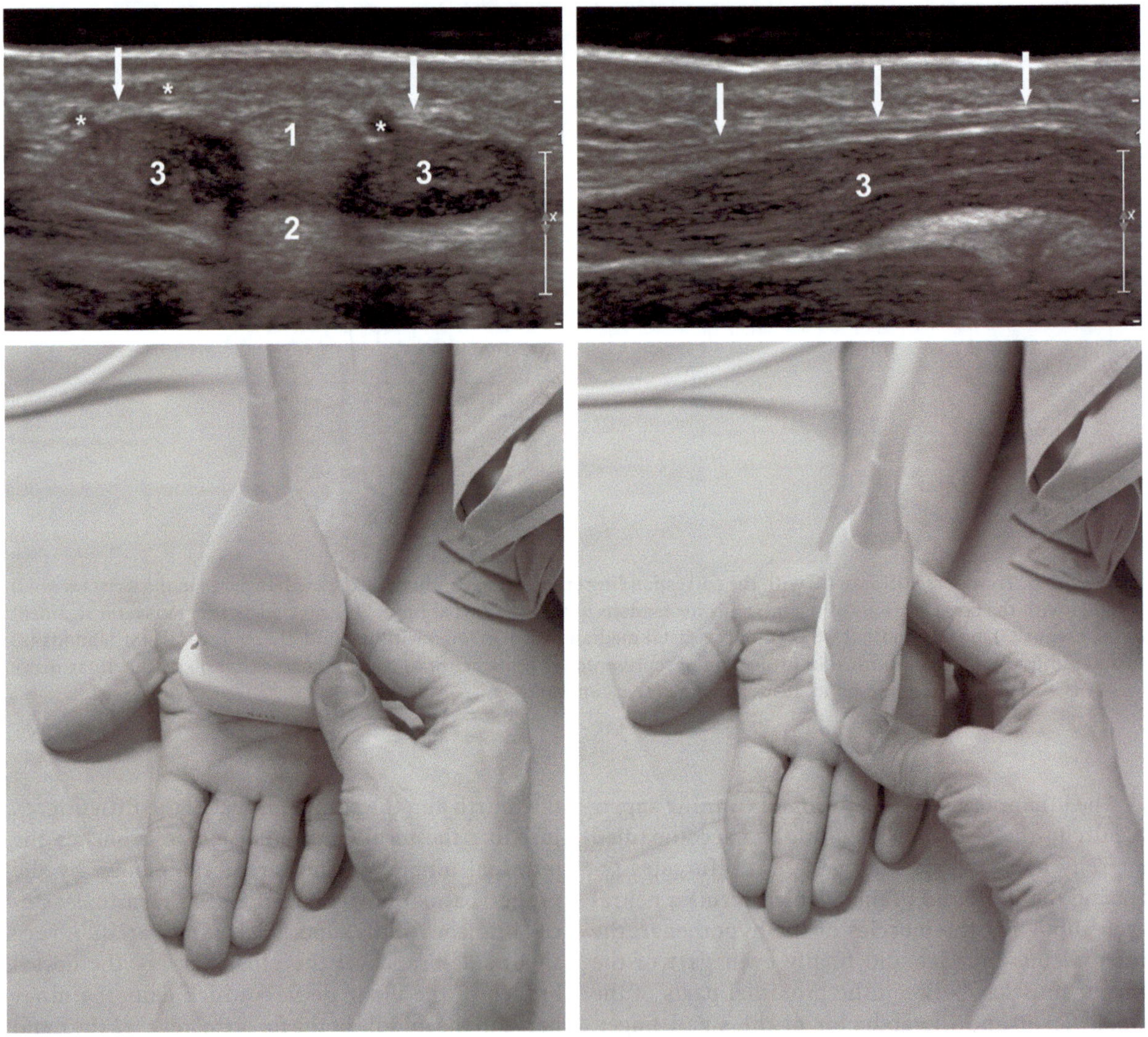

b d

Fig. 2.16a–d. Transverse US scan (**a**) with the corresponding scheme (**b**) and longitudinal US scan (**c**) with the corresponding scheme (**d**) showing the metacarpal section of the branches of the median nerve (common digital nerves, *arrows*) together with the accompanying arteries (*) (flexor tendons *1* with underlying metacarpal bone *2*; lumbrical muscles *3*)

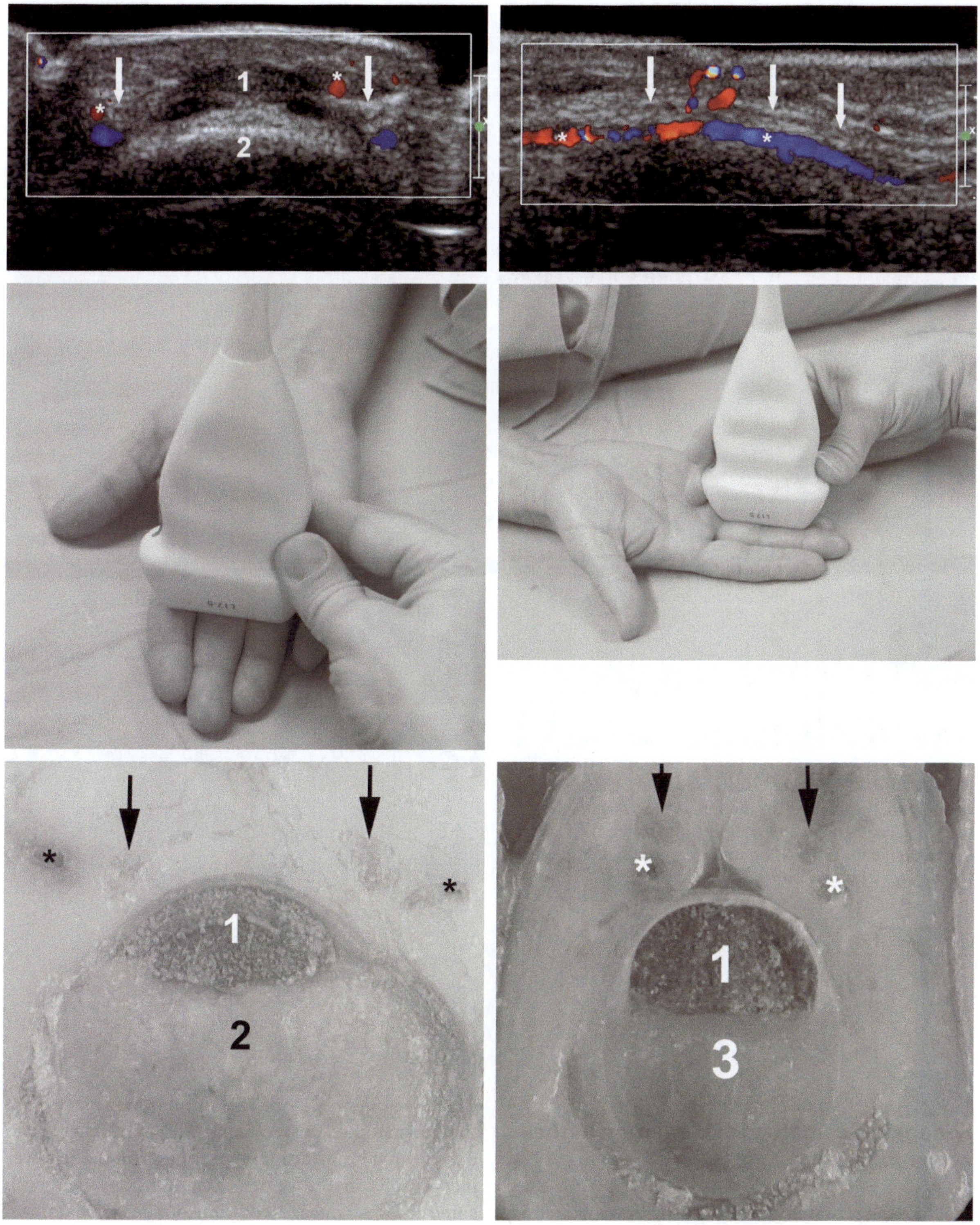

a b c d e f

Fig. 2.17a–f. Transverse US scan using Color Doppler US (**a**) with the corresponding scheme (**b**) showing the digital section of the branches of the median nerve (proper digital nerves, arrows) together with the accompanying arteries (*) (flexor tendons *1* with underlying proximal phalanx of the finger *2*. Longitudinal US scan using Color Doppler US (**c**) with the corresponding schema (**d**) showing a proper digital nerve (*arrows*) together with the closely accompanying artery (**s*). Cryosections through the proximal (**e**) and middle phalanx (**f**) of the finger showing the proper digital nerves (*arrows*) together with the accompanying arteries (*) (flexor tendons *1* with underlying proximal *2* and distal *3* phalanx). For better imaging a stand-off pad should be used

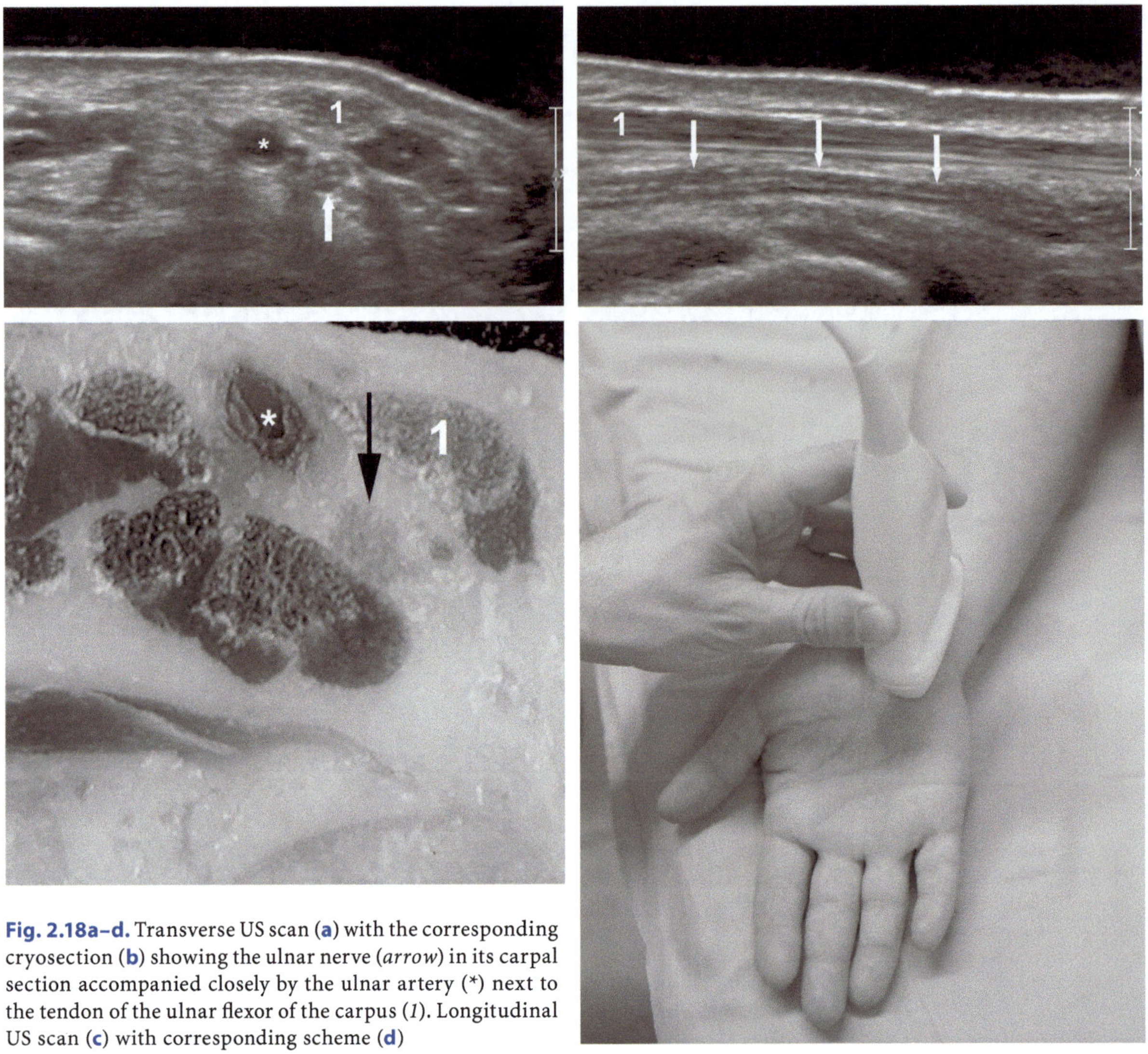

Fig. 2.18a–d. Transverse US scan (a) with the corresponding cryosection (b) showing the ulnar nerve (*arrow*) in its carpal section accompanied closely by the ulnar artery (*) next to the tendon of the ulnar flexor of the carpus (*1*). Longitudinal US scan (c) with corresponding scheme (d)

2.3 Sonographic Anatomic Correlation in the Lower Extremity

Just like the proximal extremity, the lower extremity forms paddle-like in the fetal period. It is supplied by the according neural segments (metamer segmentation) of the rump wall. In later life this ontological specialty results in the distinct distribution of the sensible dermatomes in correlation with the supplying spinal roots. For the lower extremity these are the segments L1–S3. The annular organization of the dermatomes on the rump wall is transferred to a somewhat longitudinal representation in the lower just as it is in the upper extremity, however with some kind of inward rotation of the dermatomes. The recombination of the axons with formation of the peripheral nerves itself takes place at the level of the lumbar and sacral plexus, with the ventral parts of the lower extremity supplied by the lumbar and the dorsal parts as well as the pelvic floor by the sacral plexus.

2.3.1 Nerves of the Groin and the Thigh

The most cranial nerve descending from the lumbar plexus is the sensory lateral femoral cutaneous nerve. It forms out of the ventral branches of the spinal nerves of the segments L2 and L3. It runs downward on the iliac muscle to the medial side of the anterior iliac spine and uses the very lateral part of the muscles` lacuna to get to the ventro-lateral subcutaneous space. It can be identified with sonography in the muscles' lacuna, where it enters the subcutaneous space between the sartorial and tensor fasciae lata muscle. Because of its small size its sonographic visualization may be very difficult (Fig. 2.19).

One of the biggest peripheral nerves of the human body is the femoral nerve. It contains the fascicles for the musculature and the sensibility of a great part of the ventral aspect of the lower extremity. It is the sole innervator of the knee-extensors and is responsible for the sensibility of almost the whole ventral and medial aspect of the lower extremity. The femoral nerve is usually formed out of the ventral branches of the spinal nerves of segment L1–L4. The recombination of the neural fascicles of the femoral nerve takes place within the psoas muscle, where it is split into a superficial and profound section. The proximal part of the nerve leaves the psoas muscle at its lateral border, running downward to the inguinal region in the retroperitoneum inside a groove formed medially by the psoas muscle and

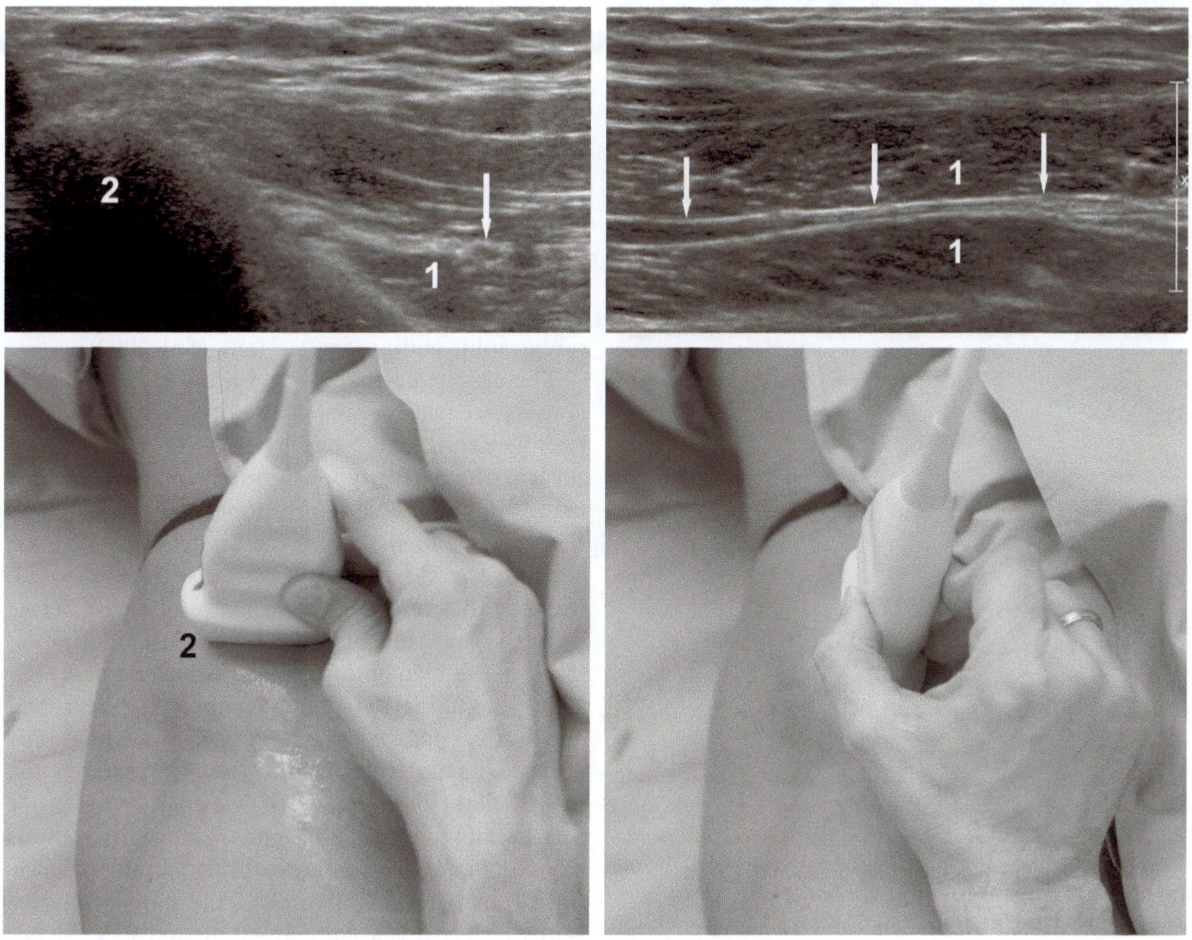

a c b d

Fig. 2.19a–d. Transverse US scan (**a**) with corresponding scheme (**b**) and longitudinal US scan (**c**) with corresponding scheme (**d**) of the lateral cutaneous femoral nerve (*arrows*) piercing through sartorius muscle (*1*) medial to the superior anterior iliacal spine (*2*) laterally by the iliac muscle. It leaves the muscles' lacuna as the most medial structure separated from the adjacent femoral artery only by the ileopectineal arch (Fig. 2.20). The latter is a thin tendinous structure, which is part of the inguinal ligament complex, and connects the inguinal ligament and the body of the iliac bone.

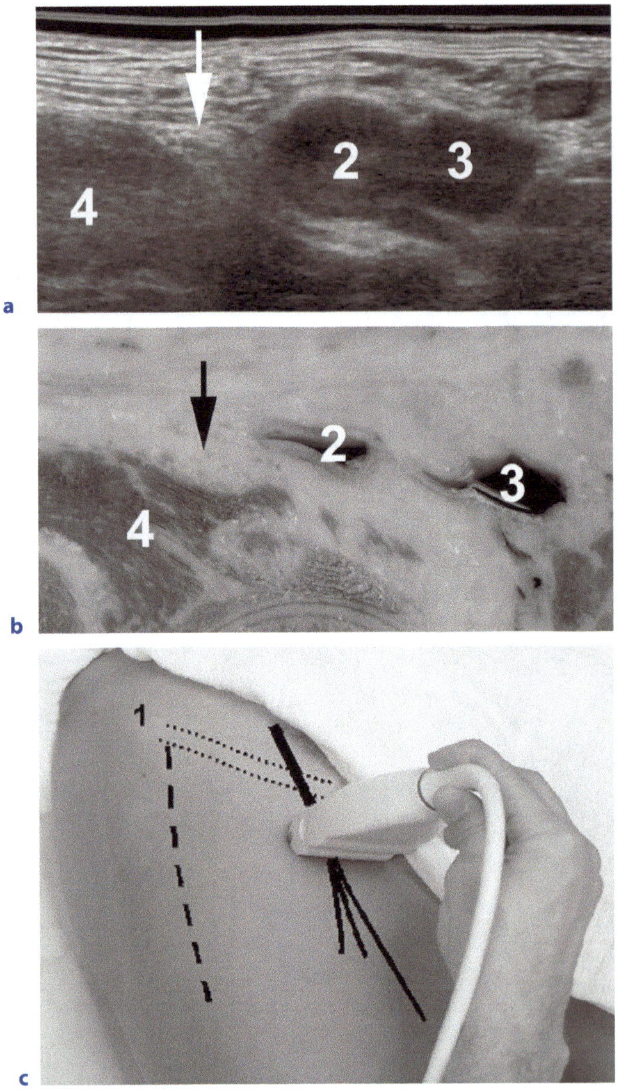

Fig. 2.20a–c. Transverse US scan (extended panoramic scan) (**a**) with the corresponding cryosection (**b**) showing the triangular cross-section of the femoral nerve (*arrow*) accompanied closely by the femoral artery (*2*) and vein (*3*) altogether on the iliopsoas muscle (*4*). **c** Scheme with skin projection of the femoral nerve (*lines*), the lateral femoral cutaneous nerve (*broken line*) and the inguinal ligament (*dotted lines*). Superior anterior iliacal spine (*1*)

After a variable distance the nerve spreads into several terminal branches: ventral and medial cutaneous nerve branches and motor branches for the supplied muscles. The main direction of the course of the femoral nerve and its branches is always parallel to the underneath lying sartorial muscle. The final branch of the femoral nerve, the saphenus nerve lies adjacent to the superficial femoral artery and perforates the vasto-adductorial membrane in its distal third of the thigh together with the descendent knee-artery, a branch of the superficial femoral artery. The saphenus nerve supplies the knee and the medial aspect of the lower leg with sensory fibers and runs subcutaneously to the region of the superficial pes anserinus. The femoral nerve is best assessed with sonography in its groin section. Here it can be found next to the pulsating femoral artery with an oval or triangular cross-sectional appearance.

The distal section of the femoral nerve in its pelvic course up to 10 cm proximal to the inguinal ligament may also be visualized with sonography after sufficient evacuation of air in the hypogastric bowel. The proximal thigh-section of the nerve may sometimes be difficult to assess due to early branching as well as to low contrast differences between the nerve and surrounding soft tissues. The saphenus nerve may only be visualized in favorable conditions in its subcutaneous course at the medial aspect of the knee. The deep muscle-supplying branches of the femoral nerve cannot be visualized with present sonographic equipment (Gruber et al. 2002).

The biggest peripheral nerve of the human body is the sciatic nerve (Fig. 2.21). In fact it consists of two big nerves combined by a common perineural sheath: the laterally positioned common fibular nerve and the medially positioned tibial nerve. The sciatic nerve forms out of the branches of the lumbar and the sacral plexus of the segments L4–S3, whereby the common fibular nerve elements derive from the branches of the segments L4–S2, and the tibial nerve elements from the branches of L4–S3 after recombination of nerve fibers in the retro- and sub-peritoneal lumbosacral plexus. The sciatic nerve exits the sub-peritoneal space through the major sciatic foramen, which is formed by the major incisura of the sciatic bone and by the sacro-spinous ligament, coursing underneath the piriform muscle (infra-piriform compartment of the major sciatic foramen). Here it is accompanied medially by the pudendal and inferior gluteal vessels and the according nerves, altogether surrounded by a considerable amount of loose connective tissue and fat. In the sub-gluteal space (only covered by the maximus gluteal muscle) it takes a slightly lateral convex course crossing the underlying small deep gluteal muscles (gemellus muscles and intern obturator muscle) and the quadratic femoral muscle (connecting the sciatic tuber and the inter-trochanteric crest of the femur). It traverses laterally to the sciatic tuber and is crossed by the gluteal vessels. In this region the nerve gets covered by proximal parts of the sciatic-crural muscles (mainly by the long head of the femoral biceps muscle), while it lies on top of the minimus and further distally magnus adductor muscle. In this region the sciatic nerve is accompanied by arterial and venous branches of the profound femoral artery (perforating vessels) which supply the sciatic-crural muscles (Graif et al. 1991).

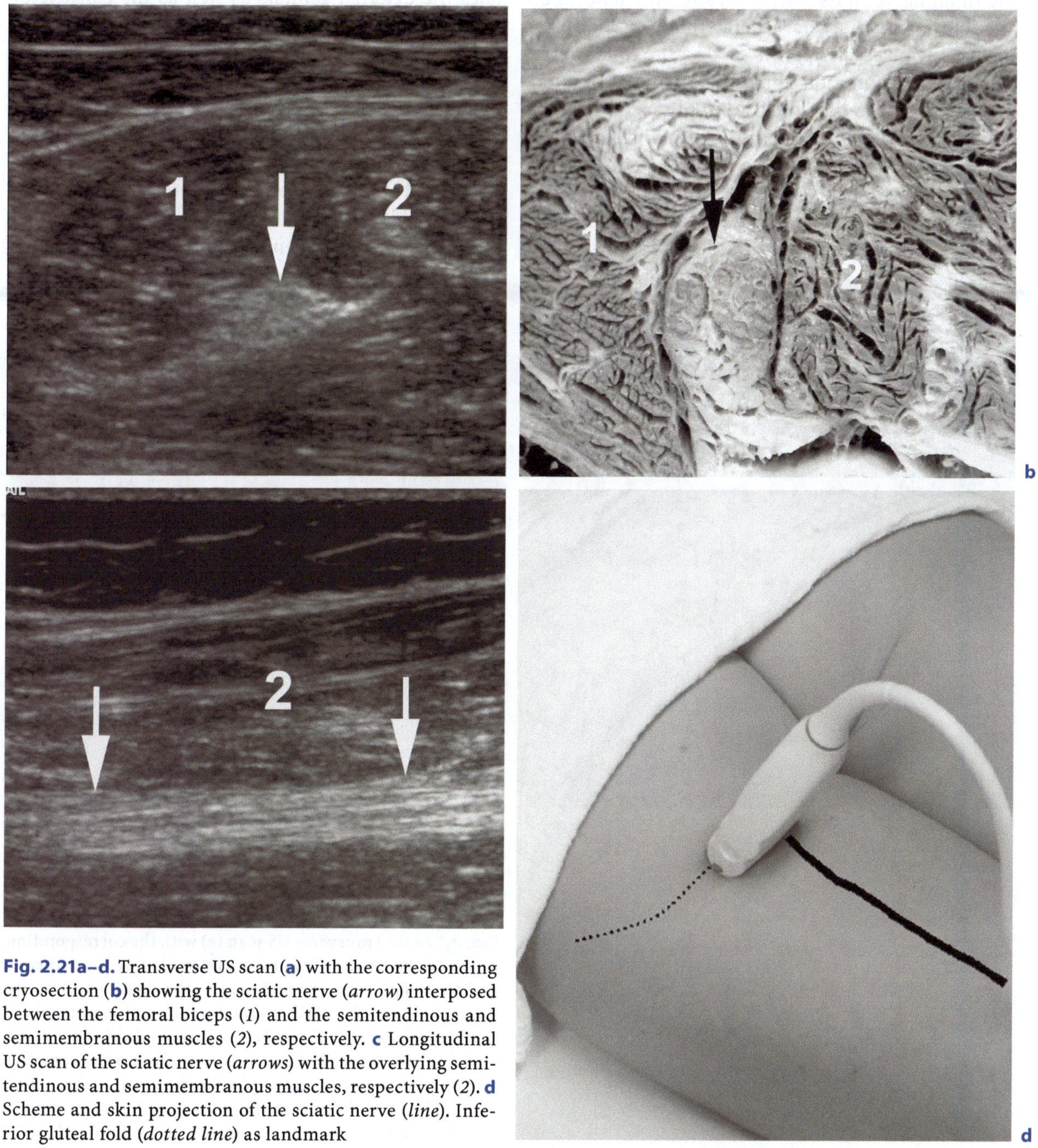

a b c d

Fig. 2.21a–d. Transverse US scan (**a**) with the corresponding cryosection (**b**) showing the sciatic nerve (*arrow*) interposed between the femoral biceps (*1*) and the semitendinous and semimembranous muscles (*2*), respectively. **c** Longitudinal US scan of the sciatic nerve (*arrows*) with the overlying semitendinous and semimembranous muscles, respectively (*2*). **d** Scheme and skin projection of the sciatic nerve (*line*). Inferior gluteal fold (*dotted line*) as landmark

In the more distal parts of the dorsal thigh the sciatic nerve divides into its intrinsic neural sections at a very individual height. These sections (the lateral common fibular nerve and the medial tibial nerve) are interposed between the two heads of the femoral biceps muscle, whereby the common fibular nerve follows the tendon of the femoral biceps muscle medially and further down dorso-medially to the tendon attachment at the head of the fibula.

After releasing the sensory sural nerve dorsally, the tibial nerve in its course through the tendinous adductorial hiatus gets accompanied medially by the popliteal vessels. In this section the tibial nerve as well as the common fibular gets almost subcutaneous only covered by the thin popliteal and crural fascia. In the very distal part of the thigh or better in the dorsal knee region the nerve gets interposed between the two heads of the gastrocnemius muscle together with the directly underlying popliteal vein and even deeper positioned artery. The sonographic identification of the sciatic nerve and the common fibular and tibial nerve, is most easily achieved at the distal third of the dorsal thigh (Fig. 2.22). After its identification in this region the sciatic nerve may be followed proximally with ease. In the gluteal region its presentation gets impaired because of the thick overlying bulk of muscle.

A very small and thin but important branch of the lumbar plexus is the pudendal nerve. It is formed out of the ventral branches of the segment S2–S4 and supplies the external genitals as well as the constrictor muscles of the urinary and intestinal tract and several muscles of the pelvic floor. It forms in the sub-peritoneal space in the sacral plexus, exits the pelvic space together with the sciatic nerve ventro-medially to it and accompanied by the pudendal artery and vein, bends around the sacro-spinous ligament to get to the medial surface of the sciatic tuber directly inferior to the anal levator muscle running within a fibro-osseous channel: the pudendal channel or channel of Al-

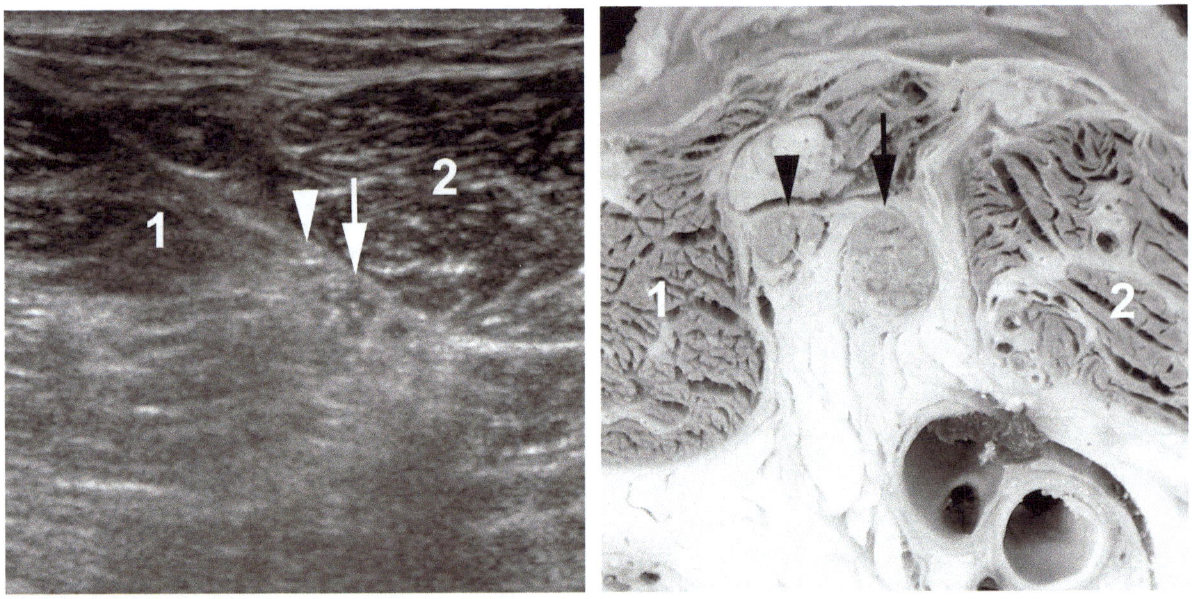

a b

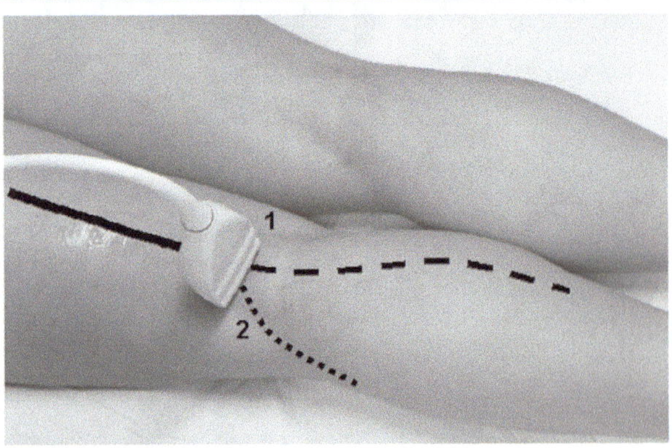

c

Fig. 2.22a–c. Transverse US scan (**a**) with the corresponding cryosection (**b**) showing the common fibular (*arrowhead*) and the tibial nerve (*arrow*) next to the distal parts of the femoral biceps (*1*) and the semitendinous and semimembranous muscles (*2*), respectively. **c** Scheme and skin projection of the sciatic nerve (*line*) and its division into the common fibular (*dotted line*) and the tibial nerve (*broken line*) with the tendons of the semimembranous and semitendinous muscle (*1*) and femoral biceps muscle (*2*) as landmarks cock (Gruber et al. 2001; Kovacs et al. 2001). A clear visualization of the complete course of the pudendal nerve with sonography is not feasible. However identification of the nerve succeeds in about 50% of subjects in the deep gluteal region. Reliable topographic relationships to the pudendal artery and bony and ligamentous landmarks however may be identified with sonography, which is important for guidance of a pudendal block (Gruber et al. 2001; Kovacs et al. 2001). The latter will be discussed in more detail in Chapter 7.

2.3.2 Nerves of the Lower Leg

Three nerves are responsible for the sensory and motor supply of the lower leg; these are the mere sensory saphenus nerve (terminal branch of the femoral nerve) for the medial aspect, the motor and sensory tibial nerve for the dorsal aspect and the motor and sensory common fibular nerve with its both terminal branches (superficial and profound fibular nerve) for the ventro-lateral aspect.

The saphenus nerve runs subcutaneously downward to the inner ankle usually accompanied dorso-medially by the saphena magna vein. It is only invariably visualized with sonography because of its small size and insufficient contrast against its surroundings.

The fibular nerve positioned medially and further distal dorso-medially to the tendon of the femoral biceps muscle bends around the dorsal and dorsolateral neck of the fibula to enter the fibular muscles (Fig. 2.23).

In this bend it divides into its terminal branches: the profound and the superficial fibular nerve. The more dorsal and caudal positioned profound fibular nerve enters the space between the dorsal lying long and the ventral lying short fibular muscle accompanied by the anterior tibial vessels medially. It supplies the two muscles and the overlying skin. The more ventral, cranial and medial positioned superficial fibular nerve enters the space between the short fibular muscle and the fibular bone to run to the ventral side of the shank between the fibular muscles and long digital extensor muscle or their tendons. Crossing the tendons of the ventral extensor musculature the superficial fibular nerve gets subcutaneous and splits up into its terminal sensory skin-branches. The common fibular nerve is easily visualized in the popliteal region and in its course around the fibular neck before it enters the fibular muscles.

The sonographic visualization of the course of both terminal branches within the fibular muscles is only possible with transducers of at least 12 MHz. The superficial fibular nerve in the ventral shank however is only invariably visualized with sonography.

The tibial nerve enters the space between the two heads of the gastrocnemius muscle in the thigh to run downward in the dorsal shank. In the proximal fourth of the lower leg, crossing the underlying oblique popliteal muscle, it perforates the proximal soleus muscle to enter the space between the superficial and profound foot flexor muscles. Usually before perforating the soleus muscle it releases multiple muscular and cutaneous branches for the dorsal shank. The subcutaneous main-branch of the dorsal shank – the sural nerve – also runs further distal, almost centrally, usually lateral to the saphena parva vein and heads for the posterior region of the outer ankle. The tibial nerve gets more and more medially oriented in the distal fourth of its course together with the accompanying posterior tibial vessels and aims for the posterior medial malleolar region (Fig. 2.24). Here the nerve is usually the most posterior structure escorted ventrally by the vessels, interposed between the loose superficial and the tense profound stratum of the retinaculum of the flexor muscles. The sonographic visualization of the tibial nerve is easiest in the distal shank but with the posterior tibial vessels as landmarks there is no problem in identification of the nerve in any section of its course.

2.3.3 Nerves of the Foot

The nerves of the foot are the terminal branches of the sciatic or better the tibial and fibular nerve, whereas the terminal endings of the saphenus nerve as end-branch of the femoral nerve reach the metatarso-phalangeal joint of the hallux at the medial foot-border.

The terminal branches of the superficial fibular nerve reach the dorsum of the foot subcutaneously, usually accompanying the tendons of the long digital extensors of the second and third toe. These very tiny nerves may only seldom be identified with sonography.

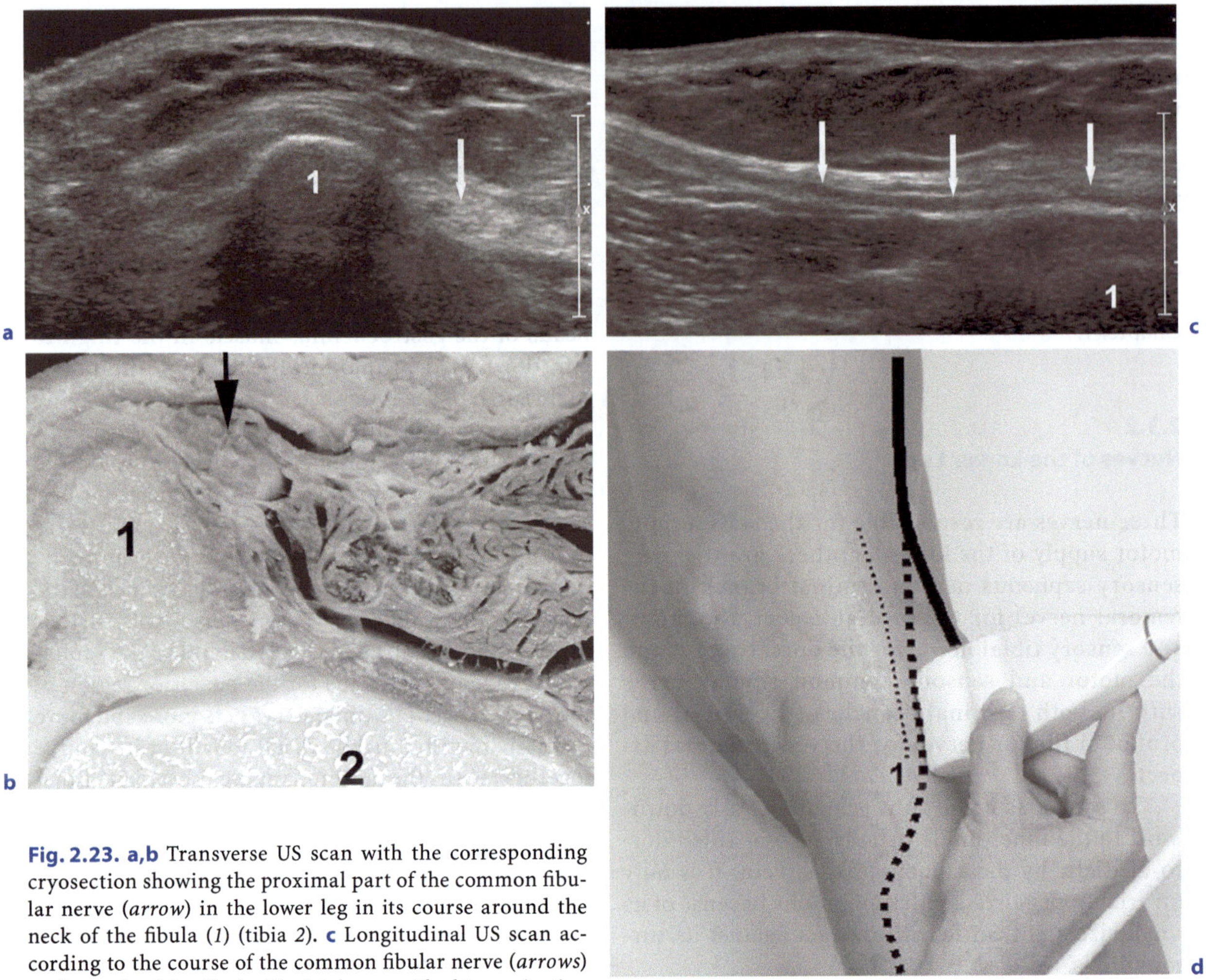

Fig. 2.23. **a,b** Transverse US scan with the corresponding cryosection showing the proximal part of the common fibular nerve (*arrow*) in the lower leg in its course around the neck of the fibula (*1*) (tibia *2*). **c** Longitudinal US scan according to the course of the common fibular nerve (*arrows*) at the neck of the fibula (*1*). **d** Scheme with skin projection of the course of the common fibular nerve (thick *dotted line*) in the lateral lower leg. Tendon of the femoral biceps muscle (thin *dotted line*), sciatic or tibial nerve, respectively, (*line*), fibular head (*1*) as landmarks

The main nerve supplying the foot with sensory and motor qualities is the tibial nerve with its both terminal branches: the medial and the lateral plantar nerve. These two branches usually form in the region of the medial malleolus. The medial plantar nerve runs planto-medially directly on the tendons and sheaths of the long flexor of the toes accompanied medially by the medial plantar vessels. The nerve divides into common and proper plantar toe nerves supplying the skin of the first to the medial surface of the fourth toe sensorial. The medial as well as the lateral plantar nerve are covered by the tight plantar fascia until it is penetrated by the common plantar finger nerves in its distal third. The subcutis of the planta is a very structured space with lobulated fatty tissue and tense connective tissue fibers, connecting the plantar fascia to the plantar skin. That is why the sonographic visualization of the terminal branches of the plantar toe-nerves is very difficult and not always achieved with sufficient clarity.

The lateral plantar nerve usually continues the course of the tibial nerve together with the now more lateral positioned main plantar vessels. It usually splits into three terminal branches for the supply of the lateral and inter-tarsal plantar intrinsic muscles, with the supply of the skin of the fibular aspect of the fourth and plantar aspect of the fifth toe, after branching into common and proper plantar toe nerves (Fig. 2.25). What has been said above for the branches of the medial plantar nerve equally applies for the sonographic visualization of these subcutaneous branches.

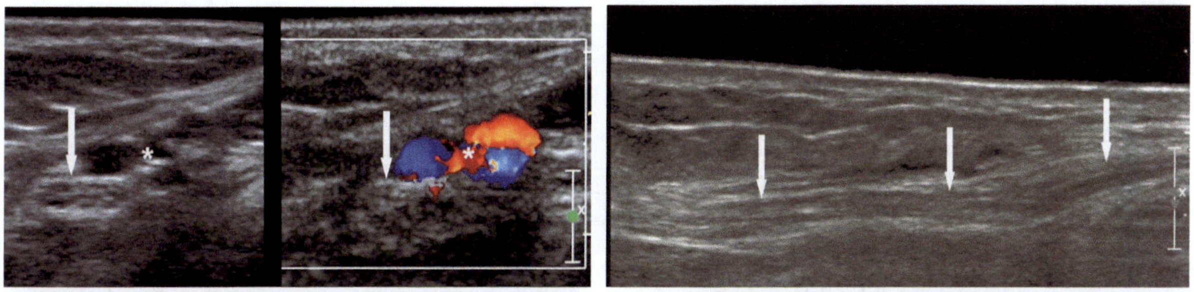

a c

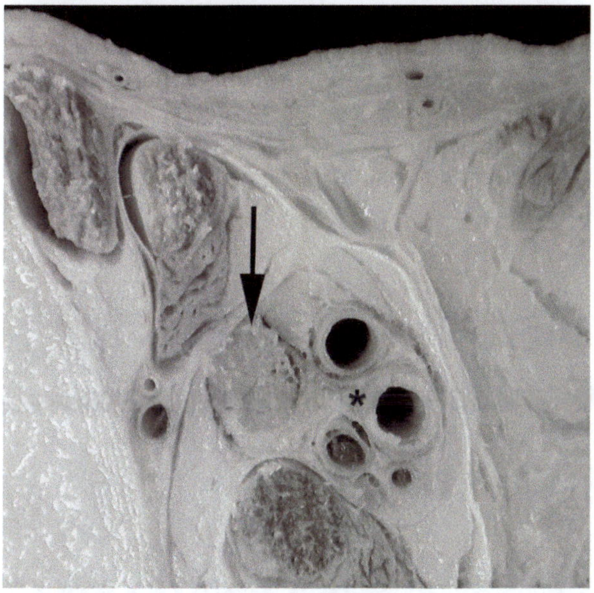

b

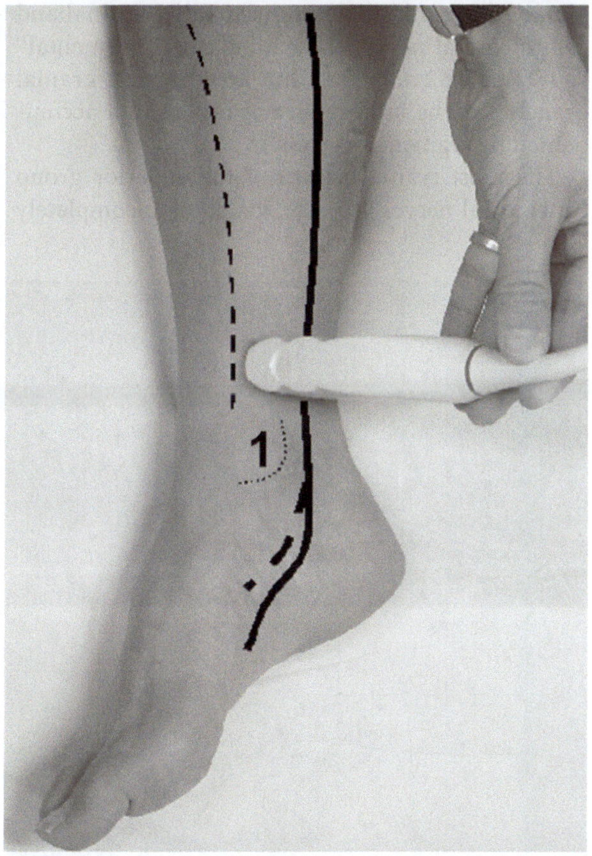

d

Fig. 2.24a–d. Transverse US scan and color US scan (**a**) with the corresponding cryosection (**b**) showing the distal tibial nerve (*arrow*) accompanied by the posterior tibial vascular bundle (*). **c** Longitudinal US scan. **d** Scheme and skin projections of the distal tibial nerve (*line*) and its terminal plantar medial (thick *broken line*) and lateral (*line*) branches: medial and lateral plantar nerve. Edge of the tibia (thin *broken line*), medial malleolus (*dotted line, 1*) as landmarks

2.4 Nerves of the Trunk

In the trunk the primordial metamer organization of the human body stays unaltered as far as peripheral nerves are concerned. The primary segmentation of the body finding its expression in the segmental organization of the vertebral column and the musculature therefore applies logically to the peripheral nerves. The usual spinal nerve exiting the intervertebral foramen splits into two main branches: the ventral root and the dorsal root. The ventral roots are mainly responsible for any motor and sensory supply of structures ventral and the dorsal roots dorsal to the respective intervertebral foramen. The thoracic nerves may be subdivided in a superior "intercostal" group (segments Th 1–Th 6) and a inferior "subcostal" group (segments Th 7–Th 12). These nerves are functionally mixed nerves (motor and sensory elements) and supply more or less the according metamer rump-wall segments (muscles as well as the overlying skin) with anterior and lateral cutaneous branches. The thoracic nerves of the superior group – the intercostal nerves – are positioned underneath the according rib together with the cranial lying segmental intercostal vessels in a space defined by the extern and intern intercostal muscles. The thoracic nerves of the inferior group show the same segmental pattern like the intercostal nerves innervating the less segmented lateral and ventral abdominal musculature and the according overlying skin, also accompanied by according segmental vessels. The most inferior of these nerves is "the" subcostal nerve (Th 12) ending in the region of the iliac crest. The nerves supplying the inguinal region of the trunk (iliohypogastric, ilioinguinal and genitofemoral nerve) show an almost "segmental" course in the rump-wall, but are the most cranial branches of the lumbar plexus and are not accompanied by segmental vessels.

The most cranial nerves of the superior group (intercostal nerves 1–3) are somehow incompletely integrated in the formation of the brachial plexus so that they release accessory sensory branches for the supply of the inner proximal upper extremity (intercostobrachial nerves).

The sonographic visualization of these segmental nerves can be performed easily for the intercostal nerves despite their smallness as they are accompanied by clearly identifiable vessels (Fig. 2.26).

The thoracic nerves of the inferior group and the "inguinal-region-trunk-nerves" of the lumbar plexus (iliohypogastric, ilioinguinal and genitofemoral nerve) are usually only visible in pathologic conditions with enlargement of the nerve, such as neuroma formation for example – the normal nerves are generally too small to be reliably assessed with sonography.

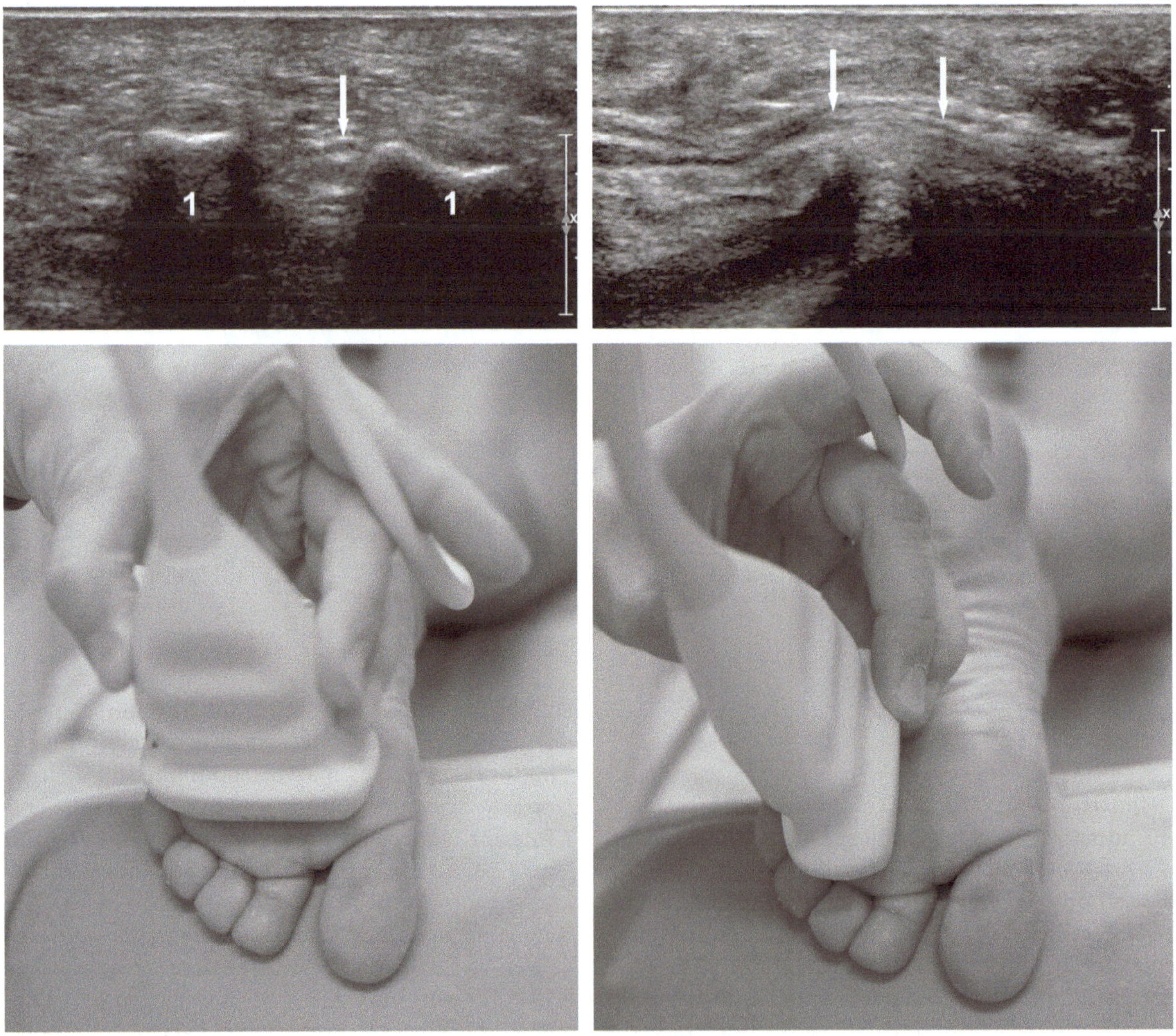

a b c d

Fig. 2.25a–d. Transverse US scan (**a**) with corresponding scheme (**b**) and longitudinal US scan (**c**) with corresponding scheme (**d**) showing a common digital nerve of the toes (*arrow*) in between two heads of metatarsal bones (*1*)

The dorsal root usually ends in a mixed segmental peripheral nerve releasing the posterior cutaneous branches – in the inferior dorsal region forming the superior and medial clunium nerves – and supplying the autochthon musculature with very fine terminal branches. The sonographic visualization of these nerves is also only achieved in the case of pathologic alterations.

a
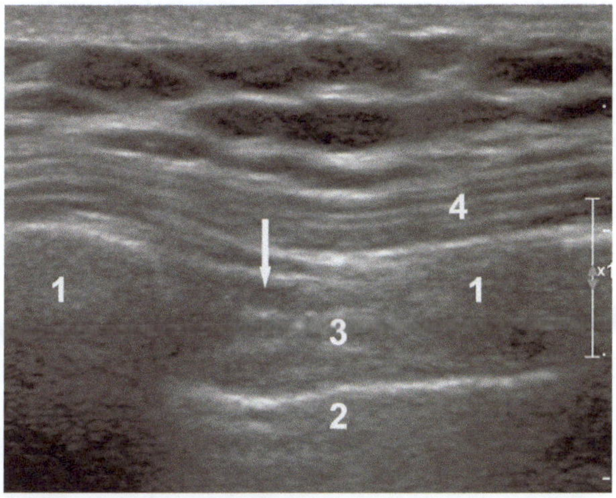

b
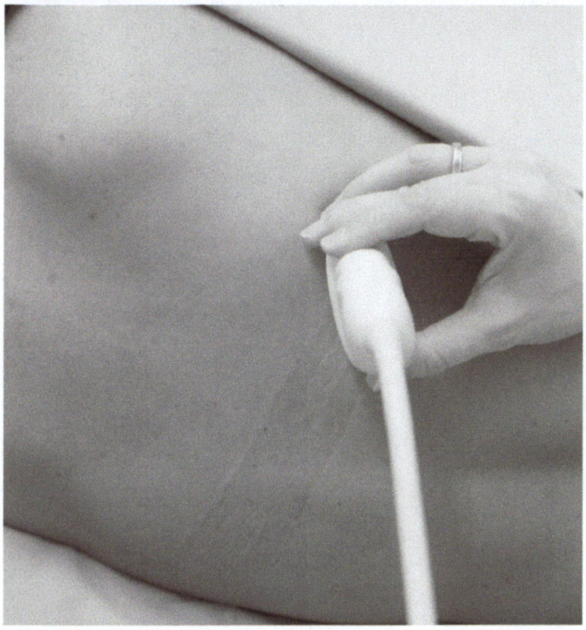

Fig. 2.26a,b. US scan (**a**) of the chest wall perpendicular to the echogenic rib bones (*1*) with acoustical shadows covering the also echogenic lung (*2*) and the cross section of an intercostal nerve (*arrow*) inferior to its according rib. Intercostal muscles (*3*) and latissimus dorsi muscle (*4*). **b** Corresponding scheme

References

Bodner G, Harpf C, Gardetto A, Kovacs P, Gruber H, Peer S, Mallhoui A (2002) Ultrasonography of the accessory nerve. Normal and pathological findings in cadavers and patients with iatrogenic accessory nerve palsy. J Ultrasound Med 21:1159–1163

Duncan I, Sullivan P, Lomas F (1999) Sonography in the diagnosis of carpal tunnel syndrome. AJR Am J Roentgenol 173:681–684

Gassner E, Schocke M, Peer S et al. (2002) Persistent median artery in the carpal tunnel – color Doppler ultrasonographic findings. J Ultrasound Med 21:455–461

Graif M, Seton A, Nerubai J, Horoszowski H, Itzchak Y (1991) Sciatic nerve: sonographic evaluation and anatomic-pathologic considerations. Radiology 181:405–408

Gruber H, Kovacs P, Piegger J, Brenner E (2001) New, simple, ultrasound-guided infiltration of the pudendal nerve: topographic basics. Dis Colon Rectum 44:1376–1380

Gruber H, Peer S, Kovacs P, Marth R, Bodner G (2002) The ultrasound appearance of the femoral nerve and cases of iatrogenic impairment. J Ultrasound Med 22:163–172

Hafferl A (1969) Lehrbuch der Topographischen Anatomie, 3. Auflage. Springer, Berlin, Heidelberg New York

Kahle W (1991) Nervensystem und Sinnesorgane, 6. Auflage. Thieme, Stuttgart

Kovacs P, Gruber H, Piegger J, Bodner G (2001) New, simple, ultrasound- guided infiltration of the pudendal nerve: ultrasonographic technique. Dis Colon Rectum 44:1381–1385

Platzer W (1982) Atlas der topographischen Anatomie. Thieme, Stuttgart

Riffaud L, Morandi X, Godey B et al. (1999) Anatomic basis for the compression and neurolysis of the deep branch of the radial nerve in the radial tunnel. Surg Radiol Anat 21:229–233

Sarria L, Cabada T, Cozcolluela R, Martinez-Berganza T, Garcia S (2000) Carpal tunnel syndrome: usefulness of sonography. Eur Radiol 10:1920–1925

Silvestri E, Martinoli C, Derchi LE et al. (1995) Echotexture of peripheral nerves: correlation between US and histologic findings and criteria to differentiate tendons. Radiology 197:291–296

Thomas SJ, Yakin DE, Parry BR, Lubahn JD (2000) The anatomical relationship between the posterior interosseous nerve and the supinator muscle. J Hand Surg [Am] 25:936–941

Von Lanz T, Wachsmuth W (1972) Praktische Anatomie, 4.Auflage. Springer, Berlin Heldelberg New York

Yang WT, Chui PT, Metreweli C (1998) Anatomy of the normal brachial plexus revealed by sonography and the role of sonographic guidance in anesthesia of the brachial plexus. AJR Am J Roentgenol 171:1631–1636

Clinical and Electrodiagnostic Work-up of Peripheral Nerve Lesions

3

Stefan Kiechl

CONTENTS

S. Kiechl, MD
Professor, Department of Neurology, Section for Electrodiagnosis (EMG/NLG), Innsbruck Medical University, Anichstrasse 35, 6020 Innsbruck, Austria

3.1 The Clinical Presentation of Nerve Lesions

Diagnostic work-up of patients with peripheral nerve lesions includes a detailed evaluation of the clinical history, a thorough search for predisposing factors and trigger events, palpation at the suspected lesion site, specific provocation maneuvers and assessment of motor deficits (distribution, muscle power and atrophy), sensory disturbances (distribution and quality) and autonomic impairment (sudomotor activity) – all embedded in a careful standard neurological examination. Motor deficits are best evaluated by a combination of manual muscle testing and functional evaluation of all individual muscles (with the hand and arm put into a normal position because wrist drop and other positioning abnormalities might pretend muscle weakness) (Labosky and Waggy 1986). Quantitative assessment of muscle strength, implicit to a proper monitoring of nerve recovery and re-innervation, may make use of a dynamometer or of the modified "Medical Research

Council (MRC) grading scale for muscle power" (Medical Research Council of the United Kingdom 1978) (Table 3.1). Neurogenic atrophy has to be differentiated from atrophy after immobilization. In the latter case the contour of the muscle is well preserved and EDX testing unremarkable.

Sensory manifestations are roughly divided into positive ones (paresthesia, pins and needle sensation, hyperpathia defined as a painful response to non-painful stimuli and neuropathic pain) and negative ones (numbness, loss of feeling, imbalance). Ascertainment of sensory deficits and a correct attribution to sensory nerve territories (Fig. 3.1) or human dermatomal maps (Foerster 1933) guides to the correct diagnosis.

Autonomic function tests like the sweat test and assessment of sympathetic skin responses, in turn, may assist in differentiating radiculopathies from plexopathies and more distal nerve lesions (Mumenthaler et al. 1998). Sudomotor sympathetic nerve fibers originate from the lateral column of the spinal cord at levels T2 to L2/3, pass the sympathetic trunk and join the brachial and lumbosacral plexus.

Table 3.1. Modified Medical Research Council (MRC) grading of muscle power

0	No contraction or movement
1	Trace of contraction
2	Active movement with gravity eliminated
3	Active movement against gravity but no resistance
3+	Active movement against gravity with transient resistance and collapse
4-	Severe weakness (examiner overcomes the muscle with minimal effort)
4	Moderate weakness (examiner overcomes the muscle with moderate effort)
4+	Slight weakness (examiner overcomes the muscle with considerable effort)
5-	Barely detectable weakness (examiner is not truly certain of weakness)
5	Normal power

3.1.1 Ulnar Nerve Compression at the Elbow – the Cubital Tunnel Syndrome

3.1.1.1 Epidemiology and Clinical Presentation

Ulnar nerve compression at the elbow is the second most common mononeuropathy of the upper extremities. As the initial clinical feature patients typically note numbness in the fifth and medial half of the fourth fingers sometimes spreading to the medial hand (Fig. 3.2). Typically sensory dis-

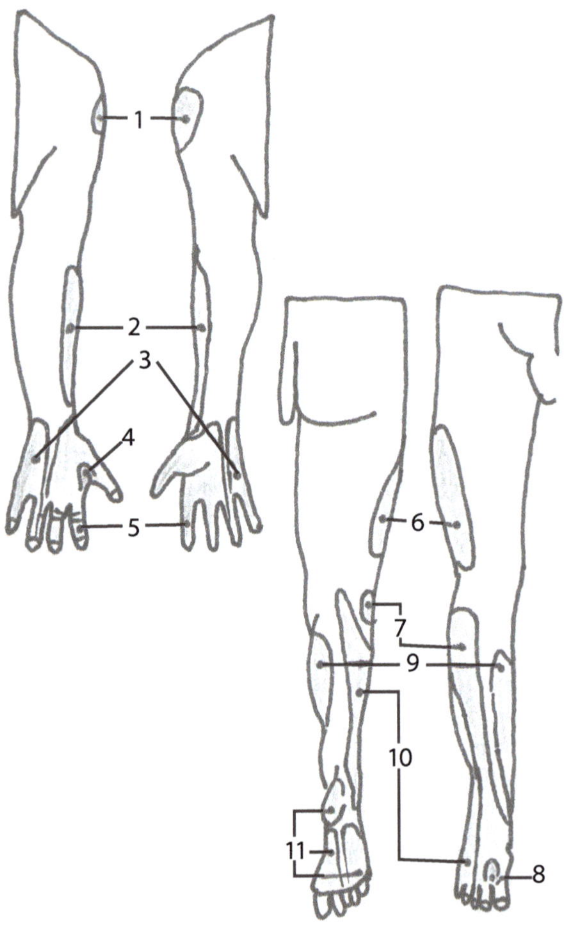

Fig. 3.1. Sensory distribution of the axillary nerve (*1*), lateral antebrachial cutaneous nerve (originating from the musculocutaneous nerve) (*2*), ulnar nerve (*3*), superficial radial nerve (*4*), median nerve (*5*), lateral femoral cutaneous nerve (*6*), superficial peroneal nerve (*7*), deep peroneal nerve (*8*), saphenus nerve (originating from the femoral nerve) (*9*), sural (*10*) and tibial nerve (*11*)

turbances do not extend much beyond the wrist. Pain and tenderness occur at the medial epicondyle and radiate along the ulnar forearm to the hand. Complaints may be provoked or enhanced by trigger situations such as resting of the elbow on a hard surface, applying external pressure to the groove, maximal flexion of the elbow or repetitive flexion and extension movements.

In the common case of progressive nerve damage, weakness of ulnar innervated hand muscles manifests and causes an abnormal posture of the hand ("ulnar clawing") as well as significant disability in the performance and fine control of finger movements. Abduction of the little finger due to paresis of the fourth interosseous muscle is recognized as the Wartenberg's sign (Mumenthaler et al. 1998). Forearm flexors (flexor carpi ulnaris and digitorum profundus muscles) are less prominently involved or even spared. Muscle wasting is best visible at the first interosseous space and hypothenar eminence. In some patients motor deficits develop insidiously without sensory symptoms.

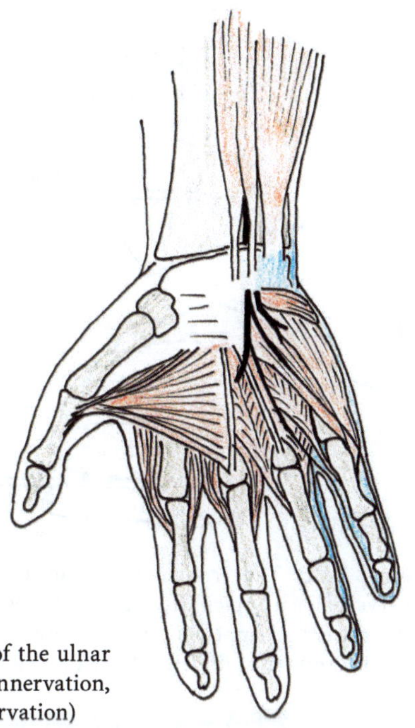

Fig. 3.2. Anatomy of the ulnar nerve (*red* = motor innervation, *blue* = sensory innervation)

3.1.1.2 Etiology

On passing through the ulnar groove at the elbow the nerve is susceptible to compression injury (Miller 1991). The precise mechanisms of nerve damage and the nature of the compressive pathology are highly heterogeneous. (1) External compression is the most common cause and derives from repeated or sustained leaning on the elbow. It may cause substantial (cumulative) nerve injury particularly in the cases of a predisposing shallow condylar groove, subluxated nerve or sustained pressure in coma or anaesthetized patients (Miller and Camp 1979). (2) Real entrapment occurs in the ulnar sulcus if the nerve is constricted by scare tissue, in the cubital tunnel ("cubital tunnel syndrome") (Campbell et al. 1991; Miller and Hummel 1980) where the ulnar nerve passes under the aponeurotic origin of the flexor carpi ulnaris muscle (1–3 cm distal to the epicondyle) or in the flexor pronator aponeurosis (more than 4 cm distal to the epicondyle). (3) Tardy ulnar nerve palsy typically develops years after fracture or dislocation of the elbow based on bony exostosis or cubita vara or valga abnormalities. Other causative bone abnormalities are advanced arthrosis, osteoarthritis or hyperostosis in Paget's disease, to name just a few. (4) Recurrent prominent dislocation of the ulnar nerve over the medial condyle can directly damage the nerve or predispose it to repetitive trauma. (5) Soft tissue masses in the condylar groove or cubital tunnel such as organized hematoma, scarring, accessory muscles (anconeus epitrochlearis) or intraneural ganglia are further potential sources of ulnar nerve compression.

3.1.1.3 Diagnosis

The diagnosis of ulnar neuropathy is – in most cases – reliably established by an experienced clinician after reviewing the patient's history (emphasis put on trigger situations) and performing a thorough neurological examination. A sensitive and highly characteristic clinical test is the Froment's maneuver (Fig. 3.3). When attempting to pinch a piece of paper between the thumb and index finger, the patient primarily utilizes the median nerve innervated long flexor of the thumb as a compensation for the ulnar hand weakness, and a typical flexed thumb posture emerges.

Other diagnoses mimicking ulnar neuropathy such as lower trunk or medial cord brachial plexus palsy, combined C8 and Th1 radiculopathy or distal ulnar nerve entrapment can be differentiated based on the pattern of sensory and motor deficits. Diagnostic work-up of patients with ulnar compression at or adjacent to the elbow should include a palpation of the ulnar nerve at the ulnar

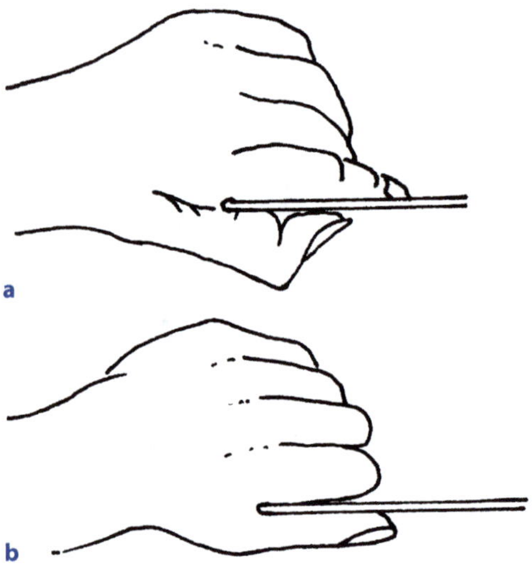

Fig. 3.3a,b. The Froment's maneuver. **a** In case of ulnar nerve palsy a typical flexed thumb posture emerges when the patient attempts to pinch a piece of paper between the thumb and index finger. **b** Maneuver in a normal subject

groove, searching for abnormal thickening, tenderness, decreased mobility or luxability. Further on, provocation tests (maximal elbow flexion for the cubital tunnel syndrome and assessment of the Tinel's sign), X-ray of the elbow and high resolution sonography of the nerve and neighboring tissues have to be performed.

Electrodiagnostic studies play a central role in evaluating suspected ulnar nerve lesions. Standard nerve conduction studies performed in a flexed elbow position are sometimes sufficient for demonstrating segmental slowing of sensory and motor fibers (focal demyelination) across the elbow (< 45 m/s or > 11 m/s difference compared to forearm nerve conduction or > 20% drop in the amplitude across the elbow) (Liveson and Ma 1992; Stoehr and Bluthardt 1993) (Fig. 3.4). Short segment stimulation (stimulation of the nerve in successive 1-cm increments) and electromyography assist in exactly localizing the lesion (Miller and Camp 1979; Campbell et al. 1992) and estimating extent and acuity of nerve damage, which is relevant to therapeutic decisions and planning of the surgical approach (Fig. 3.27). In addition, the experienced electrophysiologist is capable of detecting innervation anomalies like the forearm Martin-Gruber (Fig. 3.28) or the palmar Riche-Cannieu anastomosis between the ulnar and median nerves, and to define the origin of innervation in the various hand muscles.

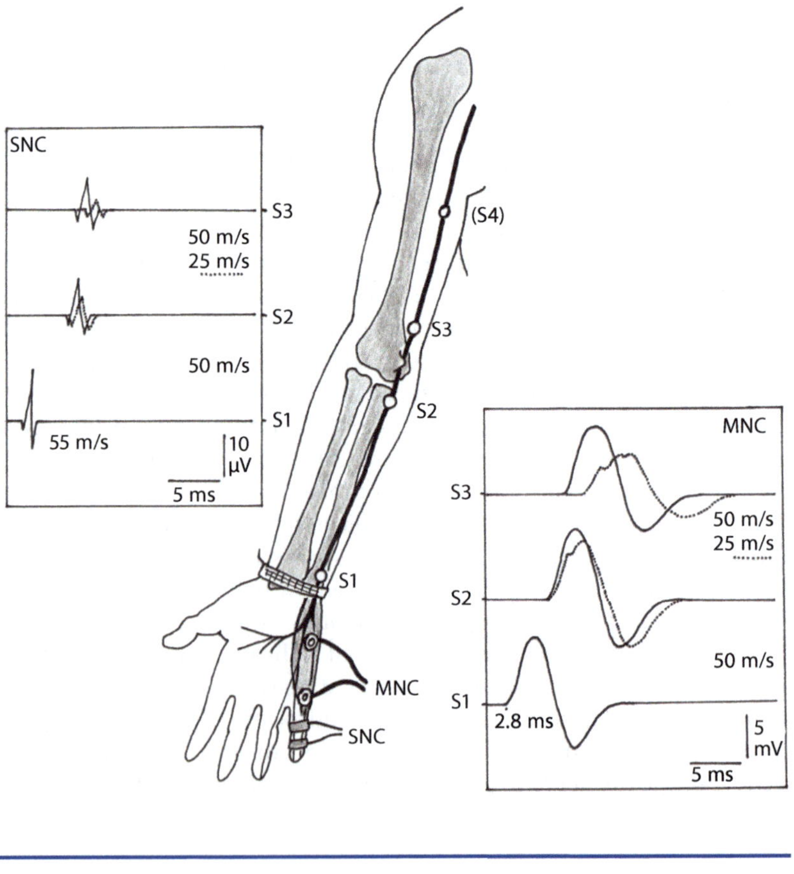

Fig. 3.4. Ulnar nerve: motor nerve conduction (*MNC*) and antidromic sensory nerve conduction (*SNC*) studies. Routinely, stimulations are performed at the wrist (*S1*), below (*S2*) and above the elbow (*S3*). Motor potentials are recorded from the abductor digiti minimi muscle (disk electrodes) and sensory potentials from the fifth finger (ring electrodes). The recordings presented are from a normal subject (*full line*) and a patient with ulnar neuropathy at the elbow (*dotted line*)

3.1.1.4 Therapy

Careful exploration for relevant trigger events and behavior related external nerve compression are crucial to a successful therapy. In such cases strict avoidance strategies are often sufficient for a reversal of symptoms and prevention of progressive nerve damage (DELLON et al. 1993). In the absence of external traumata, conservative therapy for ulnar nerve compression is limited. Steroid injection and oral anti-inflammatory drugs are not useful. A surgical procedure (release of the nerve at the ulnar groove or cubital tunnel or submuscular transposition of the nerve) (CAMPBELL et al. 1988) is reserved for patients with significant sensory-motor deficits or a severe pain syndrome. Results are generally satisfactory unless substantial damage has already manifested prior to intervention.

3.1.2 Ulnar Nerve Compression at the Wrist – the Guyon's Canal Syndrome

3.1.2.1 Etiology and Clinical Presentation

The ulnar nerve enters Guyon's canal at the level of the distal wrist crease. The canal is bordered by the pisiform bone and the hook of the hamate and the floor is formed by the transverse carpal ligament and the hamate and triquetrum bones. The roof of the canal involves the pisohamate ligament spanning the space between the pisiform bone and the hook of the hamate (Fig. 3.5). On its course through the tunnel the ulnar nerve is accompanied by the ulnar artery and vein. It divides into the superficial (predominantly) sensory branch and the deep motor branch. At the level of the pisohamate hiatus motor fibers to the hypothenar muscles leave the main trunk and supply the abductor, flexor and opponens digiti minimi muscles. Compression of the ulnar nerve in the Guyon's canal may be caused by mass lesions within the canal like ganglia, callus, lipoma or pseudoaneurysms, fractures of the hook of the hamate and external pressure related to certain occupations and sports activities (e.g. mountain biking or work with have hand tools) (BAKKE and WOLFF 1948; OLNEY and HANSON 1988; MUMENTHALER et al. 1998). Depending on the exact localization of the lesion and on the type of fibers affected, distal ulnar neuropathy may have various distinct clinical faces (OLNEY and HANSON 1988). Lesions distal to the pisohamate ligament and in the mid-palm cause a paresis and wasting of the interossei and ulnar-innervated thenar muscles with a sparing of the sensory branch and hypothenar (Fig. 3.5–1). Patients typically show claw digits, a prominent spontaneous abduction of the fifth finger and a positive Froment's sign. Lesions adjacent to the pisohamate ligament cause an additional involvement of the muscle branch to the hypothenar and thus weakness of all ulnar-intrinsic hand muscles (distal Guyon's canal syndrome) (Fig. 3.5–2). More proximal lesions affect both the deep and superficial ulnar branch leading to characteristic sensory deficit of the medial hand, digit five and ulnar half of the ring finger (palmar surface only) (Fig. 3.5–3). Occasionally, damage is restricted to the ulnar cutaneous branch resulting in sensory loss without motor deficits (Fig. 3.5–4).

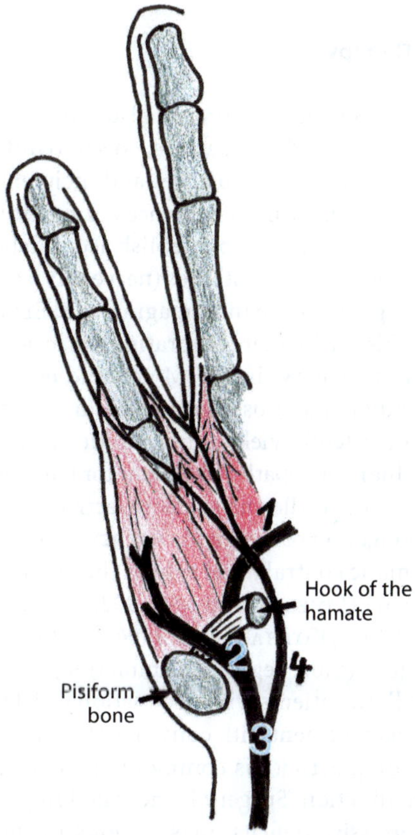

Fig. 3.5. Guyon's canal: Depending on the precise localization of the lesion four different clinical types of distal ulnar neuropathy can be differentiated: lesions distal (*1*) or adjacent to the pisohamate ligament (*2*), proximal lesions (*3*) and lesions restricted to the ulnar cutaneous branch (*4*).

3.1.2.2
Diagnosis and Therapy

Differential diagnoses include proximal ulnar neuropathies, C8 and T1 radiculopathies, lower trunk and medial cord brachial plexopathies and incipient motor neuron disease. In most instances, a careful clinical exploration allows one to establish accurately the correct diagnosis. Imaging studies (nerve ultrasonography and magnetic resonance imaging) and EDX studies are suitable for further elaborating the lesion site and the severity of nerve injury. Motor studies recording the first digital interosseous muscle are most sensitive and consistently yield abnormalities in all types of distal ulnar neuropathy (distal motor latency >4.9 and 5.3 ms with needle and surface electrode recording or prolongation of the motor latency relative to the asymptomatic contralateral side or the latency to the hypothenar) (Liveson and Ma 1992; Stoehr and Bluthardt 1993; Kothari et al. 1996; Oh 2003). Inching techniques (short segment stimulation) may be helpful as well. In patients with occupational risks a conservative management with consequent curtailing of the offending activity is commonly sufficient to restore nerve function. Surgery is indicated in patients with progressive deficits, mass lesions in the Guyon's canal and severe axonal damage without early signs of reinervation.

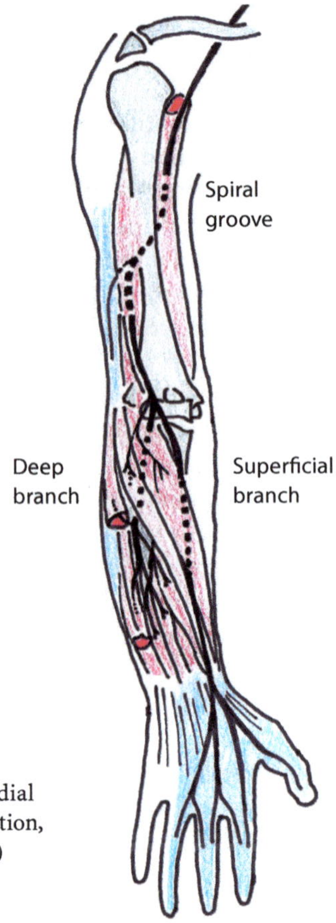

Fig. 3.6. Anatomy of the radial nerve (*red* = motor innervation, *blue* = sensory innervation)

3.1.3
Radial Nerve Compression Syndromes

3.1.3.1
Epidemiology and Clinical Presentation

Entrapment of the radial nerve may occur at various sites along its course including the upper arm and passage through the supinator muscle (Mumenthaler et al. 1998). The radial nerve receives innervation from C5 to T1 nerve roots and gives off sensory branches (posterior cutaneous nerves of arm and forearm) and muscle branches to the triceps brachii muscle before it winds around the humerus in the spiral groove. After supplying the brachio-radialis, extensor carpi radialis (long head) and supinator muscles the nerve bifurcates into the superficial (sensory) branch and the predominantly motor posterior interosseous nerve which enters the supinator muscle under the arcade of Frohse and further descends to hand and finger extensors (Fig. 3.6).

The most common type of radial neuropathy is caused by lesions at the spiral groove where the nerve is adjacent to bone and susceptible to compression (Sunderland 1945; Brown and Watson 1993). Clinically, patients are characterized by a marked wrist and finger drop and – depending on the severity of compressive nerve injury – also deficits of sensation in the distribution of the superficial radial nerve (lateral dorsal hand and dorsal aspects of the first to third and radial half of the fourth finger). Entrapment at the level of the supinator muscle called posterior interosseous neuropathy differs in its clinical presentation by the lack of sensory deficits, a partly preserved wrist extension (weak extension with radial deviation due to intact innervation of the long head of the extensor carpi radialis muscle) and the typical pain and tenderness in the region of the supinator muscle (Fig. 3.7). Pain aggravates during certain maneuvers, such as sustained extension of the middle finger or forced supination of the stretched arm.

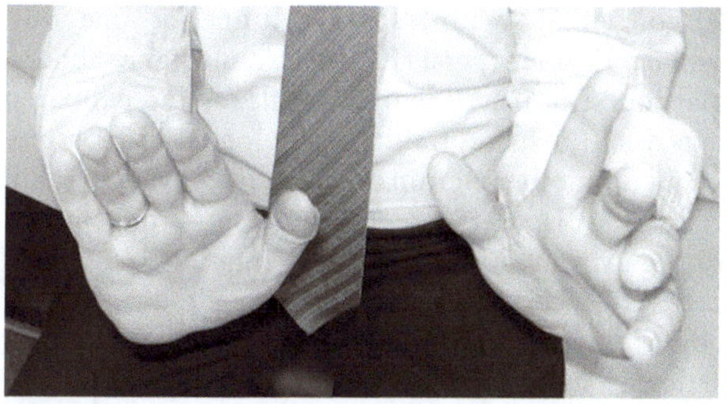

Fig. 3.7. Patient with posterior interosseous neuropathy at the left hand side showing motor deficits of finger and ulnar wrist extensors

3.1.3.2
Etiology

The most common causes for a radial neuropathy at the spiral groove are external compression (e.g. "honeymoon palsy") and fractures of the humerus with or without hematoma formation (Sunderland 1945; Brown and Watson 1993; Sturzenegger and Rutz 1991). The posterior interosseous nerve may become entrapped under the tendinous arcade of Frohse of the supinator muscle (radial tunnel) or is affected by mass lesions like ganglion cysts, lipoma or muscle hematoma (Mumenthaler et al. 1998).

3.1.3.3
Diagnosis

The correct diagnosis is usually established based on a careful neurological examination and review of the patient's history (exposure to external pressure). Differential diagnoses potentially mimicking radial neuropathy and its cardinal symptom – the wrist drop – include ischemic stroke ("central wrist drop") and C7 radiculopathy with predominantly C7 innervation of extensor muscles. EDX testing allows one to determine whether entrapment/compression has resulted in demyelination (conduction block) or severe axon loss. Nerve ultrasonography adds significantly by visualizing the causes of nerve injury other than external pressure.

3.1.3.4
Therapy

The management of radial neuropathy from external compression is primarily conservative with a strict avoidance of the offending compression. In most patients prognosis is favorable. The need for surgical intervention depends on the severity of nerve damage, clinical course and underlying cause. Whereas the decision for a surgical procedure may be straightforward in the case of compressive hematomas, dislocation of the radial nerve into the fracture gap, mass lesions in the radial tunnel and patients resistant to conservative treatment, it is much more challenging in posterior interosseous neuropathies with forearm pain but without motor deficits (Kaplan 1984).

3.1.4
Median Nerve Compression at the Wrist – the Carpal Tunnel Syndrome

3.1.4.1
Epidemiology and Clinical Presentation

The CTS is the most common entrapment syndrome of the upper extremities with an estimated incidence in the general community of 125 per 100,000 per year (Stevens et al. 1988). Typically, the dominant hand is affected first. The clinical hallmark and usually presenting feature of CTS is a pain syndrome called Brachialgia paraesthetica nocturna (Mumenthaler et al. 1998). Patients are awakened from sleep in the early morning hours, with pain radiating from the wrist proximally into the forearm and arm, and report on numbness and tingling in the hand, stiffness of fingers, and characteristic swelling sensations. All complaints rapidly resolve after repeated hand movements like shaking. Episodes of pain may exacerbate in the nights after prolonged strenuous manual work. With more severe nerve compression the patient experiences permanent paresthesia or sensory loss over the palmar thumb and digits innervated by the median nerve (Fig. 3.8), and in advanced disease weakness and wasting of part of the thenar muscles (Fig. 3.8). Significant vasomotor disturbances are comparatively rare.

3.1.4.2
Etiology

CTS arises from compression of the median nerve in the canal formed by the transverse carpal ligament and carpal bones. Under pathological circumstances tissue pressure in the carpal tunnel reaches 30 mm Hg, i.e., four times the level of normal (Szabo and Chidgey 1989). Chronic or recurrent compression of the median nerve causes focal demyelination and

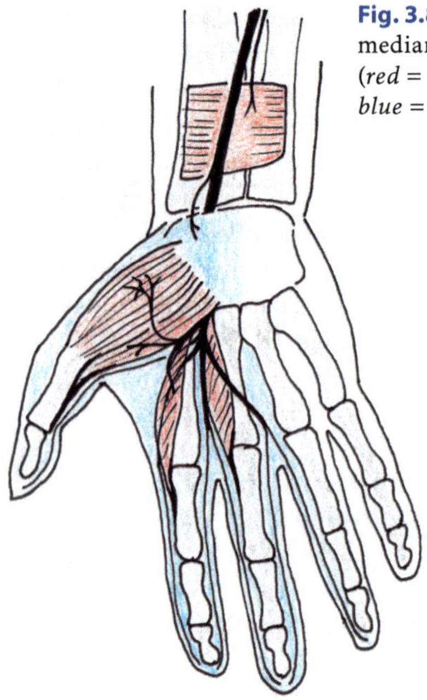

Fig. 3.8. Anatomy of the median nerve (*red* = motor innervation, *blue* = sensory innervation)

eventually axon degeneration as the pathological counterpart to the emerging clinical deficits. Temporary ischemia due to compression of vasa nervorum accounts for the reversible pain manifesting during night. Factors contributing to the development of CTS are numerous and often co-exist in individuals: (1) congenital smallness of the tunnel or anatomical peculiarities (persistent Arteria mediana, abnormal course or insertion of finger flexor and palmaris muscles); (2) susceptibility of the nerve to pressure (diabetic or other neuropathies, etc.); (3) systemic and endocrine disorders (pregnancy, hypothyroidism, acromegaly, amyloidosis, etc.); (4) reduced space in the carpal tunnel due to space occupying lesions (osteophytes, exostosis, ganglia, hematoma, tenosynovitis, articular deformities in rheumatoid arthritis, etc.) (Rosenbaum and Ochoa 1993; Stevens et al. 1992). In particular, the application of high-resolution ultrasound has expanded our knowledge on the diversity of pathological conditions underlying CTS.

3.1.4.3
Diagnosis

In most instances the diagnosis of CTS is reliably settled by an experienced clinician based on a review of the patient's history and complaints and a careful neurological examination. Clinical assessment should include the Phalen's maneuver (emergence of paresthesia in the median territory elicited by maximal passive wrist flexion for one minute (Kuschner et al. 1992; Phalen 1966) and testing for the Tinel's sign (paresthesia provoked by tapping with the finger over the carpal tunnel).

Electrodiagnostic testing is recommended when median nerve compression causes significant discomfort or sustained sensory-motor deficits. Standard nerve conduction studies usually allow to detect distal conduction abnormalities [prolonged distal motor latency (>4.0 to 4.8 ms) and reduced distal sensory nerve conduction (<45 to 55 m/s)] as indicators of nerve entrapment (Stevens 1987; Liveson and Ma 1992) (Fig. 3.9). Sensitivity of the

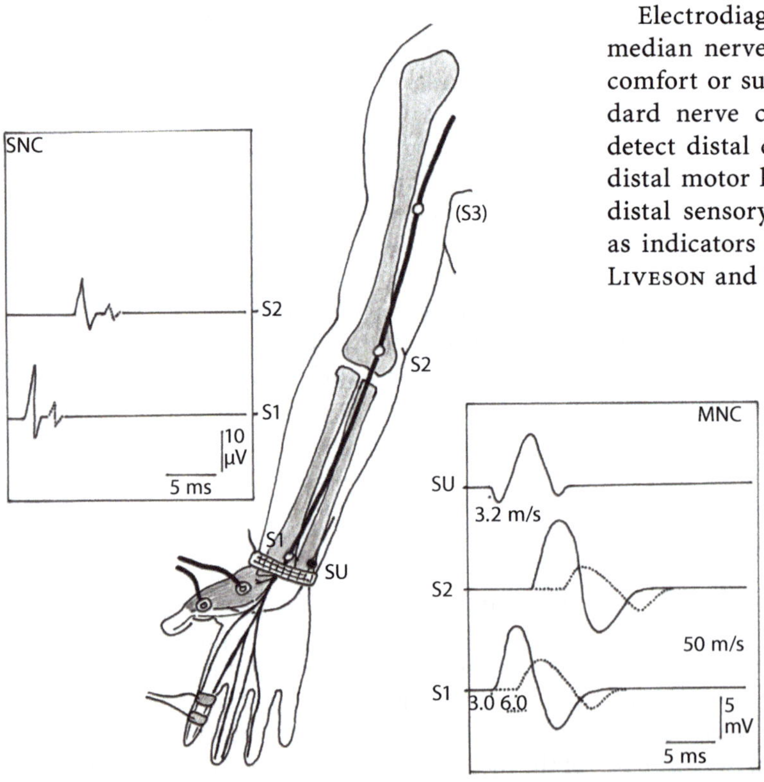

Fig. 3.9. Median nerve: motor nerve conduction (*MNC*) and antidromic sensory nerve conduction (*SNC*) studies. Routinely, stimulations are performed at the wrist (*S1*) and elbow (*S2*), and over the ulnar nerve at the wrist (*SU*). Motor potentials are recorded from the abductor pollicis brevis muscle (disk electrodes) and sensory potentials from the index finger (ring electrodes). The recordings presented are from a normal subject (*full line*) and a patient with carpal tunnel syndrome (*dotted line*)

evaluation can be improved to near 100% by more sophisticated techniques such as short-segment studies (Kimura 1979) (Fig. 3.10), palmar stimulations (Stevens 1987) and co-stimulation of the ulnar nerve for a comparison of median versus ulnar distal motor latencies (Felsenthal 1977). The latter technique creates an ideal internal control for methodological problems.

An electrophysiological work-up is particularly useful to asses the damage of the median nerve (demyelination vs axon loss) relevant to therapeutic decisions, to rule out differential diagnoses or coexistent disease, and to confirm the presence of CTS in the event of atypical complaints, pure motor deficits and prominent neuropathy.

3.1.4.4 Therapy

The mainstays of treatment are the avoidance of wrist overuse, withdrawal of provoking factors, placement of neutral wrist splints during sleep, local corticosteroid injections adjacent to the carpal tunnel (Green 1984), and – if non-surgical interventions fail or neurological deficits emerge – surgical sectioning of the volar carpal ligament. Pain and paresthesia bring most patients to medical attention before irreversible axonal loss has developed. Accordingly, overall prognosis of CTS is good to excellent in up to 80%–90% of patients given adequate management (Campbell 1998).

3.1.5 Proximal Median Nerve Compression Syndromes

3.1.5.1 Clinical Presentation, Etiology and Management

The median nerve descends medial to the humerus and anterior to the medial epicondyle to the antecubital fossa where it travels adjacent to the brachial artery towards the heads of the pronator teres muscle. After providing innervation to and passing through this muscle it gives off the anterior interosseous nerve and proceeds to the wrist. Proximal entrapment syndromes of the nerve occur at the level of medial epicondyle and the pronator teres muscle or exclusively affect the anterior interosseous nerve (Morris and Peter 1976; Suranyi 1983). The syndrome mentioned first is caused by the ligament of Struthers stretching between a bony spur and the medial epicondyle (Fig. 3.11) (Suranyi 1983). Clinically, patients may show variable weakness of pronator teres, thenar and median-innervated forearm flexor muscles and usually mild sensory deficits in a median distribution. Intense pain radiating into

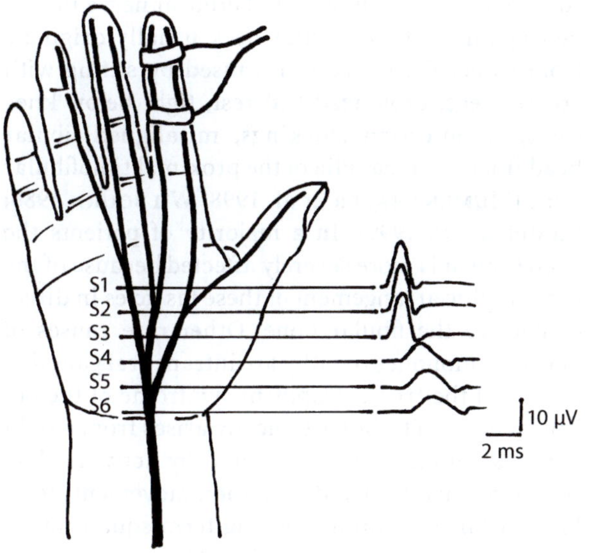

Fig. 3.10. Carpal tunnel studies: short segment stimulation

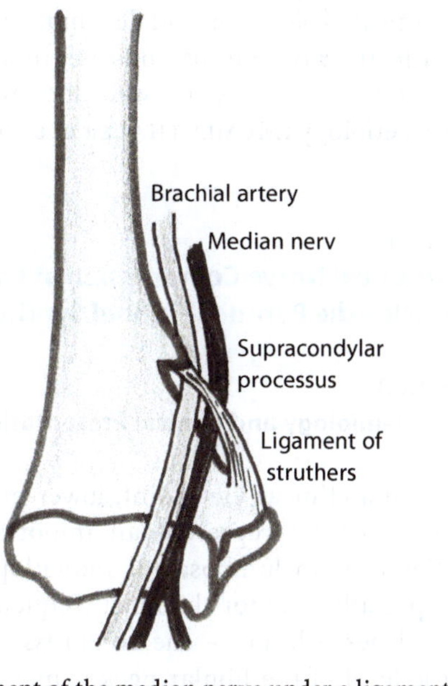

Fig. 3.11. Entrapment of the median nerve under a ligament of Struthers stretching between a bony spur and the medial epicondyle

the volar forearm is aggravated by extension and supination of elbow and forearm.

The pronator teres syndrome is characterized by similar complaints except for the sparing the pronator teres muscle and distinct provocation maneuvers (forced pronation and elbow extension). Compression may occur in the substance of the pronator teres itself or occasionally beneath at the lacertus fibrosus or sublimis bridge. The anterior interosseous syndrome in turn is hallmarked by the inability to flex the distal phalanx of the thumb and index finger and a lack of sensory disturbances (Mumenthaler et al. 1998). Compression may arise from fracture of the radius mid-shaft or anomalous fibrous bands crossing the nerve, while involvement in neuralgic amyotrophy and ischemic nerve injury represent the most common non-compressive etiologies (Wong and Dellon 1997). Overall, proximal median neuropathy is rare and diagnostically challenging because of the commonly mild and variable sensory-motor deficits. Work-up of these patients should include EDX studies, plain X-ray of the elbow and distal arm, palpation for a bony spur at the distal humerus, provocation maneuvers as outlined above and high-resolution ultrasonography of the nerve. In the case of proximal median neuropathy evoked by external compression or repetitive pronation and supination movements a conservative treatment regime (rest and prevention of sustained compression) is preferable. Patients with other causes and deteriorating symptoms, however, may benefit from surgical exploration and decompression. In patients with anterior interosseous neuropathy surgery is confined to cases with a well-documented compressive etiology (Mumenthaler et al. 1998).

3.1.6 Peroneal Nerve Compression at the Fibular Neck – the Peroneal Tunnel Syndrome

3.1.6.1 Epidemiology and Clinical Presentation

From a clinical viewpoint, lower-extremity mononeuropathies represent an important differential diagnosis to lumbosacral radiculopathies. This is especially true for the most frequent type of peroneal nerve lesion – the compression syndrome at the level of the fibular neck sometimes referred to as the "peroneal tunnel syndrome" (Mumenthaler et al. 1998).

Clinically, peroneal nerve lesions result in complete or incomplete foot drop with a weakness in foot dorsiflection and toe extension (deep peroneal branch), and ankle eversion (superficial peroneal branch). Sensory manifestations are restricted to the first web space between great and second toe (deep branch) or extend to the lateral aspect of the leg (lower two-thirds) and dorsum of the foot (superficial branch). Although peroneal nerve palsy is usually painless, some patients may complain of burning sensations in the skin area supplied by the nerve. Intense pain occurs in case of the rare, true entrapment syndrome in the peroneal tunnel (Maudsley 1967), compression of the terminal branch of deep peroneal nerve (ligamentum cruciatum at the dorsum of the foot) (Gessini et al. 1984) and represents the presenting clinical feature of the anterior compartmental syndrome of the leg caused by trauma, spontaneous bleeding into the compartment or strenuous exercise with consecutive compressive or ischemic damage to the deep peroneal nerve.

3.1.6.2 Etiology

The common peroneal and tibial nerve separate on their course through the dorsal thigh or in the popliteal fossa. The common peroneal nerve winds around the fibular neck and passes the peroneal tunnel formed by the tendinous edge of the peroneus longus muscle and the bony surface of the fibula. Near this point the nerve divides into the superficial and deep branch. Peroneal nerve mononeuropathies at the fibular neck usually originate from external compression caused by sitting with crossed legs, prolonged bed rest, tight below knee casts, compression stockings, misaligned fibular head fracture or ganglia of the proximal tibiofibular joint (Mumenthaler et al. 1998; Wilbourn 1986; Campellone 1999). In a majority of patients the deep branch is more severely affected because of the topographic arrangement of these fascicles in direct contact to the fibular bone. Other rare causes of peroneal mononeuropathy are intraneural ganglion cysts and the true entrapment syndrome of the peroneal nerve. The latter typically arises from a tight peroneal tunnel and is triggered by activities like repetitive inversion and pronation movements (e.g., long distance running) or long-term squatting for example during crop harvesting (Mumenthaler et al. 1998; Koller and Blank 1980; Kumiai 1987).

3.1.6.3
Diagnosis

Peroneal nerve lesions can usually be diagnosed on clinical grounds and by the thorough assessment of typical trigger events. Mimics like L5 radiculopathy can be differentiated by the presence of lumbar pain and the typical distribution of sensory and motor deficits. While both entities cause dorsiflexion and toe extension weakness, L5 radiculopathy additionally affects ankle inversion (tibialis posterior muscle) and hip abduction (gluteus medius muscle).

Provocation maneuvers are less helpful than in many other peripheral nerve lesions; however, pressure over the peroneal tunnel may cause local pain and the Tinel's sign may be positive as well. Standard EDX evaluation consists of motor (CAMP recorded from the extensor digitorum brevis muscle) and sensory (superficial peroneal SNAP) nerve conduction studies and electromyographic exploration of tibialis anterior and peroneal muscles as well as of L5 muscles not innervated by the peroneal nerve (e.g., tibialis posterior and gluteus medius muscles). Findings suggestive of peroneal nerve lesion at the fibular neck are a focal slowing of nerve conduction (<41 m/s) and/or conduction block (Fig. 3.12), as well as a reduced superficial peroneal SNAP in case of sensory involvement (Liveson and Ma 1992; Stoehr and Bluthardt 1993; Oh 2003). Nerve ultrasound is particularly helpful for the detection of anatomical abnormalities and intraneural ganglion cysts.

3.1.6.4
Therapy

The prognosis of a pressure palsy of the peroneal nerve at the level of the fibular neck is usually favorable with a recovery within several weeks as long as further compression is prevented. In case of significant axon loss demonstrated on EDX testing, however, the outcome is less promising. While surgery may significantly contribute to a good recovery in case of intraneural ganglion cysts, compressive scar tissue and the true peroneal tunnel syndrome, outcome after stretch and severe traumatic nerve injury remains grave (Mumenthaler et al. 1998). In cases of severe and irreversible nerve damage, posterior tibialis muscle transfer and other techniques of reconstructive surgery frequently produce satisfactory results.

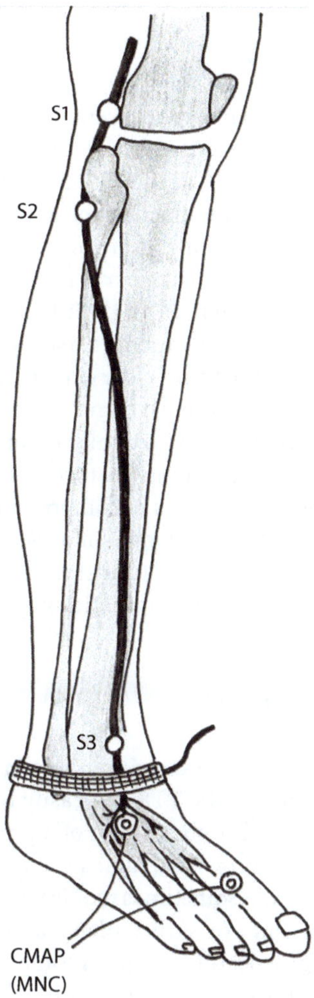

Fig. 3.12. Peroneal nerve: motor nerve conduction (*MNC*) studies. Routinely, stimulation is performed above (*S1*) and below the fibular neck (*S2*) and at the dorsum of the foot (*S3*). Motor potentials (*CMAPs*) are recorded from the extensor digitorum brevis muscle (disk electrodes)

3.1.7
Tibial Nerve Compression – the Tarsal Tunnel Syndrome

3.1.7.1
Epidemiology and Clinical Presentation

The tarsal tunnel syndrome (TTS) (Keck 1962; Mumenthaler et al. 1998) is less frequent than peroneal nerve compression and entrapment syndromes of upper extremities. The disorder is insidious in onset and mostly unilateral. Patients complain of burning pain at the plantar side of the foot which sometimes radiate to the calf and typically increase while walking (DeLisa and Saeed 1983). Pain is often accompanied by paresthesia and foot numbness in the distribution of one or all of the terminal sensory branches. Sensory manifestations may worsen by foot eversion. Paresis of small foot muscles with development of "claw digits" and abnormal posture of the foot is rare.

3.1.7.2
Etiology

The tibial nerve descends behind the medial malleolus and passes under the flexor retinaculum ("laciniate ligament") to the plantar side of the foot, where it divides into the calcaneal, medial and lateral plantar branches. In the tarsal tunnel, roofed by the flexor retinaculum, the nerve is prone to compression injury (Goodgold et al 1965; Oh and Meyer 1999). In a majority of patients tarsal tunnel syndrome is idiopathic with no clear precipitating factors detectable. The second most common cause is entrapment due to scare tissue or articular deformities originating from previous trauma (distortion or fracture of the ankle). Further sources of compression are an accessory flexor digitorum longus muscle and space occupying lesions within the tunnel such as lipoma, varicose veins, ganglia, non-traumatic exostosis or neoplasm.

3.1.7.3
Diagnosis

If fully expressed (characteristic sensory and motor deficits), the TTS can easily be diagnosed on clinical grounds only. In case of a pure pain syndrome, however, a correct diagnosis may be much more demanding and sometimes requires ancillary, e.g., radiological testing. In such patients a positive compression test (provocation of typical complaints by manual pressure applied on the tarsal tunnel for 30 s) may be helpful. Standard electrodiagnostic testing consists of the measurement of distal motor latencies to abductor hallucis and/or abductor digiti minimi muscles and electromyographic exploration of the muscles of the sole. Unilateral prolongation of the motor latency (>7 ms to the abductor digiti minimi muscle) and/or emergence of severe chronic or acute damage on electromyography strongly supports the diagnosis (Goodgold et al. 1965) (Fig. 3.13). However, normal results are not contradictive to the presence of TTS (sensitivity 50%–80%) (Liveson and Ma 1992). Interpretability of electrodiagnostic testing may be difficult in the events of coexisting neuropathy or severe damage of the nerve root S1. The procedure with the highest diagnostic sensitivity is an anesthetic nerve block.

Finally, an orthopedic examination is mandatory to distinguish TTS from numerous differential diagnoses such as stress fractures, bursitis, inflammatory arthritis or plantar fasciitis. It has to be considered that some of these conditions may affect tibial nerve function in terms of a (non-compressive) local irritation.

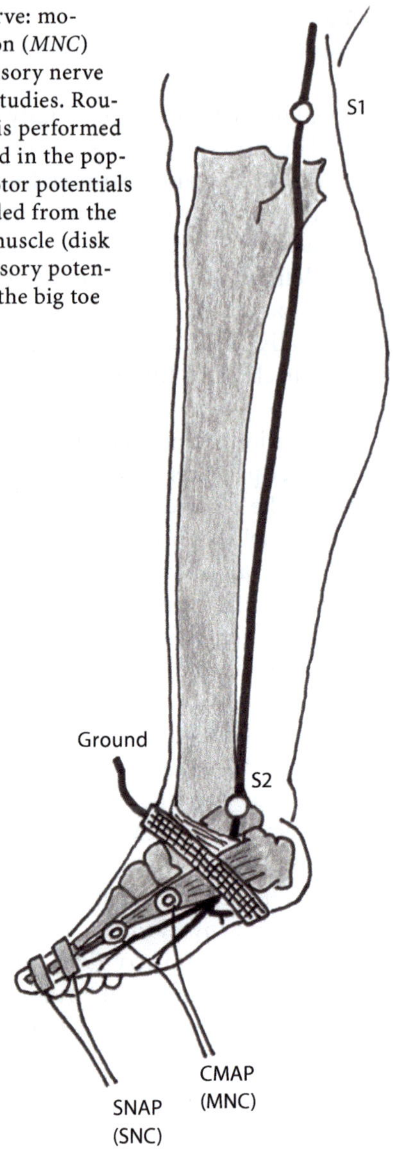

Fig. 3.13. Tibial nerve: motor nerve conduction (*MNC*) and antidromic sensory nerve conduction (*SNC*) studies. Routinely, stimulation is performed at the ankle (S1) and in the popliteal fossa (S2). Motor potentials (*CMAPs*) are recorded from the abductor hallucis muscle (disk electrodes) and sensory potentials (*SNAPs*) from the big toe (ring electrodes)

3.1.7.4
Therapy

Potential sources of external compression like badly fitting shoes should be eliminated. Local corticosteroid injections are sometimes helpful. If TTS produces substantial discomfort or sensory-motor deficits and conservative treatment options fail, operative release of the flexor retinaculum is the therapy of choice. Outcome after surgery is favorable in about three quarters of patients (Mondelli et al. 1998). A minority of patients develop chronic pain syndromes with features of reflex sympathetic dystrophy.

3.2 An Introduction to Electrodiagnosis

3.2.1 Basic Principles

Standard electrodiagnostic (EDX) examination consists of nerve conduction studies, recording of late responses and needle electromyography (Guidelines in Electrodiagnostic Medicine 1999). On performing EDX testing a few contraindications have to be considered (Table 3.2).

3.2.1.1 Nerve Conduction Studies

The study of nerve conduction entails depolarizing the nerve fibers with an electric stimulus and subsequent recording of evoked motor or sensory responses by means of various types of surface electrodes (Fig. 3.14). In particular, if responses are very small and the initial deflection cannot be reliably assessed, recording with needle electrodes from atrophic muscles or sensory nerves may be more appropriate. The stimulus is applied at the skin surface with the cathode held distally and the ground is best placed between the stimulation and recording site.

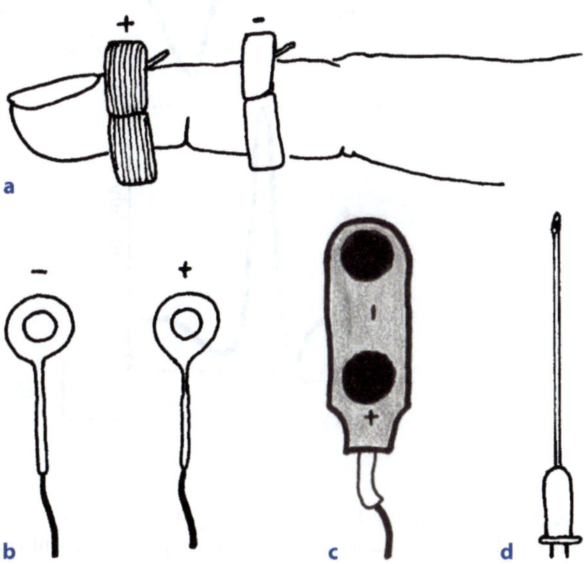

Fig. 3.14. a Ring electrodes for antidromic sensory nerve conduction studies. **b** Disk electrodes for motor and orthodromic sensory nerve conduction studies and F-wave recording. **c** Stimulator and **d** concentric needle electrode respectively, for standard electromyography

Motor nerve conduction studies: according to the tendon insertion the active recording electrode is fixed on the centre of the muscle belly usually resembling the end plate region and the reference electrode placed over the insertion of the tendon (Fig. 3.15).

Table 3.2. Contraindications to electrodiagnostic (EDX) testing

Electromyography
Any kind of coagulation disorder rendering patients at risk of muscle hemorrhage such as hemophilia, oral anticoagulation (INR > 1.7) or dose-adjusted intravenous heparin therapy
Wounds or infected skin covering the muscles of interest
Nerve conduction studies
Pacemakers: proximal stimulation at Erb's point (brachial plexus) or axilla ipsilateral to a pacemaker may cause dysfunction of the technical device

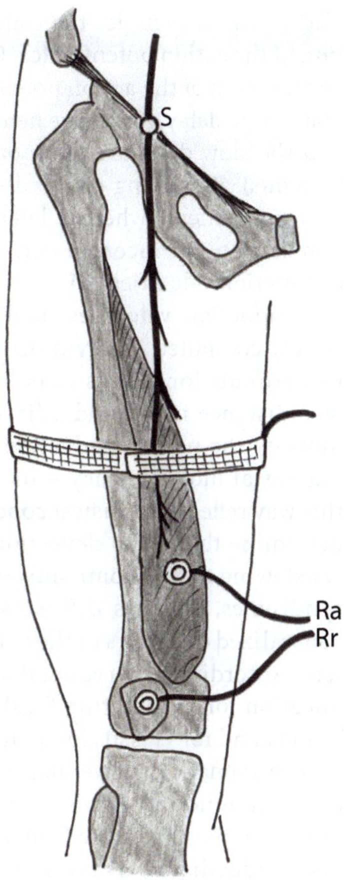

Fig. 3.15. Belly-tendon method of electrode placing in femoral nerve studies. The active recording electrode (*Ra*) is fixed on the centre of the muscle belly resembling the end plate region and the reference electrode (*Rr*) is placed over the insertion of the tendon

If properly performed, this technique produces a biphasic motor potential with an initial negativity and steep upward deflection from baseline. The M-response results from summation of the muscle fiber action potentials and is termed compound muscle action potential (CMAP) if virtually all nerve and muscle fibers depolarize (Fig. 3.16). To ensure sufficient stimulation of the nerve, the current applied is slowly increased until the generated motor response does no longer grow in size, and a final recording is performed with an electric stimulus 20% above this level (= supramaximal stimulation). Standard machine settings are a gain of 5 mV/division (y-axis of the screen – amplitude), sweep duration of 2–5 ms/division (x-axis of the screen) and a duration of the electrical impulse of 200 ms. Routinely, the following parameters of the M-response are assessed.

Latency: the latency is the time elapsing between onset of the stimulus and the initial negative deflection from baseline (in milliseconds = onset latency) (Fig. 3.16a). It includes the time required for initiation of the action potential (ca. 0.1 ms), orthodromic propagation of the action potential to the motor end plate, time delay across the neuromuscular junction and the slow depolarization of given muscle fibers (3–5 m/s). Reporting of the distal motor latency is very convenient, whereas latencies from proximal stimulation are incorporated in the calculation of conduction velocities (CVs).

Conduction velocities: motor CVs (in m/s) are simply computed by dividing the distance between two stimulation points (tape measurement of surface distance in a standardized limb position – in mm) by the nerve conduction time (proximal minus distal motor latency – in ms). CVs assessed in this way reflects the fastest conducting axons, which determine the initial deflection of the CMAPs. Focal slowing of CVs commonly occurs in entrapment syndromes, whereas diffuse slowing is typical of generalized disorders of the peripheral nervous system. Accordingly, nerve conduction studies find application for pinpointing focal (compressive) nerve lesions and for classifying polyneuropathies as primarily axonal or demyelinating. It has to be considered that mild slowing is not specific for demyelination but may also arise from selective loss of large, fast conducting fibers prone to pressure damage.

Amplitude: CMAP amplitudes are measured as base-to-peak amplitudes (initial negative component of the potential) (Fig. 3.16a) or, less commonly, as peak-to-peak amplitudes. Amplitudes mirror the number and synchrony of depolarizing muscle fibers. Low CMAP amplitudes upon distal stimulation are either a consequence of motor axon loss or distally located conduction blocks.

Duration: CMAP duration is measured from the initial deflection from baseline to the first baseline crossing and serves as a measure of synchrony (Fig. 3.16a).

Sensory nerve conduction studies: these are technically more demanding because sensory nerve action potentials (SNAPs) are small – in the range of 1–50 μV (Fig. 3.16b). The SNAP is a compound potential representing the summation of the individual nerve action potentials of all sensory axons. It is recorded directly from the nerve with two ring or disk electrodes placed in a line over the nerve (interelectrode distance 3–4 cm) and the gain set to 5–20 μV/division. Signal averaging is often necessary to suppress background noise and other artifacts. Other technical requirements resemble those described for

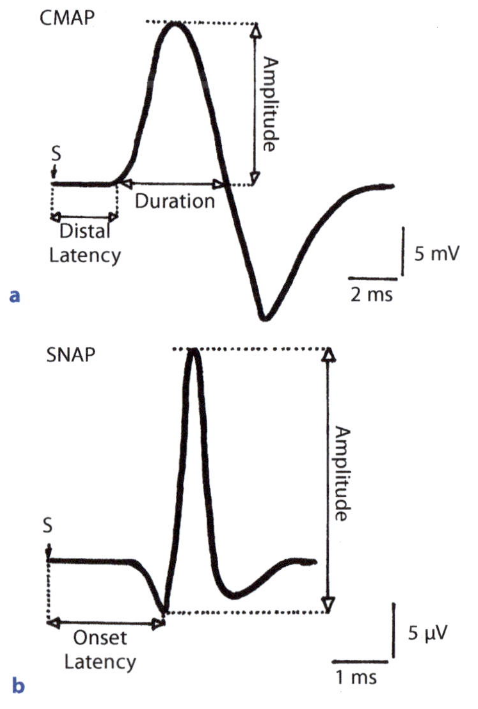

Fig. 3.16. a Compound muscle action potential (*CMAP*). It represents the summation of all the underlying muscle fiber action potentials and is biphasic with an initial negative deflection. The latency, amplitude and potential duration are routinely assessed. **b** Sensory nerve action potential (*SNAP*). It represents the summation of all the underlying sensory fiber action potentials and is bi- or triphasic. The onset latency and amplitude are routinely assessed

motor nerve conduction studies except for a usually much lower stimulation threshold.

SNAPs are bi- or triphasic and characterized by the following parameters.

SNAP amplitude: in most laboratories peak-to-peak amplitudes (Fig. 3.16b) are assessed. Low SNAP amplitudes may result from technical factors (edema, incorrect placement, etc.), axon loss or asynchrony of conduction velocities in demyelinating disorders. Due to the phenomena of temporal dispersion and phase cancellation SNAPs elicited by proximal stimulation are much lower in amplitude while the duration of the potential (distance between onset and first baseline crossing) is increased.

SNAP latency: so-called onset latencies are routinely used and represent the time interval from stimulus to the initial negative deflection of biphasic potentials or the initial positive peak of triphasic potentials (Fig. 3.16b). Unlike motor conduction studies, distal conduction velocities can be calculated with only one stimulation by dividing the distance between the active recording electrode and stimulation point by the onset latency. Assessment of proximal conduction velocities matches the procedure described for motor nerves. As a rule, sensory nerve conduction studies are more sensitive than motor studies in detecting focal and generalized neuropathies.

Stimulation and recording procedures: both antidromic (stimulation towards the sensory receptors) and orthodromic (stimulation away from the sensory receptors) sensory studies are available (Fig. 3.17). Whereas conduction velocities are the same with either method, amplitudes are generally higher in the antidromic potentials because recording electrodes are closer to the nerve. Because of this advantage and the ease of application, preference is usually given to the antidromic technique unless SNAPs are superimposed by a volume-conducted motor potential and the onset of the potential cannot be identified.

Reliability and external influences: fast saltatory conduction of peripheral nerves depends on a mature nerve architecture. Accordingly, motor and sensory conduction velocities markedly increase in the first years of life parallel to advancing myelination, and decrease after age 60 due to slow axon and myelin degeneration in higher ages. Apart from age, nerve conduction is influenced by the skin temperature (0.7–2.4 m/s for each degree centigrade) (Liveson and Ma 1992). In many laboratories temperature is measured and, if necessary, corrected by heating or computational adjustment. Reproducibility studies yielded measurement errors ranging from some 5% (~3 m/s) (intra-observer reliability) up to 10% (~6 m/s) if weeks are allowed to elapse between examinations and the examiner changes (long-term inter-observer reliability) (Gassel 1964; Honet et al. 1968). This inaccuracy is inherently related to the complex methodological requirements of EDX studies and should find consideration when interpreting alterations of nerve conduction over time.

3.2.1.2
Late Responses – the F-wave

Nerve conduction studies are appropriate for assessing peripheral nerves up to Erb's point (upper extremities) and the gluteal fold/inguinal ligament (lower extremities) but are not applicable to the very proximal nerve segments (plexus) and nerve roots. Recording of late responses especially the F-wave permits one to close this gap (Eisen et al. 1977). After routine (supramaximal) motor nerve stimu-

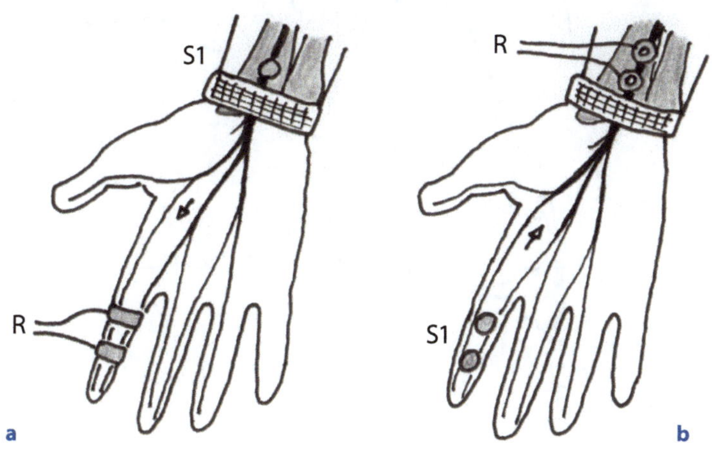

Fig. 3.17. a Antidromic (stimulation towards the sensory receptors) sensory studies. **b** Orthodromic (stimulation away from the sensory receptors) sensory studies. Amplitudes of SNAPs are generally higher in the antidromic potentials (*S1* site of stimulation, *R* site of potential recording)

lation the action potential conducts distally to the neuromuscular junction eliciting the CMAP or M-response and proximally towards to anterior horn cells (via the motor nerve roots) where it triggers a backfiring of a small and variable subpopulation of these cells (Fig. 3.18). This action potential again spreads distally and causes a second low-amplitude response (1%–5% of the CMAP). Strictly speaking, the F-wave is no reflex, since both the efferent and afferent loops are purely motor without an intervening synapse (Fig. 3.18).

The technical equipment and recording set-up is the same as in standard motor nerve conduction studies except for an increase in gain (100–200 µV) and sweep speed (5–10 ms). In clinical routine 10–20 responses are recorded, which typically vary in latency and amplitude owing to the continuously changing population of anterior horn cells involved in the generation of this potential (Fig. 3.19). The minimal F-wave latency reflecting conduction of the fastest motor fibers (normative values depend on body height) and the F-wave persistence (normal, 80%–100%) are the best standardized and most reliable measures obtainable from F-wave studies (Fig. 3.19).

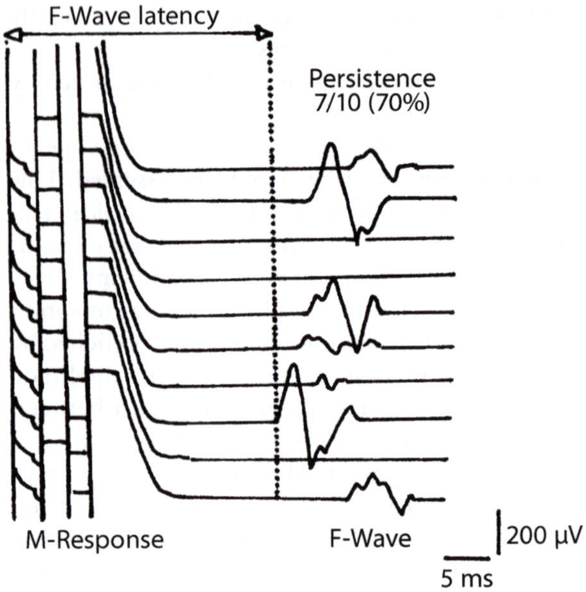

Fig. 3.19. F-wave measurements: the minimal F-wave latency is the shortest of the 10 responses, representing the largest, fastest conducting fibers. The F-wave persistence is the number of responses obtained per number of stimulations (70% in this case)

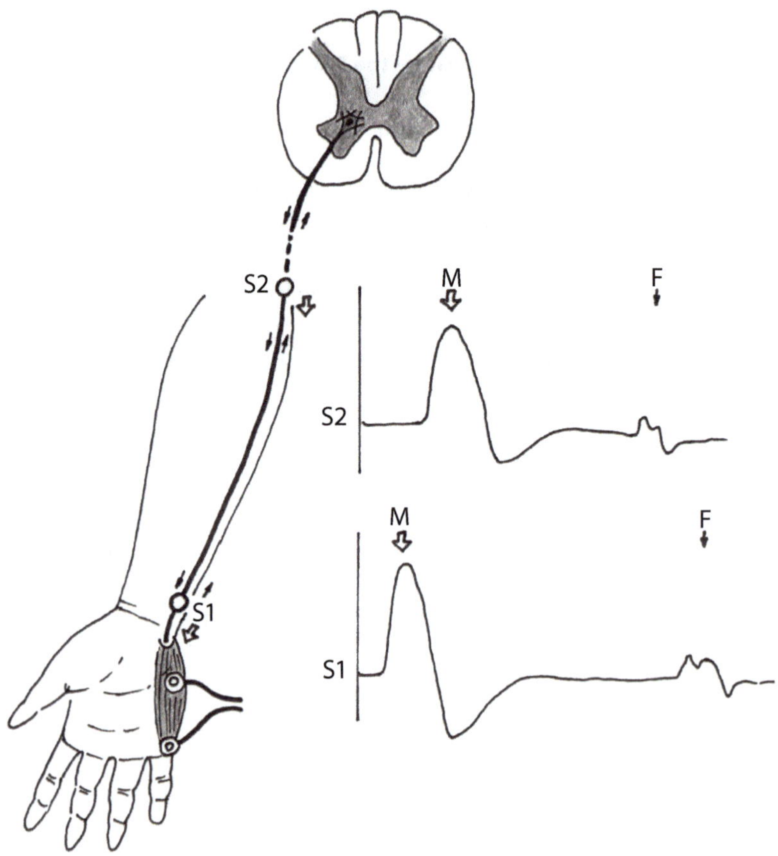

Fig. 3.18. F-response circuitry: the direct muscle response (*M*) occurs from orthodromic travel. The F-wave (*F*) is derived by antidromic travel to the anterior horn cells, back firing of some anterior horn cells, and orthodromic travel down to the muscle. With proximal stimulation (*S2*) the latency of the M-response increases but the F-wave latency decreases

If nerve conduction velocities are unremarkable, a prolonged F-wave latency and/or inconsistent response are strongly suggestive of proximal nerve lesion, e.g., plexus palsy. Otherwise, F-waves can be adjusted for distal conduction abnormalities by calculation of corrected F-waves. On interpreting F-wave parameters several limitations have to be considered. F-wave responses are often not recordable from nerves with severe axonal damage and difficult to obtain from muscles supplied by the nerve roots L2–L4 and C5–C7. In addition, sensitivity of the test for assessing abnormalities confined to a single nerve root is low.

3.2.1.3
Needle Electromyography

As with the nerve conduction studies, needle electromyography has to be individualized for each patient based on the clinical problem and results of the ongoing evaluation. Conduction of EMG, especially the correct placing of the needle and sampling of muscles (Fig. 3.20), and interpretation of the recordings obtained, are a challenging part of the EDX examination.

Usually, concentric bipolar needle electrodes are used containing both the active (wire in the centre of the needle) and reference electrode (shaft) (Fig. 3.14). The ground electrode is placed to the limb being investigated to suppress background noise. Insertion of the needle into the muscle may produce some discomfort. If performed skillfully, however, the examination is usually well tolerated even when numerous muscles are sampled.

The EMG examination is routinely composed of three stages – recording of rest activity, analysis of voluntary MUAPs and registration of the interference pattern during maximal muscle contraction. Electrical signals from the muscle are displayed on the screen and simultaneously presented acoustically over a loudspeaker.

Rest activity: normal muscle does not show any activity at rest (= spontaneous activity) expect for the end plate region where end plate noise (irregular monophasic negative potentials) and end plate spikes (irregular biphasic potentials with an initial negative deflection) occur (Fig. 3.21a). Pathological spontaneous activity in terms of fibrillation potentials and positive waves manifest in denervated muscle at the second to third week. Both signals have the same significance but differ in configuration. Fibrillations (fib.) are brief triphasic spikes with an initial positive deflection (duration 1–5 ms, amplitude

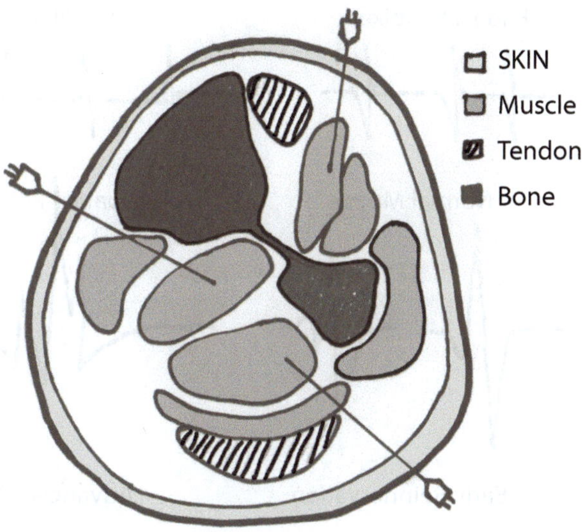

Fig. 3.20. Needle EMG: correct placement of the needle is mandatory for a reliable examination as exemplified for the lower calf

10–20 μV) and a regular firing pattern, whereas positive waves (pw.) have a brief initial positive signal followed by a long negative phase (Fig. 3.21a). There are two common ways of quantifying the density of pathological spontaneous activity also inferred to as denervation activity. Either it is graded on a scale ranging from 0 to 3 (0 no fib./pw., + persistent single fib./pw., ++ moderate numbers of fib./pw. in two areas, +++ many fib./pw. in all areas tested) or depicted as the number of recording sites in a muscle where fib./pw. emerge relative to the number of areas examined (e.g. 7 of 10 or “7/10”).

Analysis of voluntary MUAPs: a motor unit consists of all muscle fibers (usually five to several hundreds) supplied by a single motor neuron. Physiologically, the territories of motor units show a broad overlap and cover an area of 5–10 mm (Fig. 3.22a).

MUAPs recorded during needle EMG represent the compound action potential of all muscle fibers of a single motor unit, weighted towards the fibers nearest to the needle (Fig. 3.23). The morphology of MUAPs (duration, amplitude and phases) reflects the architecture of given motor units and thus permits a reliable differentiation of myopathic and neuropathic processes (Figs. 3.21b and 3.22d,e). By definition, the MUAP duration is measured from the initial deflection of the potential towards the final return to baseline (in ms). The MUAP amplitude denotes the distance between the maximum positive and

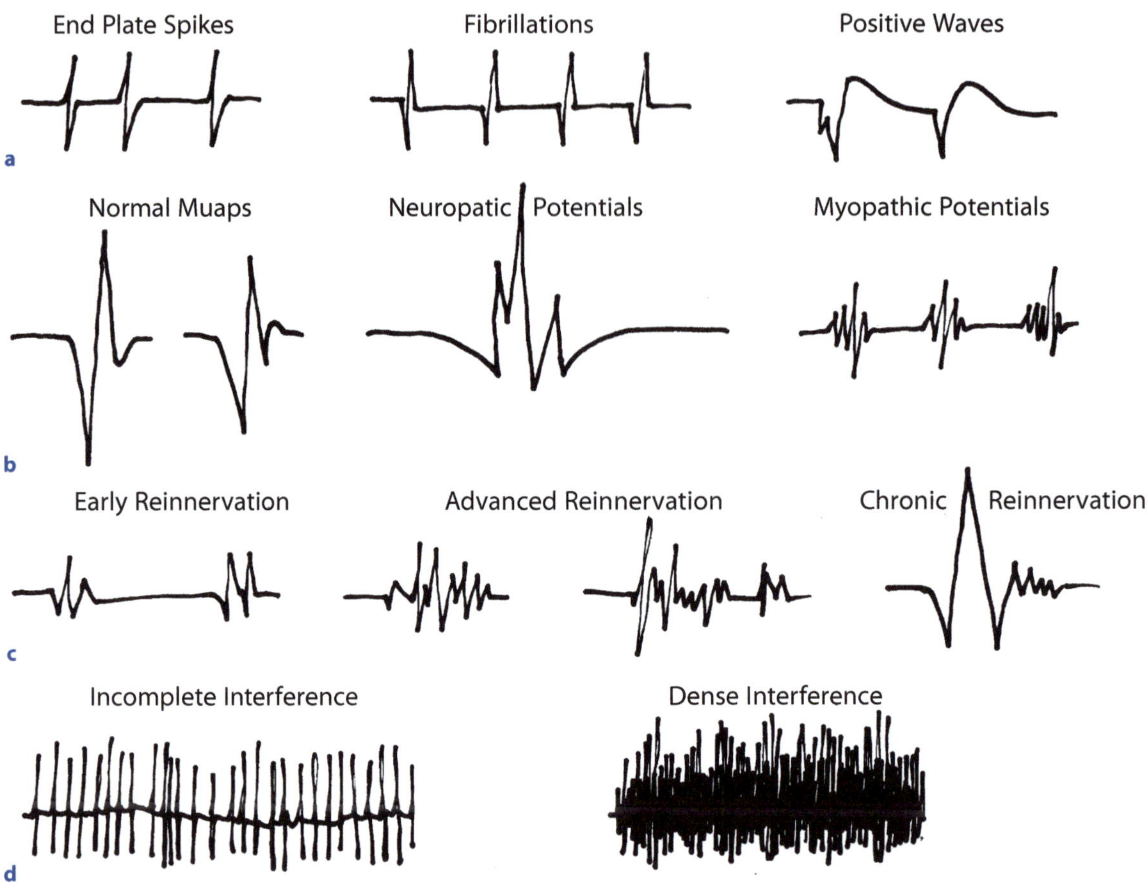

Fig. 3.21a–d. Needle electromyography. **a** Physiological and pathological spontaneous activity (recording of rest activity). **b** Normal, neuropathic and myopathic MUAPs. **c** Early, advanced and chronic reinervation potentials. **d** Incomplete and complete interference during maximal muscle contraction

negative peaks (in mV) and MUAP phases are calculated by counting the number of baseline crossings (Fig. 3.23). As a standard, 10–20 distinct MUAPs are recorded from each muscle with the needle placed within or close to the motor unit (rise time < 0.5 ms), and analyzed on a quantitative or qualitative basis. Because MUAP configuration varies substantially in various muscles and changes with advancing age, examinations will yield valid interpretations only if performed by an experienced electromyographer.

Long-duration high-amplitude MUAPs result from prominent enlargement of motor units, which is usually the consequence of axon loss and collateral sprouting of the remaining intact nerve fibers, and therefore characteristic of chronic neuropathic disorders (Figs. 3.21b and 3.22e). Short-duration low-amplitude MUAPs are the hallmark of myopathic disorders and originate from a loss or atrophy of muscle fibers and / or blockage of end plates (Figs. 3.21b and 3.22d). Polyphasia in turn (number of baseline crossings of a MUAP > 5) is a non-specific abnormality occurring both in neurogenic diseases and myopathies (Fig. 3.23). It depends primarily on the synchrony of muscle fiber firing and to a second instance on the architecture of the motor unit.

In early reinervation processes thinly myelinated axonal sprouts form new neuromuscular junctions to denervated muscle fibers, which corresponds with the emergence of low-amplitude desynchronized MUAPs on EMG ("early reinervation potentials") (Figs. 3.21c and 3.22b). Over time, MUAPs continuously grow in size, number of phases and duration ("advanced reinervation potentials"), the myelin of sprouts mature and depolarization of muscle fibers synchronizes, thereby producing an increase in the amplitude along with a decrease in the number of phases and potential duration ("chronic reinervation potential") (Figs. 3.21c and 3.22c,e).

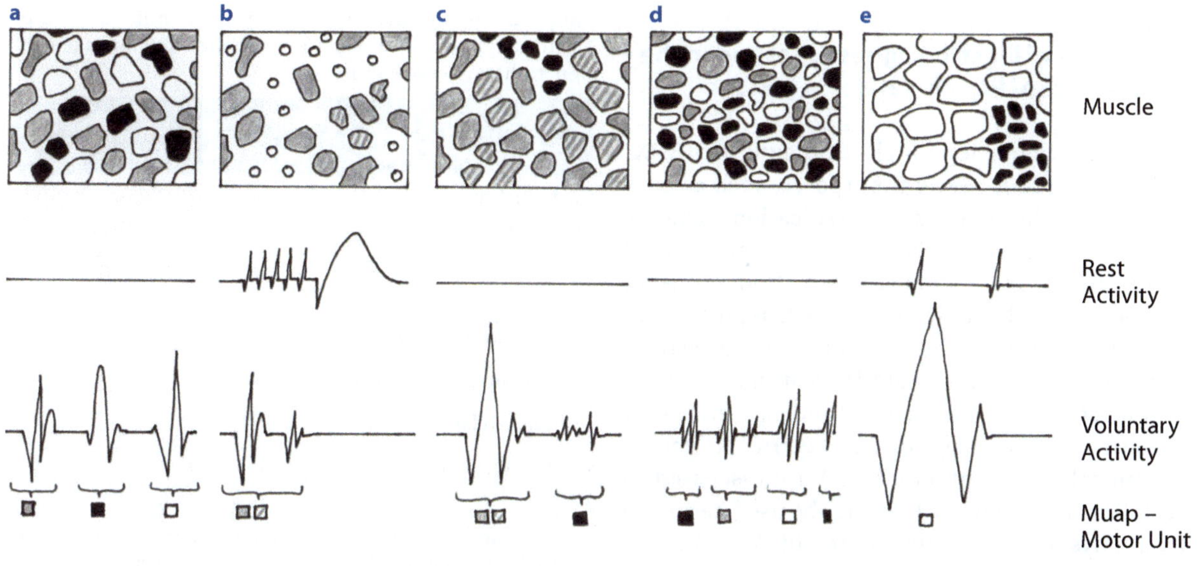

Fig. 3.22a–e. Architecture of motor units and corresponding electromyography findings. **a** Normal muscle. The territories of three motor units (*black*, *gray* and *white*) show a broad overlap. Morphology of the corresponding three MUAPs is unremarkable. **b** Axonotmesis of two of the three motor axons. Muscle fibers supplied by these axons are denervated (spontaneous activity). The intact third (*gray*) axon shows collateral sprouting – one of two main mechanisms of regeneration – and has formed new end plates to three additional muscle fibers (*gray-white*). Accordingly the MUAP shows a late component. **c** Advanced stage of reinervation. Meanwhile the gray motor axon has formed end plates to most denervated muscle fibers (*gray-white*). As a consequence the size of the motor unit has substantially increased and a typical long-duration high-amplitude MUAP is recordable on electromyography (neuropathic potential). In addition the black motor axon has again reached the muscle by true axonal sprouting from the lesion site, and formed first endplates to a few muscle fiber (early reinervation potential). **d** Myopathy. Short-duration low-amplitude MUAPs are the typical electromyography finding and originate from a loss or atrophy of muscle fibers. **e** Severe chronic neurogenic damage with a grouped atrophy of muscle fibers and giant potentials on electromyography. Such findings are typical of motor neuron diseases and chronic reinervation processes

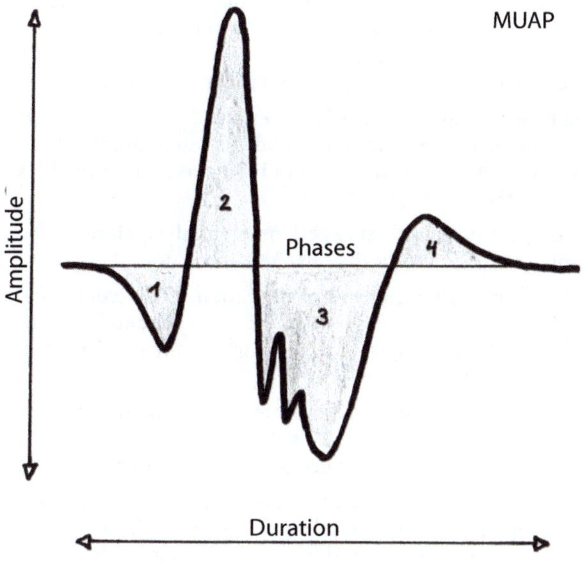

Fig. 3.23. Motor unit action potential (*MUAP*) measurements – amplitude, duration and phases

Interference pattern: during maximal contraction MUAPs normally overlap creating a "dense" or "complete" interference pattern with no single MUAPs being distinguishable given an appropriate sweep speed of 50–100 ms (Fig. 3.21d). An incomplete interference pattern is either due to poor central motor activation (central nervous system disorders) or, more frequently, due to reduced recruitment of MUAPs in the case of severe axon loss (neurogenic disorder) or manifestation of conduction blocks (Fig. 3.21d). A mild fall in the number of elicitable motor units is compensated for by a higher firing frequency of the remaining intact units. In myopathy an early (increased) recruitment of many motor units is seen already if the muscle is activated with small force.

3.2.2 Significance of Electrodiagnostic Testing in the Management of Peripheral Nerve Lesions

In peripheral nerve lesions electrodiagnostic (EDX) studies are used for several purposes, such as confirmation of the diagnosis, classification of nerve injury, localization of the lesion site, assessment of the underlying pathology, detection of nerve anastomosis and monitoring of regenerative processes (GUTIERREZ and ENGLAND 2002). Relevancy, strengths and limitations of EDX testing, its potential impacts on case management and its significance in relation to other diagnostic procedures especially the clinical evaluation (Table 3.3) are discussed in the following chapters. Commonly used terms in electrophysiology are summarized in Table 3.4.

Table 3.3. Significance of the clinical examination and of electrodiagnostic studies in the evaluation and management of peripheral nerve lesions

	Clinical assessment	NCS/EMG
Establishment of the diagnosis	+++	+
Assessment of the severity of nerve damage	+	+++
Localization of nerve damage	++	++
Follow-up and prognosis	++	+++
Etiologic classification	+	(+)
Detection of innervation anomalies	(+)	+++

+++ method of choice, ++ substantial contribution, + substantial contribution in selected patients, (+) usually not helpful; NCS, nerve conduction studies; EMG, electromyography

Table 3.4. Commonly used terms in electrodiagnostic (EDX) testing

Neurapraxia	Least severe type of nerve lesion with the continuity of axons preserved and clinical deficits being attributable to local demyelination and manifestation of (reversible) conduction abnormalities (Fig. 3.25). Electrophysiological characteristics: slowing of nerve conduction and emergence of conduction blocks
Axonotmesis	More severe type of nerve lesion with disruption of axons and surrounding endoneurinal sheets but maintenance of per- and epineurium (Fig. 3.25). Electrophysiological characteristics: denervation activity and axonal damage on electromyography
Neurotmesis	Most severe type of nerve lesion with complete disruption of axon, endo-, peri- and epineurium. *Electrophysiological characteristics:* extensive denervation activity and no voluntary muscle activity
Nerve entrapment	Nerve compression at sites where it passes through a narrow space often termed "tunnel"
Wallerian degeneration	Arises from severe nerve injury (axonotmesis or neurotmesis) and is characterized by axonal enlargement and breakdown (fragmentation of axon and myelin) with subsequent phagocytosis of the entire axonal material distally to the site of injury (Fig. 3.26). This degenerative process takes up to 4 (7) days and is immediately followed by slow axonal regeneration
Denervation activity	Consists of fibrillation potentials and positive waves – occurs on needle EMG after acute axonal nerve damage and represents a spontaneous depolarization of denervated muscle fibers. Fibrillations are brief spikes (duration 1–5 ms) and positive waves brief spikes followed by a slow negative phase. Both potentials manifest at rest (Fig. 3.21a)
F-wave	Late motor response triggered by an antidromic motor nerve action potential which results in a backfiring of a small sub-population of anterior horn cells (Fig. 3.18 and 3.19)
Distal motor latency	Time interval (in ms) between electric stimulation and initial deflection of the compound muscle action potential from baseline (Fig. 3.16a). It is composed of the nerve conduction to the neuromuscular junction, time delay across the neuromuscular junction and the synchronized depolarization of muscle fibers
CMAP	= "Compound muscle action potential" – summation of the action potentials of all muscle fibers. CMAPs are recorded in motor nerve conduction studies (Fig. 3.16a). With the tendon-belly method of electrode placing the CMAP is biphasic with an initial steep negative deflection
MUAP	= "Motor unit action potential" – is recorded while the patient is asked to slightly contract the sampled muscle (needle EMG). MUAPs represent the electrical signal generated by all muscle fibers supplied by a single axon (motor unit) and are assessed for duration, amplitude, phases and recruitment pattern (Fig. 3.23). Analysis of MUAP morphology allows a classification as normal, neuropathic or myopathic

3.2.2.1
Diagnosis of Peripheral Nerve Lesions

In most instances the correct diagnosis can be established based on the clinical pattern of motor and sensory deficits, localization and radiation of pain and eventually vegetative disturbances. A thorough review of the patient's medical history with emphasize on potential trigger events, demonstration of a Tinel's sign (TINEL 1915) at the site of suspected entrapment and results of provocation tests may serve to further substantiate the diagnosis. In some patients, however, diagnostic inaccuracies remain and EDX testing can substantially contribute to the classification of peripheral nerve lesions. Such pitfalls are often related to one of the following differential diagnoses:

- Plexus palsy vs polysegmental radiculopathies: differentiation can easily be achieved by the simple principle that SNAPs are diminished or absent in post-ganglionic damage (plexus) (LEVIN 2002; MA et al. 1984) but normally preserved in preganglionic i.e. root lesion (Fig. 3.24). Sometimes electromyography of paravertebral muscles is required as a supplementary test.
- Peripheral vs central paresis: radial, ulnar and peroneal nerve palsy is sometimes mimicked by small cortical or subcortical brain lesions along the pyramidal tract. In case of a peripheral origin documentation of conduction abnormalities or axonal damage allows an accurate classification.
- Pure pain syndromes (e.g. non-paretic compression of the radial nerve under the arcade of Frohse (ROSENBAUM 1999) or TTS without sensory-motor deficits): EDX testing may yield evidence of sub-clinical nerve damage and thus guide to the correct diagnosis.

3.2.2.2
Severity of Peripheral Nerve Lesions

The clinical impression alone is often insufficient for an early and adequate estimation of the severity of nerve damage – especially in the clinically relevant case of severe motor deficits. A reliable differentiation between neurapraxia and partial or total axonotmesis (GUITIERREZ and ENGLAND 2002; SEDDON 1943) is a domain of electrophysiology and crucial to all therapeutic decisions (Fig. 3.25). Both conditions may produce an identical amount of clinical weakness when the same number of motor fibers are involved. Whereas in neurapraxia impulses cannot pass across the lesion site due to a myelin disorder, in axonotmesis the nerve stump distal to the lesion undergoes degeneration and phagocytosis (Wallerian degeneration) (LUBINSKA 1977; GUTIERREZ and ENGLAND 2002; MUMENTHALER et al. 1998) (Fig. 3.26).

The electrophysiological hallmarks of neurapraxia are a synchronized or desynchronized slowing of nerve conduction (Fig. 3.25). In addition, conduction studies may identify typical conduction blocks or yield evidence of severe proximal conduction abnormalities. The latter phenomenon is characterized

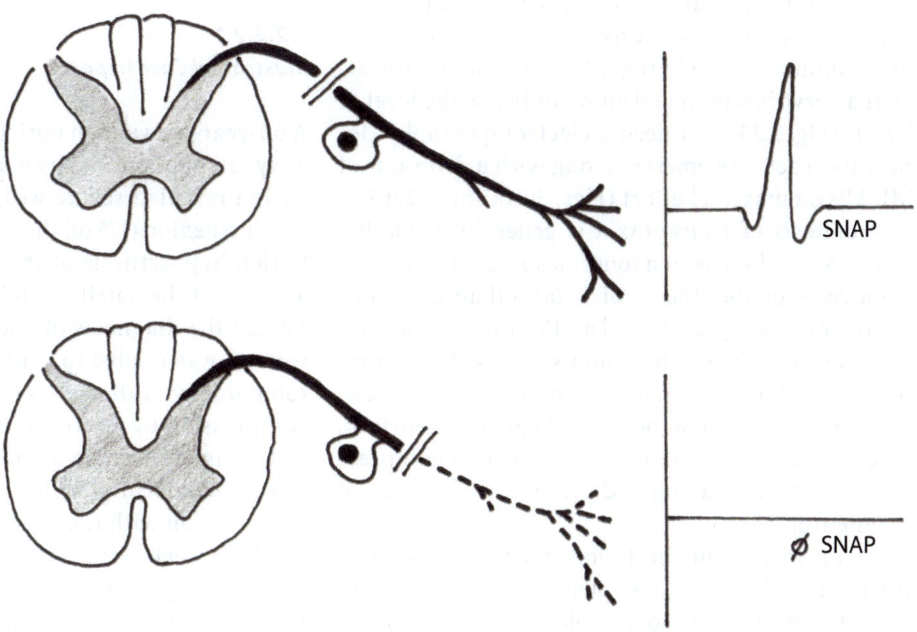

Fig. 3.24a,b. Sensory nerve conduction studies in nerve root (**a**) and peripheral nerve lesions (**b**). The dorsal root ganglia are bipolar cells whose central processes form the sensory roots, and the distal processes continue as the peripheral sensory nerve fibers. In the case of a root lesions (**a**) the distal sensory nerve does not degenerate and normal *SNAPs* are elicited because the lesion is proximal to the ganglia

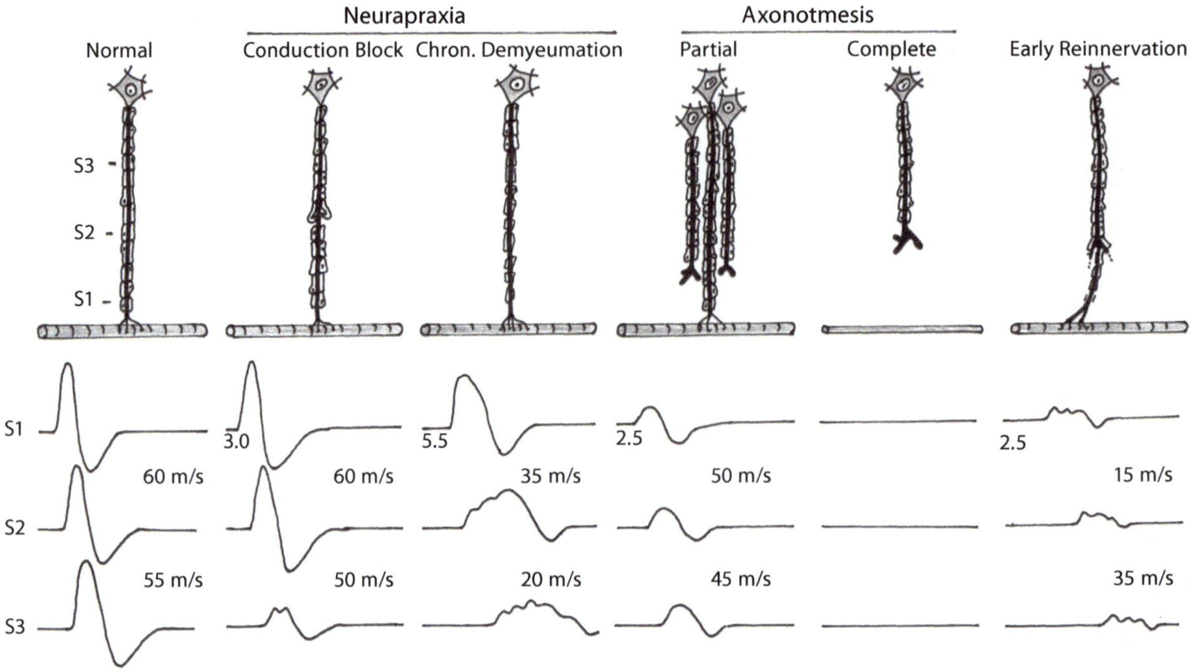

Fig. 3.25. Typical abnormalities of nerve conduction studies in neurapraxia (chronic demyelination and conduction blocks), partial and complete axonotmesis and reinervation after axonotmesis

by a (near) normal motor response to electric nerve stimulation despite high-grade paresis, and absent or inconsistent F-wave responses. Conduction blocks are variably defined by a >30%–50% loss in the amplitude of the CMAP without substantial increase in the potential duration (<20%) on sequential nerve stimulation (OH et al. 1994) (Fig. 3.25). Acute axonal nerve damage (axonotmesis), in contrast, results in low-amplitude CMAPs regardless of whether the affected nerve is stimulated above or below the level of lesion (Fig. 3.25). On needle electromyography denervation activity emerges along with a drop-out of MUAPs on maximal effort (Figs. 3.21a and 3.22b).

Prognosis of neurapraxia is generally favorable (Table 3.5), whereas in axonotmesis functional outcome relies on the efficacy of distal collateral sprouting of nerve fibers preserved and/or on adequate axonal sprouting from the lesion site (Fig. 3.22), both of which are influenced by factors such as the regeneration distance, intactness of the epi-/perineurium, mechanism of nerve damage, evidence of compressive disorders, scarring and presence or absence of polyneuropathy.

As an important limitation, there is no way to distinguish between complete axonotmesis and neurotmesis by electrophysiological means. High resolution nerve ultrasound or MRI usually qualify for accurately assessing discontinuity of the damaged nerve.

An illustrative example showing, how EDX studies assist in the therapeutic management is given below.

3.2.2.2.1
Illustrative Case Report

A 60-year-old women noticed leg weakness immediately after abdominal hysterectomy. Clinical examination revealed severe weakness of knee extension and hip flexion (1/5 on the Medical Research Council Scale), hypoesthesia at the anteromedial thigh and absence of the patellar tendon reflex allowing to establish the diagnosis of a femoral nerve lesion. The woman was unable to walk without aid. Computed tomography of the pelvis was performed to rule out compression by a retroperitoneal hematoma.

Comment: Iatrogenic injury of the femoral nerve during pelvic surgery most commonly arises from compression with the lateral retractor blade.

Three weeks after surgical intervention first EDX testing was performed. Remarkably, inguinal stimulation of the diseased femoral nerve elicited a near normal motor response in spite of high-grade paresis [CMAP recorded from the vastus medialis head of the quadriceps muscle (Fig. 3.15) 8 mV vs 10.5 mV at the normal side], and electromyography disclosed low-density denervation activity restricted to parts of the vastus lateralis muscle (fibrillation potentials 2/10).

Comment: this finding clearly indicates presence of a proximal conduction block as the main mechanism of muscle weakness – and an overall good prognosis. Because conduction blocks frequently restore spontaneously over a period of up to 3–6 weeks early explorative surgery is usually not performed.

In this patient, however, the further clinical course was unfavorable without any improvement in muscle strength over the following three months. Results of control EDX studies remained virtually unchanged except for a disappearance of pathological spontaneous activity and beginning reinervation in the vastus lateralis muscle. Magnetic resonance imaging of the pelvis did not reveal any pathological finding. Ultrasonography, however, showed segmental thickening of the nerve 8 cm rostral to the inguinal ligament as indirect evidence of nerve compression.

Comment: if blockage of nerve conduction is maintained over several months the conditions is termed "persistent conduction block". Such abnormalities are either of immunological origin, which can be ruled out in our patient, or are caused by constrictive scare tissue. Operative exploration was performed. The nerve was found constricted in scar tissue at the location identified by ultrasonography, and carefully released. Two days after successful neurolysis the conduction block has partly resolved and the woman was able to walk again. At a follow-up 3 months later muscle strength and knee jerk have normalized.

Comment: it is a frequent experience that conduction blocks promptly disappear after elimination of the causative compressive pathology.

3.2.2.3
Localisation of Peripheral Nerve Lesions

A thorough clinical examination usually permits a crude localization of nerve lesions. The precision for localization is high in classic entrapment syndromes (e.g., CTS or TTS) and in segments of peripheral nerves at which numerous branches divide from the main trunk in a consistent order, but comparatively low in most other instances.

EDX testing is particularly useful in assessing the exact site of a nerve lesion. Both a focal slowing of nerve conduction and emergence of conduction blocks have a high significance towards localization. In superficially located nerves suitable for short-segment stimulation such phenomena can be assessed with a precision of 5–10 mm (Figs. 3.10 and 3.27). This applies to most nerves of the upper extremities, the distal sensory branches of the sciatic nerve as well as the peroneal and tibial nerves at their course through the popliteal fossa or behind the fibular neck, respectively. In other nerves precision towards localization is much lower and only in the range of several centimeters.

In analogy to EDX studies, nerve ultrasound is capable of assessing the site of peripheral nerve lesions in a majority of patients. Both diagnostic modalities are complementary in that conduction studies may reveal abnormalities in nerve segments with a normal sonographic appearance and, vice versa ultrasound may document substantial pathologies in the absence of electrophysiological peculiarities. In this context it is worth mentioning that the nerve conduction velocity assessed by standard surface recording always reflects the speed of the fastest conducting axons. In compression syndromes propagation of the pressure within the nerve cross-section is often inhomogeneous and some fascicles may be even spared.

A special challenge is the differentiation between traumatic brachial plexus palsy and avulsion injury of nerve roots. In the latter disorder complex reflex studies utilizing cutaneous silent periods permit a reliable classification provided that there is at least minimal residual motor function in the affected arm and the patient is able to cooperate. In the more common case of a combination of both conditions, however, EDX testing mostly fails to give a clear diagnosis and CT-myelography or magnetic resonance imaging are the diagnostic golden standard in this situation (Levin 2002).

3.2.2.4
Etiology of Peripheral Nerve Lesions

Nerve ultrasound and other radiological techniques are the method of choice for assessing the nature of compressive and intraneural pathologies (scare tissue, ganglia, anatomical variants, neoplasm, etc.). In case of external compression (e.g., classic pressure palsy) essential information on the eliciting event has to be drawn from a thorough exploration of the patient's medical history and clinical inspection of the lesion site.

Contribution of EDX testing to this particular issue is restricted to the exclusion of non-compressive mononeuropathies such as focal manifestations of systemic nerve disorders (e.g., multiplex and other asymmetric neuropathies, motor neuron disease, multiple neurofibroma in neurofibromatosis, etc.) and immunological diseases of the peripheral nerve (motor neuropathy with conduction blocks). Sometimes entrapment syndromes emerge on the basis of predisposing polyneuropathies which can reliably be assessed by clinical and electrophysiological examinations.

3.2.2.5 Detection of Innervation Anomalies

Inconsistent anastomoses between nerves and true innervation anomalies are important sources of clinical misinterpretation and thus merit short consideration.

The most frequent anomaly is the Martin-Gruber anastomosis (Fig. 3.28) occurring in up to 30% of healthy subjects (Kimura et al. 1976; Wilbourn and Lambert 1976). It entails a forearm crossover of nerve fibers from the median to the ulnar nerve. The exchanged fibers usually supply hypothenar and/or thenar muscles. A further accessory communication between both nerves may exist in the palm of the hand known as the Riche-Cannieu anastomosis (Riche 1897). From a clinical perspective, presence of a nerve anastomosis may cause marked deviations of the innervation pattern from normal and accordingly obscure the clinical presentation of entrapment syndromes. For example, severe carpal and cubital tunnel syndrome with advanced axon loss may exist in the absence of motor deficits. In general, innervation of intrinsic hand muscles is much less consistent than commonly assumed – ranging from an all-ulnar to all-median hand (Rowntree 1949).

Electronically, the presence of a Martin-Gruber anastomosis is indicated by a lower amplitude of the CMAP on distal than on proximal stimulation and by changes in the configuration of the motor response. Special focus should be on the initial deflection of the motor response from baseline and a composition of the potential of two components. If recognized, complex stimulation studies can determine the exact course of the anastomosis and the (motor) innervation afforded by the shunting fibers. Detection of innervation anomalies is equally important for diagnostic and therapeutic purposes.

3.2.2.6 Follow-up of Peripheral Nerve Lesions

Patients with axonal nerve damage may or may not be subject to immediate surgery (Table 3.5). In the latter, more common case, short-term follow-ups aim at estimating the extent of expectable spontaneous recovery as a basis for the decision on a potential, later surgical intervention. The longer the elapsed time interval since nerve injury, the more accurate is such a prognostic assessment. On the other hand, if surgery is delayed by more than 3–6 months endoneural tubes undergo shrinkage and obliteration and the probability of satisfactory remission gradually declines. Given these opposite requirements optimal timing of follow-up examinations is a challenging task in each individual patient.

Table 3.5. Prognosis of peripheral nerve lesion

Neurapraxia	Prognosis is usually favorable with spontaneous recovery being expectable within 3–6 weeks after onset – or earlier if nerve compression is transient and mild. In a minority of patients, however, conduction abnormalities (especially conduction blocks) do not resolve or even worsen due to shrinking scare tissue. In selected cases surgical intervention may become necessary
Axonotmesis (partial/complete)	Prognosis is in part favorable but regeneration may take months or even years. An individual prognostic evaluation based on the extent of damage, regeneration distance and various other factors influencing the capacity of nerve regeneration (see Sect. 3.2.2) is mandatory for an optimal therapeutic management. In some patients early operative intervention improves the probability of regular reinervation, other, however, have more benefit from withholding surgery. In the case of an initially conservative therapy a rigorous clinical and electrophysiological monitoring is recommended (for details see Sect. 3.2.2)
Neurotmesis	Because prognosis of spontaneous regeneration is definitely poor, surgical repair with adaptation of the nerve endings (end-to-end suture) or bridging of a potential gap with autogenously sural nerve grafts is warranted as early as practicable

Clinical follow-up should include a detailed registration of the extent and course (onset and dynamics) of motor and sensory recovery, and a testing for the Tinel's sign along the nerve trunk, which gives a good impression of the velocity of axonal sprouting. Reinervation starts in the muscles next to the nerve lesion and progresses distally. In addition to regeneration of the transacted axons, recovery may arise from distal collateral sprouting of remaining intact axons (GUTIERREZ and ENGLAND 2002; MUMENTHALER et al. 1998) (Figs. 3.22, 3.25 and 3.26).

Electromyography is particularly useful in the follow-up of patients, because disappearance of denervation activity and emergence of early reinervation potentials precede clinically visible motor recovery by up to 4–8 weeks (Fig. 3.21c). Accordingly, serial electromyography helps to speed up the decision process. If no clinical and/or electromyographic evidence of functional reinervation becomes evident, patients are usually subject to surgery. Further control evaluations at longer intervals are recommended and may serve as a basis for rehabilitation programs and social reintegration.

3.2.2.7 Diagnostic Work-up in Patients with Peripheral Nerve Lesions

A thorough neurological examination by an experienced clinician is the mainstay in optimal management of peripheral nerve lesions and a necessary basis for the interpretation of all ancillary diagnostic procedures. A decision pathway for a cost-effective application of methodologically complex examinations is depicted in Figure 3.29. Guidelines for an optimal timing of EDX studies are summarized in Table 3.6.

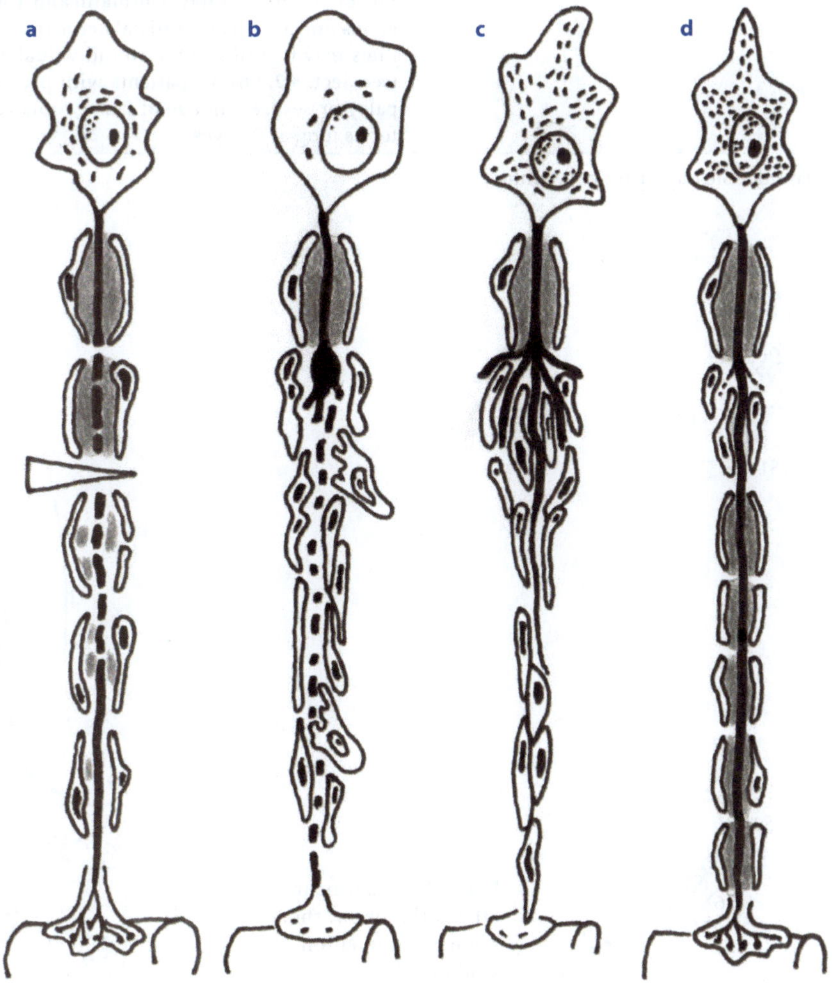

Fig. 3.26a–d. Wallerian degeneration. **a** Axonotmesis – the site of nerve transaction is indicated by the arrow. **b** Within 4–7 days axonal enlargement and breakdown (fragmentation of axon and myelin) with subsequent phagocytosis of the entire axonal material distally to the site of injury emerges. **c** The degenerataive process is followed by slow axonal regeneration (sprouting). **d** Late stage of reinervation, which is favorable in this case. (Modified reproduction with permission from Mumenthaler M, Schliack H. Läsionen peripherer Nerven. Thieme Verlag, Stuttgart New York)

Table 3.6. When to time electrodiagnostic (EDX) studies

Day[a] 1 to 6:	Generally not useful	Nerve conduction studies and electromyography provide no prognostic and little diagnostic information. Examinations in this time period should be reserved for the solving a few well-defined clinical problems (e.g. differentiation between painful peroneal nerve lesion in vasculitis and L5 radiculopathy)
Day[a] 7 to 14 (21)	Exceptionally indicated	Wallerian degeneration has now finished. Amplitudes of the compound muscle action potentials and sensory action potentials allow a crude estimation of the degree of axonal damage. However, since CMAPs can only be recorded from superficial (distal) muscles and the various fibers of a nerve are often not uniformly affected, accuracy of the prognostic evaluation has its limitations even in the hand of an experienced electrophysiologist. Therefore, EDX studies should only be scheduled in this time interval, if early surgical intervention is being considered
Day[a] > 14 (21)	Adequate time for examination	In case of acute axonal damage denervation activity has now developed. Detection and quantification of fibrillation potentials and positive waves on electromyography and supplementary NCSs permit a precise assessment and localization of nerve damage in almost all patients. This information serves as a basis for a reliable prognostic evaluation
Follow-up examinations	At 3 to 6 months	Standard intervals for follow-up are 3 to 6 months. Shorter periods may be adequate if the therapeutic decision depends on the results of serial EMG examinations (monitoring of spontaneous regeneration) or if the lesions is distal and the regeneration distance short. Axonal sprouting at the site of injury (axon transaction) along intact endoneural tubes occur at an average rate of 1–2 mm per day (Gutmann and Young 1944) provided that the growing axons find access to the distal nerve trunk (Figs. 3.26). Expected nerve growth rates may be utilized for an individual adjustment of examination intervals (see Sect. 3.2.2.6). In patients with proximal nerve lesions especially plexus palsy or severe damage of nerve roots regenerative processes may be active for as long as 2–3 years

[a]Days denote days after nerve injury

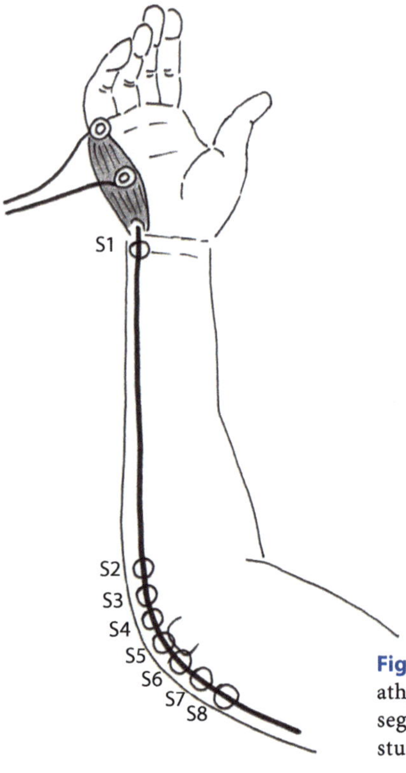

Fig. 3.27. Ulnar neuropathy at the elbow: short segment stimulation studies

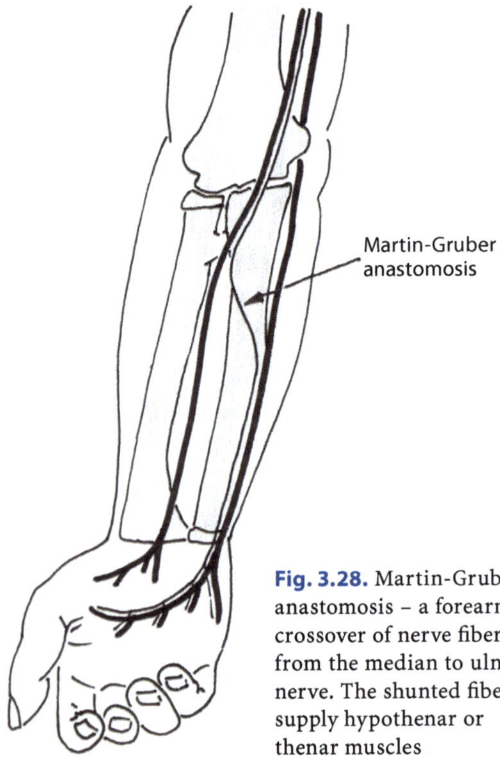

Fig. 3.28. Martin-Gruber anastomosis – a forearm crossover of nerve fibers from the median to ulnar nerve. The shunted fibers supply hypothenar or thenar muscles

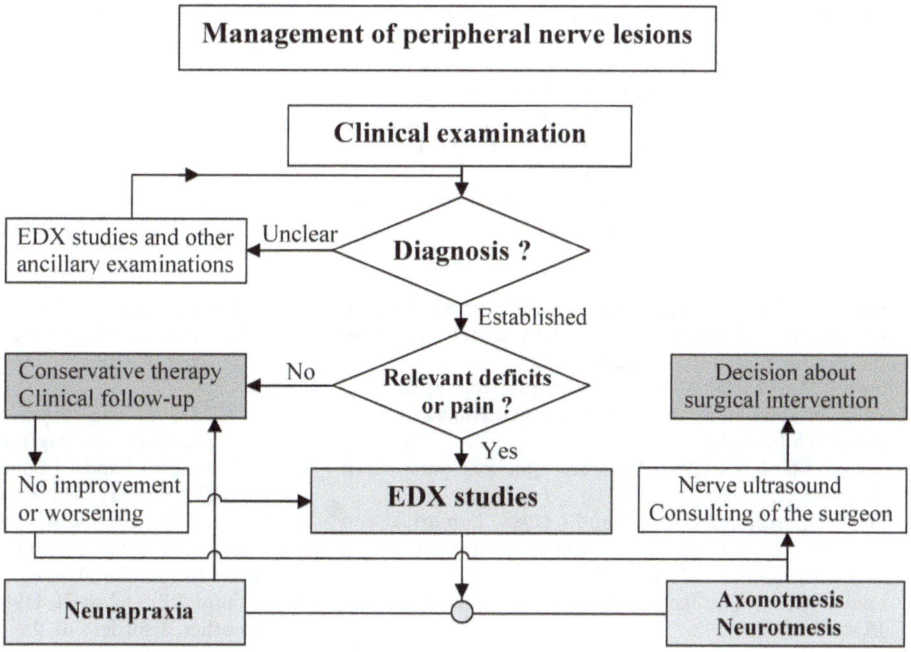

Fig. 3.29. Management of peripheral nerve lesion

If surgical intervention is being considered, EDX testing and nerve ultrasound should be performed. Both examinations are not alternative procedures but highly complementary regarding strengths and limitations, and may substantially contribute to the final therapeutic decision and – choice of the surgical approach. A high level of diagnostic and localization security, as required in the pre-operative setting, is met if the clinical appearance and results of both aforementioned diagnostic modalities fit well together.

References

Bakke JL, Wolff HG (1948) Occupational pressure neuritis of the deep palmar branch of the ulnar nerve. Arch Neurol Psychiatry 60:549

Brown WF, Watson BV (1993) Acute retrohumeral radial neuropathies. AAEM case report 27. Muscle Nerve 16:706–711

Campbell WW (1998) Entrapment neuropathies. In: Gilchrist J (ed) Prognosis in neurology. Butterworth-Heinemann, Boston, pp 307–312

Campbell WW, Sahni KS, Pridgeon RM et al. (1988) Intraoperative electroneurography: management of ulnar neuropathy at the elbow. Muscle Nerve 11:75–81

Campbell WW, Pridgeon RM, Riaz, G et al. (1991) Variations in anatomy of the ulnar nerve at the cubital tunnel: pitfalls in the diagnosis of ulnar neuropathy at the elbow. Muscle Nerve 14:733–738

Campbell WW, Pridgeon RM, Sahni KS (1992) Short segment incremental studies in the evaluation of ulnar neuropathy at the elbow. Muscle Nerve 15:1050–1054

Campellone JV (1999) Peroneal neuropathy from antithrombotic stocking. J Clin Neuromusc Dis 1:14–16

DeLisa JA, Saeed MA (1983) The tarsal tunnel syndrome. Muscle Nerve 6:664–670

Dellon AL, Hament W, Gittelshon A (1993) Nonoperative management of cubital tunnel syndrome: an 8-year prospective study. Neurology 43:1673–1677

Eisen A, Schomer D, Melmed C (1977) The application of F-wave measurements in the differentiation of proximal and distal upper limb entrapments. Neurology 27:662–668

Felsenthal G (1977) Median and ulnar distal motor and sensory latencies in the same normal subject. Arch Phys Med Rehabil 58:297–302

Foerster O (1933) The dermatomes in man. Brain 56:1–39

Gassel MM (1964) Sources of error in motor nerve conduction studies. Neurology 14:825

Gessini L, Jandolo B, Pietrangeli A (1984) The anterior tarsal syndrome. Report of four cases. J Bone Joint Surg Am 66:786–787

Goodgold J, Kopell HP, Spielholz NI (1965) The tarsal tunnel syndrome. N Eng J Med 273:742–745

Green DP (1984) Diagnostic and therapeutic value of carpal tunnel injection. J Hand Surg 9:850–854

Guidelines in Electrodiagnostic Medicine (1999) American Association of Electrodiagnostic Medicine. J Muscle Nerve, Suppl S5–S12

Gutierrez A, England JD (2002) Peripheral nerve injury. In: Katirji B, Kaminski HJ, Preston DC et al. (eds) Neuromus-

cular disorders in clinical practice. Butterworth-Heinemann, Boston
Gutmann E, Young JZ (1944) The re-innervation of muscle after various periods of atrophy. J Anat 78:15–43
Honet JC, Jebsen RH, Perrin EB (1968) Variability of nerve conduction velocity determinations in normal persons. Arch Phys Med Rehabil 49:650–654
Kaplan PE (1984) Posterior interosseous neuropathies: natural history. Arch Phys Med Rehabil 65:399
Keck C (1962) The tarsal tunnel syndrome. J Bone Joint Surg 44A:180–182
Kimura J (1979) The carpal tunnel syndrome: localization of conduction abnormalities within the distal segment of the median nerve. Brain 102:619–635
Kimura J, Murphy MJ, Varda DJ (1976) Electrophysiological study of anomalous innervation of intrinsic hand muscles. Arch Neurol 33:842
Koller RL, Blank NK (1980) Strawberry pickers' palsy. Arch Neurol 39:320–324
Kothari MJ, Preston DC, Logigian EL (1996) Lumbrical and interossei recordings localize ulnar neuropathy at the wrist. Muscle Nerve 19:170–174
Kumiai D (1987) The facts of Katmandu: squatter's palsy. JAMA 257:28
Kuschner SH, Ebramzadeh E, Johnson D et al. (1992) Tinel's sign and Phahlen's test in carpal tunnel syndrome. Orthopedics 15:1297–1302
Labosky DA, Waggy CA (1986) Apparent weakness of median and ulnar motors in radial nerve palsy. J Hand Surg 11A:528
Levin KH (2002) Cervical radiculopathies. In: Katirji B, Kaminski HJ, Preston DC et al. (eds) Neuromuscular disorders in clinical practice. Butterworth-Heinemann, Boston
Liveson JA, Ma DM (1992) Laboratory reference for clinical neurophysiology. Davis Company, Philadelphia
Lubinska L (1977) Early course of Wallerian degeneration in myelinated fibers of the rat phrenic nerve. Brain Res 130:47–63
Ma MD, Wilbourn AJ, Kraft GH (1984) Unusual sensory conduction studies. American Association of Electromyography and Electrodiagnosis, Rochester
Maudsley R (1967) Fibular tunnel syndrome. J Bone Joint Surg 49B:384–389
Medical Research Council of the United Kingdom (1978) Aids to the examination of the peripheral nervous system. MRC, Pendragon House, London
Miller RG (1991) Ulnar neuropathy at the elbow. AAEM case report 1. Muscle Nerve 14:97–101
Miller RG, Camp PE (1979) Postoperative ulnar neuropathy. JAMA 242:1636–1639
Miller RG, Hummel EE (1980) The cubital tunnel syndrome: treatment with simple decompression. Ann Neurol 7:567–569
Mondelli M, Giannini F, Reale F (1998) Clinical and electrophysiological findings and follow-up in tarsal tunnel syndrome. Electroencephalogr Clin Neurophysiol 109:418–425
Morris HH, Peter BH (1976) Pronator teres syndrome: clinical and electrophysiological features in seven cases. J Neurol Neurosurg Psych 39:461–464
Mumenthaler M, Schliack H, Stoehr M (1998) Läsionen peripherer Nerven und radikuläre Läsionen. Thieme Verlag, Stuttgart New York
Oh SJ, Kim DE, Kuruoglu HL (1994) What is the best diagnostic index of conduction block and temporal dispersion? Muscle Nerve 17:489–493
Oh SJ, Meyer RD (1999) Entrapment neuropathies of the tibial (posterior tibial) nerve. Neurol Clin 17:593–615
Oh SJ (2003) Clinical electromyography. Nerve conduction studies. Lippincott Williams and Wilkins, Philadelphia
Olney RK, Hanson M (1988) Ulnar neuropathy at or distal to the wrist. AAEE case report 15. Muscle Nerve 11:828–832
Phalen GS (1966) The carpal tunnel syndrome: seventeen years' experience in diagnosis and treatment of six hundred fifty-four hands. J Bone Joint Surg 48A:211–228
Rich P (1897) Le nerf cubital et les muscles de le'éminence thenar. Bull Mem Soc Anat Paris 5:251
Rosenbaum RB (1999) Disputed radial tunnel syndrome. Muscle Nerve 22:960–967
Rosenbaum RB, Ochoa JL (1993) Carpal tunnel syndrome and other disorders of the median nerve. Butterworth-Heinemann, Boston
Rowntree T (1949) Anomalous innervation of the hand muscles. J Bone Joint Surg 31B:505
Seddon HJ (1943) Three types of nerve injury. Brain 66:237–239
Stevens JC (1987) Electrodiagnosis of carpal tunnel syndrome. AAEE minimonograph 26. Muscle Nerve 10:99–113
Stevens JC, Sun S, Beard CM et al. (1988) Carpal tunnel syndrome in Rochester, Minnesota, 1961 to 1980. Neurology 38:134–138
Stevens JC, Beard M, O'Fallon WM et al. (1992) Conditions associated with carpal tunnel syndrome. Mayo Clin Proc 67:541–548
Stoehr M, Bluthardt M (1993) Atlas der klinischen Elektromyographie und Neurographie. Kohlhammer, Stuttgart Berlin Köln
Sturzenegger M, Rutz M (1991) Die Radialisparesen: Ursachen, Lokalisation und Diagnostik. Nervenarzt 62:722–729
Sunderland S (1945) Traumatic injuries of the peripheral nerves – simple compression injuries of the radial nerve. Brain 68:56–72
Suranyi L (1983) Median nerve compression by Struthers' ligament. J Neurol Neurosurg Psych 46:1047–1049
Szabo RM, Chidgey LK (1989) Stress carpal tunnel pressures in patients with carpal tunnel syndrome and normal patients. J Hand Surg 14:624–627
Tinel J (1915) Le signe du „fourmillement" dans les lésions des nerfs périphériques. Presse Méd 23:385–396
Wilbourn AJ (1986) Common peroneal mononeuropathy at the fibular head. Muscle Nerve 9:825–836
Wilbourn AJ, Lambert E (1976) The forearm median-to-ulnar nerve communication: electrodiagnostic aspects. Neurology 26:368
Wong L, Dellon AL (1997) Brachial neuritis presenting as anterior interosseous nerve compression. J Hand Surg 22:A536–539

Nerve Compression Syndromes

4

Gerd Bodner

CONTENTS

G. Bodner, MD
Professor, Department of Radiology, St. Bernards Hospital, Europort 1–4, Gibraltar

4.1 Introduction

The future is bright for sonography of peripheral nerve compression. Recent soft- and hardware development of sonographic equipment and transducers now working up to 17 MHz, has boosted the capability of sonography to investigate common and uncommon peripheral compression syndromes. Sonography of the peripheral nerves is now developing into an extremely valuable tool as an adjunct to neurological investigations. Observing the development of the use of sonography throughout the medical fields such as anesthetics and peripheral neurology we feel that sonography is taking its valuable place in non-invasive diagnosis of peripheral neuropathy.

Generally speaking neuropathy caused by extrinsic compression may occur anywhere in the body and affect a variety of peripheral nerves. Special anatomic conditions, however, may result in an increased risk for the development of so-called entrapment neuropathies at certain locations. There are several such conditions: Nerves may travel through narrow passageways together with tendons and vessels. Osteofibrous tunnels in the upper or lower limb, for example, are spaces superficially confined by tight fibrotic retinacula and at the bottom either by bone or musculotendinous structures. The retinacula, which are anchored on bony ridges or osseous prominences on either side of the tunnel, prevent dislocation of the structures contained inside. Nerves traveling inside such tunnels may be affected by chronic external wear and tear often of uncertain origin or by the presence of abnormal tissue inside the tunnel such as an ulnar artery aneurysm inside Guyon's canal for example.

A nerve may also be compromised by an abnormally tight ligament or an anatomic muscle or vessel variant running across the nerve in an oblique course, such as the ulnar nerve within the ulnar sulcus or the femoral cutaneus lateral nerve when piercing the inguinal ligament. Nerve compression may also occur secondary to trauma or surgery at certain sites, such as the posttraumatic tarsal tunnel syndrome, with development of neuropathy in a previously asymptomatic individual due to narrowing of the tarsal tunnel caused by malaligned fractures or callus formation.

Regardless of which underlying mechanism results in a compression syndrome, the reaction of a nerve to external compression has some common features. Chronic irritation of a nerve due to stretching or persistent compression is thought to interfere with the local intraneural microvasculature (Stewart 1993). Ischemia due to compression of the vasa nervorum and venous congestion results in epineural and endoneural edema. As the disease progresses to a more chronic state, fibrotic reactions in the nerve sheath result in further compromise to the fascicles.

Sonographic findings in patients with entrapment neuropathies reflect these pathophysiological reactions. Changes in echotexture and in shape and alignment of nerves may be detected. The nerve commonly shows an abrupt change in diameter, with flattening at the site of direct compression. This sonographic sign was first described for the detection of median nerve compression in the carpal tunnel by Buchberger et al. (1991) and is now also considered to be a reliable measure for entrapment neuropathy in other locations (Chiou et al. 1998; Martinoli et al. 1996, 2000; Sarria et al. 2000; Bodner et al. 2001). Proximal to the level of nerve entrapment localized enlargement of the nerve with swelling of fascicles is an expression of vasocongestion and edema (Martinoli et al. 2002; Nakamichi and Tachibana 2007; Peer et al. 2002). An increase in intraneural and perineural flow signals in color Doppler or power Doppler images is commonly seen and represents the hypervascular state seen in nonspecific, reactive inflammation (Martinoli et al. 2000; Mallouhi et al. 2006). Changes in echotexture accompany a general change in nerve diameter with loss of fascicular discrimination at the site of maximum compression and flattening of the nerve, and swelling of individual fascicles or often coalescence of fascicles to a single large hypoechoic cord at the level of edema and vasocongestion. The longer the nerve compression persists, the more severe the sonographic changes appear.

However, care should be taken not to misinterpret normal flattening of a nerve or fusiform appearance of a peripheral nerve with a sonographic pathological feature, since peripheral nerves at typical locations show flattening because the are branching or they show normal fusiform thickening, such as the ulnar nerve at the ulnar groove.

In comparison with MRI, which is the only competing imaging modality for the work-up of nerve compression syndromes, sonography is low cost and generally available. At the same time sonography causes no discomfort, is quickly performed and easily adjusted to a patient's complaints in static as well as dynamic examinations. The latter are an important adjunct to the standard evaluation of peripheral nerve diseases, and especially valuable for the diagnosis of functional disorders such as the snapping triceps syndrome with ulnar nerve dislocation (Jacobson et al. 2001). This functional evaluation is beyond the abilities of MRI. A huge advantage of sonography in comparison with MRI is its ability to image longer nerve segments in a single study and its superior resolution. The development of high frequency probes working with up to 17 MHz allow the detection of even the smallest superficial nerves such as the lateral femoral cutaneus nerve, or the superficial peroneal nerve. In contrast to these benefits, the quality of the information provided by sonography is strongly user-dependent and the time to achieve a sufficient level of expertise in examination technique and interpretation of results is probably longer than for MRI.

The next sections discuss the most common typical clinical and sonographic features and rare peripheral nerve compression syndromes in more detail.

Generally speaking neuropathy caused by extrinsic compression may occur anywhere in the body and affect a variety of peripheral nerves. Special anatomic conditions, however, may result in an increased risk for the development of so-called entrapment neuropathies at certain locations. These conditions are multiple:

- Nerves may travel through narrow passageways together with tendons and vessels. Osteofibrous tunnels in the upper or lower limb, for example, are spaces superficially confined by tight fibrotic retinacula and at the bottom either by bone or musculotendinous structures. The retinacula, which are anchored on bony ridges or osseous prominences on either side of the tunnel, prevent dislocation of those structures contained inside. Nerves travelling inside such tunnels may be affected by chronic external wear and tear, often of uncertain origin, or by the presence of abnormal tissue inside the tunnel such as an ulnar artery aneurysm inside Guyon´s canal for example.
- A nerve may also be compromised by an abnormally tight ligament or an anatomic muscle or vessel variant, which runs across the nerve in an oblique course.
- At the forefoot compression of the interdigital nerve against the transverse intermetatarsal ligament, favored by forefoot deformities or clothing habits, may lead to development of Morton's metatarsalgia.
- Nerve compression may also occur secondary to trauma or surgery at predilected sites, such as posttraumatic tarsal tunnel syndrome, with development of neuropathy in a previously asymptomatic individual due to narrowing of the tarsal tunnel caused by malaligned fractures or callus formation.

4.2 Accessory Nerve Syndrome

4.2.1 Introduction

Accessory nerve syndrome is a rare compression syndrome in the neck area. The nerve can be injured along its course from the skull base to where the nerve enters the trapezius muscle. Injury to the accessory nerve results in instability to the shoulder with winging of the scapula. Pain and reduced mobility of shoulder and arm elevation is always present in this type of nerve injury.

4.2.2 Anatomy

The accessory nerve is a motoric nerve formed by fusion of a cranial and a cervical root. The nerve trunk exits from the skull base through the jugular foramen and divides into two branches: The internal branch fuses with the vagal nerve. The external branch of the accessory nerve is mainly a motor nerve containing some sensory nerve bundles, arising from C1–C3 spinal roots. It runs between the occipital artery and the internal jugular vein, and passes underneath the digastricus muscle and the sternocleidomastoideus muscle. This area is called the lateral cervical triangle, which is bordered ventrally by the sternocleidomastoideus muscle, dorsally by the trapezius muscle and caudally by the clavicle (Fig. 4.1). In the lateral cervical triangle the accessory nerve has a superficial course directly beneath the superficial cervical fascia, adjacent to a group of between five and ten superficial lymph nodes. The nerve enters the

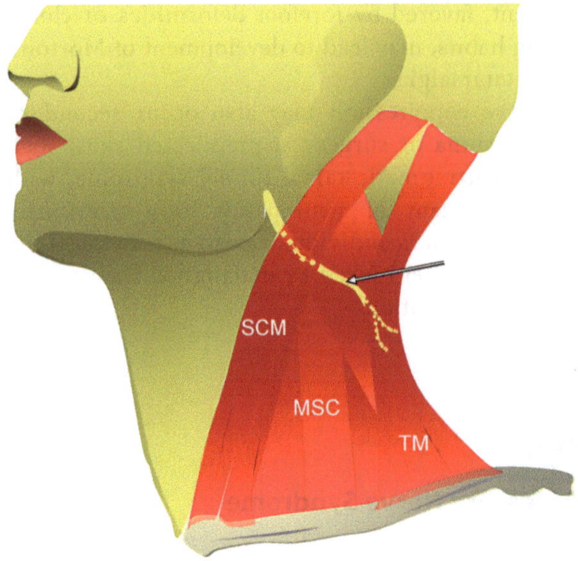

Fig. 4.1. Accessory nerve. The anatomical course of the accessorius nerve, arising from C1–C3 spinal roots. The nerve emerges beneath the sternocleidomastoideus muscle (*SCM*) and becomes superficial at the lateral cervical triangle, entering and innervating the trapeze muscle (*TM*)

trapezius muscle at the ventral side of the muscle and innervates the muscle together with branches of the cervical plexus.

4.2.3 Etiology and Clinical Signs

Iatrogenic accessory nerve lesions occur most often after lymph node biopsy at the lateral cervical triangle (Nason et al. 2000). Because of its superficial course the nerve is easily injured during this procedure (Kierner et al. 2000). Other accessory nerve lesions are associated with neck dissection, whiplash injury or direct nerve trauma (Terrel et al. 2000; Harpf et al. 1999; Wiater and Bigliani 1999; Miyata and Kitamura 1997; Bodack 1998). Glass cut injury or gun shot injury have also been reported to cause accessory nerve palsy (Vandewеyer et al. 1997).

The trapezius muscle is one of the major muscles, which stabilizes the scapula during rotation, elevating the upper limb and retracting the scapula. Consequently accessory nerve palsy causes dysfunction, weakness and pain of the trapezius muscle. The patient normally presents with a dropping shoulder, winging of the scapula and weakness at forward elevation.

4.2.4 Diagnosis

Early diagnosis is usually delayed because of unclear clinical signs, as atrophy of the trapezius muscle is not easily visualized on early clinical inspection. Electrodiagnostic testing is currently the only method to diagnose accessory nerve palsy.

4.2.5 Sonography

Sonographic diagnosis of accessory palsy is mainly based on the evaluation of the echogenicity of the trapezius muscle to assess denervation, which is easily recognized by the hyperechoic texture and the loss of muscle volume (Fig. 4.2). Comparison with the non-affected contralateral side is essential. According to our experience in nerve palsy caused by whiplash injuries no abnormalities along the accessory nerve can be found. In cases of direct trauma or lymph nodes biopsy and nerve dissection nerve swelling or scar tissue can be visualized (see also Chap. 5).

4.2.6 Therapy

Depending on the type of injury the appropriate treatment is chosen. Treatment of nerve dissection includes microsurgical nerve reconstruction within 12 months; otherwise the motoric end plate of the affected muscle is permanently damaged. When primary nerve reconstruction is not accomplished due to delayed diagnosis or in cases of normal appearance of the accessory nerve, surgical procedures have to include rearrangement of the muscle insertion on the scapula.

4.3 Thoracic Outlet Syndrome

4.3.1 Introduction

Thoracic outlet syndrome (TOS) is a rare compression syndrome of the neurovascular bundle at the thoracic outlet region (Roos 1996). Historically, a

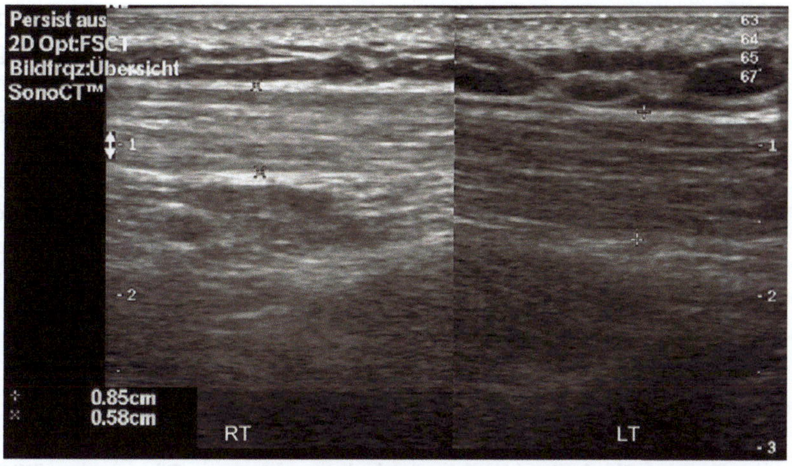

Fig. 4.2. Accessory nerve palsy. Longitudinal 12-MHz scans shows an atrophic, hyperechoic trapeze muscle with hyperechoic echotexture and loss of muscle volume at the right side (*RT*), compared to the normal trapeze muscle on the left side (*LT*)

similar case description was already reported in the second century AD by Galen describing a cervical rib, whereas in the beginning of the 19th century Murphy (Murphy 1905) and Adson reported further cases of cervical ribs and new therapeutic approaches. In the 1940s Wright first described neurovascular compression during prolonged hyperabduction of the arm. The term thoracic outlet was first created by Peete et al. in 1956. It is caused by anatomical abnormalities or acquired changes in the soft tissues and bony structures in the scalene region. The brachial plexus is the most frequently affected structure, followed by the subclavian vein and artery. Patients clinically present with pain, numbness, paraesthesia, muscle atrophy and Raynaud's Syndrome.

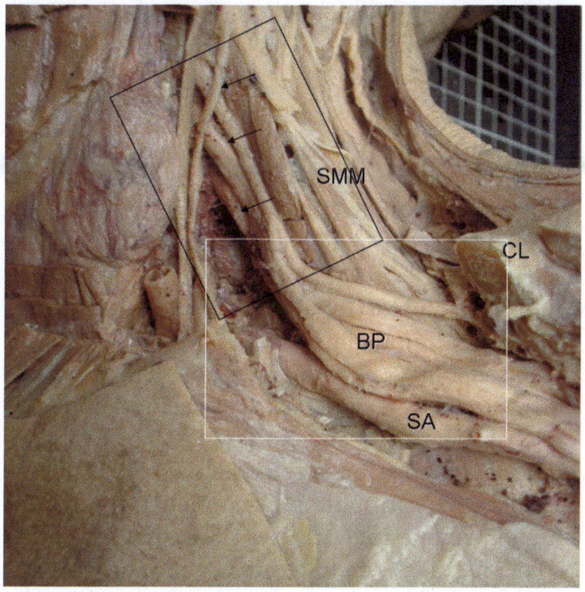

Fig. 4.3. Brachial plexus. Anatomical dissection the left neck area showing the *black box* covering the anterior scalene space and the *white box* covering the costoclavicular space. The nerve roots (*arrows*) are running distally, forming the brachial plexus (*BP*),adjacent to the subclavian artery (*SA*). *SCM*, sternocleidomastoideus muscle; *CL*, partially resected clavicle

4.3.2 Anatomy

The brachial plexus is formed by the nerve roots from C4 to T1. Running distally the brachial plexus and the subclavian vessels can be compressed mainly in three different spaces: (1) at the anterior scalene space, (2) at the costoclavicular space and (3) at the pectoralis minor space.

The anterior scalene space is confined anteriorly by the anterior scalenus muscle, the median scalene muscle posteriorly, the first rib and sternocleidomastoideus muscle (Fig. 4.3). Most neurogenic compression occurs in this space; compression of the neurovascular bundle in this space is also known as the anterior scalene syndrome. The costoclavicular space is confined by the clavicle, the upper scapula, the first rib and the scalene muscles. In this space vascular and neurogenic compression are frequently caused by functional changes or anatomical abnormalities also known as the costoclavicular syndrome. In the pectoralis minor space the neurovascular bundle runs beneath the pectoralis minor muscle and the coracoid process. Anterior and lateral elevation of the arm may stretch the relatively fixed neurovascular bundle, causing compression and stretching (hyperabduction syndrome).

4.3.3 Etiology and Clinical Signs

Although its incidence is still debated in the literature, this type of compression syndrome is relatively frequent, affecting 3–80 cases in 1000; the gender ratio is 3:1 in favour of females. Normally the thoracic outlet is a sufficiently wide space to allow the brachial plexus, the subclavian artery and vein to pass between the chest wall, the first rib and the scalene muscles.

The most frequent structure affected is the brachial plexus followed by vascular compression; the lower roots are more prone to compression than the upper roots. Clinical symptoms include weakness, atrophy, pain, hand swelling, even headache and chest pain. Arterial compression results in intermittent ischemia and Raynaud-like symptoms. Subclavian aneurysms just distal from the compression have been observed. Venous compression may cause thrombosis of the subclavian and axillary vein.

The anterior scalene syndrome, also called Naffziger syndrome (Naffziger and Grant 1938), is characterized by pain and tingling in the forearm and hand similar to that occurring in cervical rib syndrome. A hypertrophic anterior scalene muscle, a scalenus minimus muscle or fibrous bands between the muscles may cause compression of the brachial plexus and subclavian artery against the first thoracic rib (Urschel and Kourlis 2007). Exercise-induced compression of the brachial plexus attributed to a hypertrophic scalenus muscle has been found in competitive athletes (Baltopoulos et al. 2008). Vascular symptoms are usually rare.

The costoclavicular syndrome is caused by the presence of a cervical rib, an anomalous first rib or by a hypertrophic transverse process, although the presence of a cervical rib does not necessarily confirm the diagnosis. Functional anatomy and bad posture play a more important role as causative elements. Clinical findings are similar to the scalenus muscle regarding the neurological findings. Vascular symptoms are predominant in this type of compression. Arterial TOS is caused by emboli arising from subclavian artery stenosis or aneurysms. Venous TOS presents with arm swelling, cyanosis and pain due to subclavian vein obstruction, with or without thrombosis (Sanders and Hammond 2002).

The neurovascular bundle may be compressed as it passes beneath the pectoralis minor tendon during arm abduction, also known as the hyperabduction syndrome. Typically this is an occupational disease affecting those who perform repetitive arm movements. Clinical findings are vague; pain, swelling and numbness are the main findings. Elevation of the arm and increased inspiration trigger and aggravate the clinical findings. Differential diagnosis of TOS includes cervical radiculopathy, brachial neuritis (Parsonage-Turner Syndrome), intrinsic and extrinsic tumors and others.

4.3.4 Diagnosis

Diagnosing TOS can be very challenging and time-consuming. In most cases, the physical examination findings are normal and the sensory examination is often unreliable. Provocative tests, such as the Adson, costoclavicular and hyperabduction maneuvers are also unreliable. Diagnosis is usually made after evaluating a combination of clinical tests, electroneurographic tests (ENG, EMG) and diagnostic imaging (Gillard et al. 2001). Diagnostic imaging methods include X-ray of the neck, dynamic sonography, color Doppler sonography, dynamic phlebography, dynamic angiography, dynamic multislice CT angiography and dynamic MRI angiography. Dynamic images include neutral arm position and hyperabducted arm position at 90° and 120°. The final diagnosis of TOS is frequently deleted due to its inconsistent clinical presentation.

4.3.5 Sonography

Plane X-ray of the neck may well show a hyperplastic transverse process or a cervical rib, but obviously absence of visualization of the nerve roots (Fig. 4.4a). Sonography enables not only an assessment of the presence of a cervical rib (Blankstein et al. 2006), but also shows the relationship between the cervical rib and the nerve roots, as seen in one of our patients with left-sided severe shoulder and severe arm pain, which was exacerbated during rotational head movement (Fig. 4.4a–d). However, apart from assessing the cervical rib and the nerve roots, sonography is currently unable to give important information on the neurogenic TOS in the costoclavicular and pectoralis minor space; in particular, possible fibrous bands or accessory scalene muscles

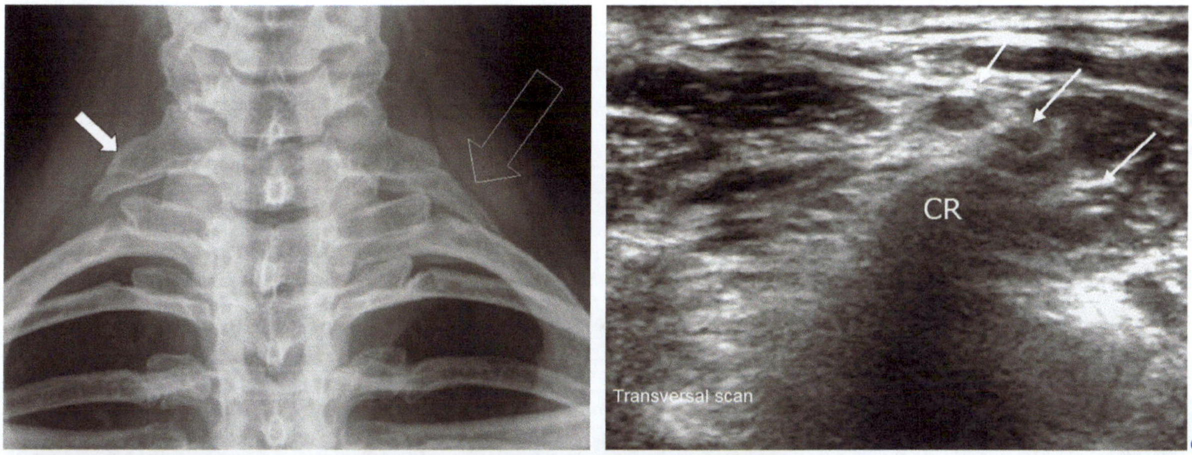

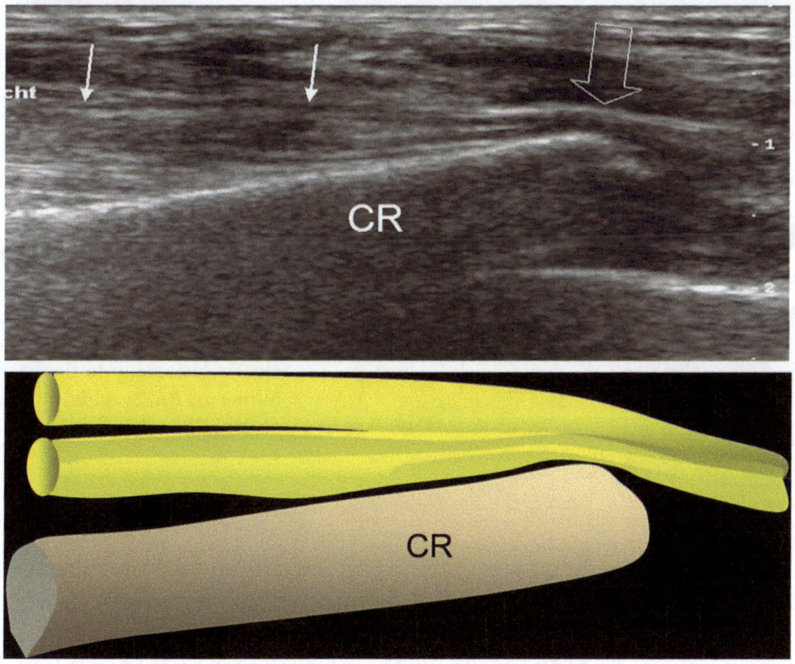

Fig. 4.4a–d. Cervical rib and hypertrophic costotransversal process. **a** Anteroposterior X-ray of the cervical spine illustrates a hypertrophic costotransversal process on the right side (*small arrow*) and a cervical rib on the left side (*large arrow*). **b** Longitudinal 15-MHz scan along the left cervical rib (*CR*) demonstrates a nerval root (*small arrows*) riding on the edge of the end of the cervical rib. The affected nerve segment is flattened (*large arrow*). **c** Corresponding schematic drawing illustrates the nerve flattening due to the tight relationship between the nerve and the cervical rib. **d** Transverse sonogram across the end of the cervical rib (*CR*) demonstrates the close relationship of the nerve roots (*arrow*) with the cervical rib. Forced rotation of the head showed snapping of the single nerve roots over the end of the cervical rib (not shown)

cannot be clearly visualized. MRI is currently the most appropriate imaging method for assessing the entire thoracic outlet space.

Color Doppler sonography has proved to be helpful in the diagnosis of vascular TOS (Demondion et al. 2006; Longley et al. 1992) by showing an increase in the maximum systolic velocity in the costoclavicular space. Venous obstruction or cloth formation can also be seen with sonography. Abnormal sonographic findings, however, should be interpreted cautiously since, according to Stapleton et al. (2007), abnormal sonographic findings during hyperabduction arm position can also be found in individuals without any clinical features of TOS.

4.3.6 Treatment

Treatment of TOS greatly depends on the type and duration of TOS. First attempts to treat TOS should always start with a conservative approach such as avoiding hyperabduction, accounting especially for the neurological TOS (Bahm 2007). Surgery for neurogenic TOS in patients with cervical ribs should include both cervical and first rib resection (Sanders et al. 2007). Arterial TOS is seen less frequently than the neurogenic form; however, in most cases it requires surgical treatment. Vascular procedures include resection and replacement of the subclavian artery aneurysms, decompressive procedures performed through a supraclavicular and infraclavicular approach. Decompression is achieved by cervical rib excision or combined cervical and first rib excision. The complication rate among surgical decompression is up to 45%, including brachial plexus injuries. Baltopoulos et al. (2008) recently described successful scalenectomy in athletes.

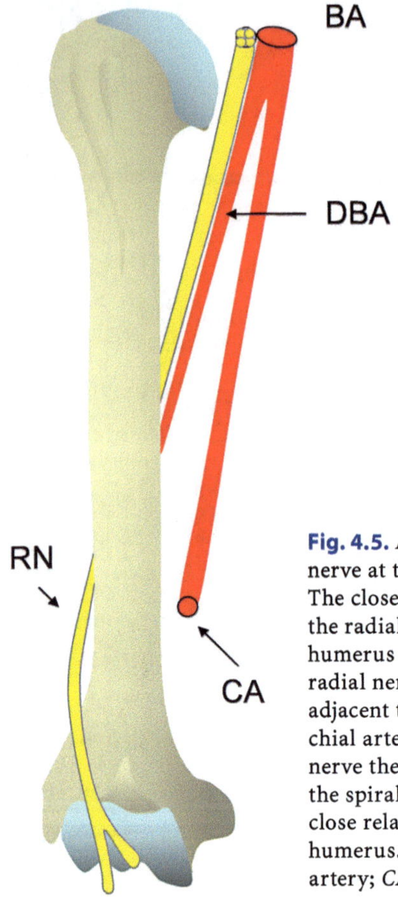

Fig. 4.5. Anatomy of radial nerve at the humerus area. The close relationship of the radial nerve to the humerus is shown. The radial nerve runs distally, adjacent to the deep brachial artery (*DBA*). The nerve then runs around the spiral groove in a close relationship to the humerus. *BA*, brachial artery; *CA*, cubital artery

4.4 Radial Nerve Compression

4.4.1 Introduction

The radial nerve at the upper arm can be compressed while passing through the spiral groove where the nerve is in close relationship to the dorsal aspect of the humerus (radial compression of the spiral grove) (Fig. 4.5). After dividing into the superficial and deep branch, the deep branch penetrates the supinator muscle where the nerve is susceptible to compression (supinator syndrome). The superficial branch runs distally and, because of its superficial course, the nerve is prone to compression and direct trauma (Wartenberg disease).

4.4.2 Anatomy

The radial nerve is the largest branch of the posterior cord of the brachial plexus and contains cervical root contributions from C4–C8. The nerve consists of between five and eight fascicles with motoric and sensory components, which supply the muscles of the extensor compartments, i.e. the triceps muscle, the lateral part of the brachialis muscle, the brachioradialis muscle, the forearm extensors and the dorsolateral area of the hand. After exiting the axillary area the nerve runs distally at the posterior and lateral aspect of the humeral shaft, accompanied by the brachial artery, between the muscle bellies of the medial and the long head of the triceps muscle. Approximately 10 cm proximal to the lateral epicondyle of the humerus, the radial nerve penetrates the lateral intermuscular septum and enters the anterior space of the upper arm, where it lies volarly to the brachialis muscle and dorsally to the brachioradialis muscle. Just anterior to the lateral epicondyle, the nerve bifurcates into the sensory or superficial radial nerve and the motor or deep radial nerve components (posterior interosseous nerve) (Fig. 4.6).

The local anatomy of the radial tunnel is key to understanding the supinator syndrome. Immediately after its origin, the deep branch enters the "radial tunnel", an outlet formed by muscles and aponeuroses. The floor is formed by the anterior capsule of the humeroradial joint together with the deep layer of the supinator muscle. The roof is built by the arcade of Frohse (Fig. 4.6), defined by the fibrous adherence between the brachialis and brachioradialis muscle in front of the radial head, the medial edge of the extensor carpi radialis brevis muscle and the superficial layer of the supinator muscle. The brachioradialis and extensor carpi radialis longus muscle form the anterolateral wall. The medial wall includes the biceps tendon resting on the brachialis muscle.

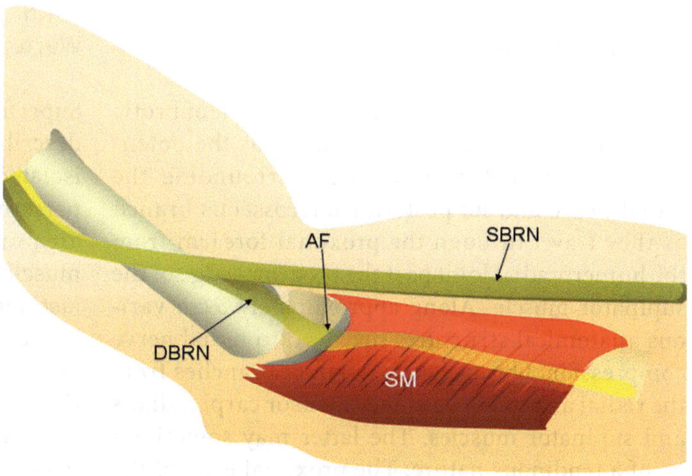

Fig. 4.6. Anatomy of radial nerve at the cubital area. The illustration demonstrates the course and division of the radial nerve slinging down from the spiral groove, splitting into the superficial branch of the radial nerve (*SBRN*) and the deep branch of the radial nerve (*DBRN*), then later enters the supinator muscle (*SM*), passing the arcade of Frohse (*AF*)

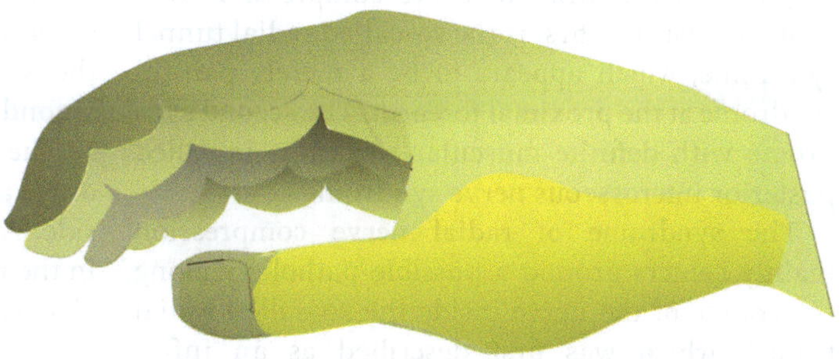

Fig. 4.7. Superficial radial nerve innervation. The sensory innervation supplied by the superficial branch of the radial nerve is demonstrated

Between the two layers of the supinator muscle the DBRN passes the "radial tunnel" and extends downward as the dorsal interosseus nerve between the superficial and deep layers of the extensor muscles of the forearm supplying both muscle groups.

The superficial branch courses over the pronator teres muscle, along the brachioradialis muscle and passes through a fascial layer. The nerve then runs closely to the radial artery to reach the skin of the forearm and dorsolateral area of the thumb (Fig. 4.7).

4.4.3 Radial Nerve Compression at the Spiral Groove

The radial nerve has a close anatomic relationship to the humerus in the spiral groove. In traumatic humerus fracture associated with radial nerve palsy we distinguish the primary lesions that occur with the event of the trauma and secondary lesions that appear within the healing process of the humerus fracture. The nerve can be impinged by fracture fragments or muscles which are dissected or simply oedematous due to intrafascicular hematoma. In secondary nerve palsy the nerve can be surrounded or displaced by callus or riding on a loose metal plate (Bodner et al. 2001) (see Chap. 5).

A frequent external radial nerve compression syndrome among chronic drinkers is caused by the abnormal position of the upper limb, when the arm is stretched across a hard support. This syndrome is commonly referred to as "Saturday night nerve palsy". Other causes for nerve compressions may be ganglia at the elbow (Ogino et al. 1991) or an anomalous triceps muscle (Wilhelm 1985), which can impinge on the nerve or strain the nerve during arm motion or muscle contraction. Other rare cases of radial nerve palsy are tumors, lymph node metastases and persistent pressure from crutches (Phalen et al. 1971).

4.4.4 Supinator Syndrome

The radial tunnel is not a bony or osteofibrotic tunnel in its true sense. It is defined as the potential space created by structures surrounding the radial nerve and its posterior interosseous branch as they travel through the proximal forearm from the humeroradial joint past the proximal edge of the supinator muscle. Along approximately 5 cm various anatomical structures may lead to radial nerve compression: fibrous bands, a fan of branches from the radial artery, edges of the extensor carpi radialis and supinator muscles. The latter may sometimes be of a tendinous nature. The proximal edge of the supinator muscle, known as the arcade of Frohse, is tendinous in about half the population (Spinner 1968). At the "radial tunnel" two distinct and probably completely different nerve compression syndromes exist. The first is the so-called radial tunnel syndrome, which appears to be a merely painful syndrome at the proximal forearm. The second syndrome with definite muscular weakness is called posterior interosseous nerve syndrome.

The syndrome of radial nerve compression mainly centers around a possible pathology along the course of the nerve inside the so-called radial tunnel, which was first described as an infrequent cause of persistent tennis elbow (Roles and Maudsley 1972). This syndrome is known as the supinator syndrome, radial tunnel syndrome or posterior interosseous nerve paralysis. This type of nerve palsy is often misdiagnosed as lateral epicondylitis. It should be mentioned that the radial tunnel syndrome is heavily disputed in the literature (Kalb et al. 1999; Rosenbaum 1999). Today there is some evidence that misdiagnosis of radial nerve compression may have occurred in several cases, and even postsurgical improvement of a patient's symptoms is not considered evidence of the true existence of radial tunnel disease by some authors (Rosenbaum 1999). Sonography may prove helpful in this regard with direct demonstration of radial nerve compression and subsequent structural changes inside the nerve bundle (Bodner et al. 2002; Martinoli et al. 2004). Other extrinsic compression syndromes of the radial nerve may occur due to external forces or coexisting pathology such as ganglia at the elbow or musculoskeletal tumors.

4.4.5 Wartenberg Syndrome

Superficial radial nerve compression was first described by Wartenberg in 1932. He called this isolated superficial radial neuropathy "cheiralgia paresthetica", describing nerve compression at the area underneath the tendon of the brachioradialis muscle. Various surgical procedures at the wrist, but also tenovaginitis De Quervain and drug infusion at the radial side of the wrist may cause this type of neuropathy. Clinically patients present with dysesthesia and paresthesia over the area of the thumb, without any motoric deficiency, frequently having a major negative impact on quality of life, especially when the dominant hand is affected (Lanzetta and Foucher 1995; Zöch and Aigner 1997).

The superficial branch runs across the supinator muscle and reaches the skin passing through the antebrachial fascia reaching the skin at the area of the wrist. The nerve supplies the skin of the first, second and radial half of the third finger.

The nerve is at risk especially in surgical procedures and intravenous infusion placed on the radial side. A typical clinical sign is sensory disturbance in the region of the thumb; there is no motoric deficiency.

4.4.6 Clinical Considerations

The clinical work-up of a patient with radial nerve palsy includes a detailed physical and neurological examination. As a general guideline sensory and motor radial deficiency relates to a proximal (axillary) compression. Motor radial deficiency, sparing the triceps muscle, appears in compression syndromes at the spiral groove. Weakness of finger extension, sparing the extensor carpi radialis, supports the presence of a compression syndrome of the deep branch of the radial nerve.

Electroneurographic examination is currently the method of choice to indicate the level of nerve compression and to assess functional nerve recovery. In most cases of radial nerve palsy, conduction studies show activity and therefore integrity of the nerve. Follow-up EMG can assess the amount of recovery. Nerve conduction tests, however, are unable to differentiate the cause of nerve compression, for example if the nerve is dissected in traumatic lesions, impinged or severely encased by callus. In these cases no, or only minimal, neurological activity can be measured. It is important, however, to diagnose the cause of the nerve compression at an early stage, as irreversible degeneration of the motor end plate of the muscle may occur after 6–12 months. According to the literature, a nerve without signs of recovery should undergo surgical inspection. The lack of information from electroneurographic testing regarding integrity of the nerve calls for a noninvasive method such as sonography to accurately visualize the nerve itself.

The radial tunnel syndrome is characterized by pain and tenderness in the region of the radial tunnel, with an increase in pain during certain maneuvers, such as resisted extension of the middle finger or resisted supination with extension of the elbow. These maneuvers contract the extensor carpi radialis and/or supinator muscle with possible impingement of the radial nerve. Patients with radial tunnel syndrome differ clinically from patients with true compression neuropathies in so far as they do not show any prominent focal tenderness, any neurological deficit or pathological findings during electrodiagnostic testing (Rosenbaum 1999).

The posterior interosseous nerve syndrome, or "true neurogenic radial tunnel syndrome" (Rosenbaum 1999), manifests with muscle weakness typically sparing the extensor carpi radialis (no wrist drop!), but during wrist extension the hand may deviate radially because of weakness of the extensor carpi ulnaris. There is impairment of finger extension at the metacarpophalangeal joints, as well as reduced function of the abductor pollicis longus, and extensor pollicis longus and brevis muscle. This clinical syndrome may be caused by a variety of structures compressing the nerve along the radial tunnel and compression at the arcade of Frohse is most common. As stated above purely sensory deficit at the dorsolateral hand without motoric deficiency is typical for Wartenberg syndrome (Fig. 4.7).

4.4.7 Sonography

Using a 5- to 17-MHz broad-band linear array the radial nerve is easily detected in a transverse scan at the lateral aspect of the mid-humerus, and can be followed upward or downward from this level (Foxall et al. 2007; Bodner et al. 2002; Martinoli et al. 2004; Rossey-Marec 2004). In addition color Doppler sonography allows visualization of the accompanying deep brachial artery, which may serve as a guideline for identification of the nerve. The nerve consists of between four and eight hypoechoic tubular structures (fascicle groups) surrounded by an echoic rim. The nerve's normal transverse diameter ranges from 4.0 to 4.2 mm and the normal anteroposterior diameter ranges from 2.3 to 3.5 mm. The nerve changes its form from a more rounded shape at the proximal part to oval at the central part and rounded again at the distal part of the humerus. At the level of the lateral condyle between the brachioradialis and brachialis muscle, the nerve splits into two branches, the deep and superficial branches, which may also be assessed with sonography (Bodner et al. 2002; Chien et al. 2003; Nakamichi and Tachibana 2007).

As with any injured peripheral nerve, the radial nerve also shows swelling proximal to the damaged segment. On sonography the damaged nerve appears hypoechoic with loss of its regular dotted pattern. In cases of "Saturday night" palsy sonography shows spindle-like swelling at the area of compression (Fig. 4.8). The impingement of the deep branch of the radial nerve at the level of the supinator muscle can be detected with sonography. In our own case series of four patients with a supinator syndrome, sonography enabled clear visualization of an edematous nerve with a caliber change proximal to the supinator muscle in all cases. The echotexture of the affected nerve was hypoechoic and rich vascularity was seen at the superficial epineurium (Fig. 4.9a–c).

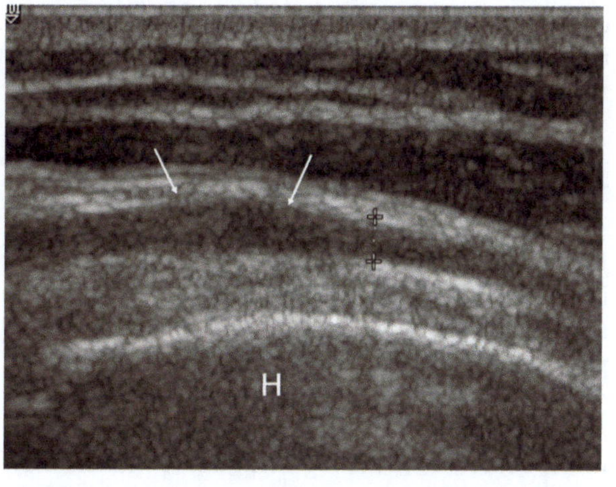

Fig. 4.8. Saturday night palsy. Longitudinal 15-MHz scan along the radial nerve at the spiral groove shows a spindle-like swelling of the radial nerve (*arrows*). Caliber measurements show normal nerve caliber. *H*, humerus

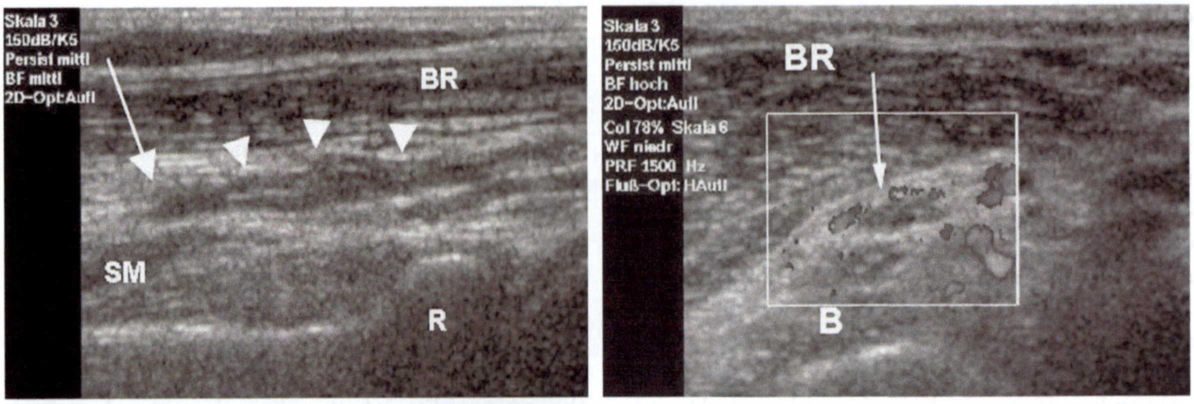

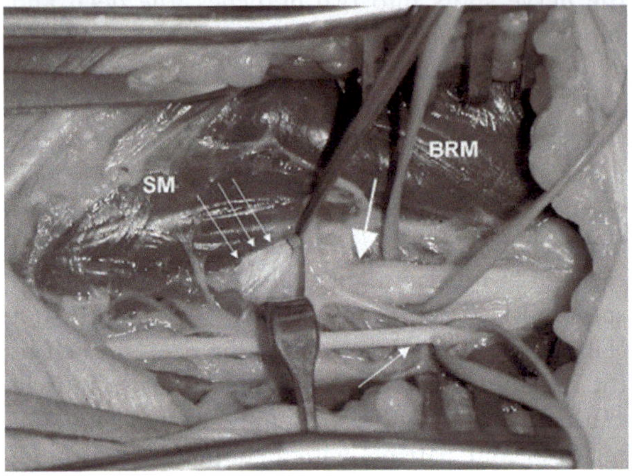

Fig. 4.9a–c. Longitudinal sonogram (**a**) in a patient with clinical evidence of supinator syndrome shows a hypoechoic tubular structure (*arrowheads*) with reduction in nerve diameter (*arrow*) at the entry point into the supinator muscle (*SM*). *BR*, brachioradialis muscle; *R*, radial head. Transverse sonogram (**b**) shows a hypoechoic structure corresponding to the deep radial nerve branch which is surrounded by multiple vessels. Intraoperative nerve inspection (**c**) shows an edematous deep branch of the radial nerve (*arrow*) at the level of the arcade of Frohse (*arrows*). *Small arrow*, normal superficial branch of radial nerve; *SM*, supinator muscle; *BR*, brachioradialis muscle

High frequency probes working with 15–17 MHz allow visualization of the superficial radial branch in its entire length and therefore also assessment of minute pathological changes within the affected nerve or assessment of any extrinsic or intrinsic causative compressing elements such as ganglia, thrombophlebitis or i.v.-related nerve damage.

4.4.8 Therapy

In cases with proven radial nerve compression inside the radial tunnel surgical decompression is advocated (Ritts et al. 1987). While the normal patient work-up implies clinical and electrodiagnostic follow-up examinations for at least 6 weeks and surgery if no improvement of deficits is achieved under conservative management, this rationale may change with the introduction of sonography. If an underlying anatomical and surgically treatable cause for radial nerve paralysis is detected early surgery may be advocated based on sonographic findings. In patients suffering from Wartenberg syndrome sonographic-guided injection of a minimal amount of cortisone proves to be therapeutic. In cases of nerve entrapment at the brachioradialis tendon surgical tendon splitting is advocated (Lanzetta and Foucher 1995).

4.5 Median Nerve Compression

The median nerve is formed by the fibers of the lateral medial cords. At the upper arm the nerve runs lateral to the brachial artery to the mid humerus, then crosses over and reaches a more superficial and medial anatomic position. At the upper arm no defined areas of compression are known; however, the nerve, because of its superficial course, is prone to direct trauma.

Compression of the median nerve above the wrist is rare, accounting for approximately 1% of compression syndromes in the upper limb (Nigst and Dick 1979). Two distinct syndromes are known, i.e. pronator syndrome and anterior interosseus nerve syndrome.

By far the most common compression neuropathy is found at the carpal tunnel. At this site the median nerve travels through a narrow passage together with the flexor tendons and is therefore subject to entrapment if any coexisting condition results in a further decrease in the space beneath the flexor retinaculum.

4.5.1 Compression Syndromes Above the Wrist

4.5.1.1 Pronator Syndrome

Pronator syndrome is a rare compression syndrome of the median nerve, first described in 1951 by Seyffarth. It affects the median nerve at the cubital fossa mostly in men in their fifth decade. The predilected space of compression is where the median nerve pierces the two heads of the pronator teres muscle and crosses under the deep and superficial flexor tendons (Fig. 4.10).

The sites of compression include the lacertus fibrosus, the Struthers ligament, the pronator teres and the proximal arch or the flexor digitorum superficialis.

A variety of anatomical abnormalities and functional etiologies have been named to cause this syndrome: Anatomical abnormalities include fibrous bands, thickened lacertus fibrosus and accessory muscles (Johnson et al. 1979; Lacey and Soldatis 1993). Functional or dynamic compression have been described in repetitive supination or elbow extension, during this maneuver the nerve gets squashed between the muscle bellies. Delayed diagnosis of this syndrome is very common since clinical signs are vague although, in contrast to the CTS, this syndrome involves the thenar muscles and the wrist and flexor muscles. In addition the sensory impairment also involves the dorsal and volar side of the hand. Clinically patients complain of pain in the proximal volar forearm and the distal arm; pain is often exacerbated with activity, especially against resistance. Contrary to carpal tunnel syndrome nocturnal pain is uncommon. Tinel's sign along the median nerve at the level of the pronator teres is frequently positive; pain and musculo-neurological impairment can be triggered by a stressing test, putting resistance to forced supination.

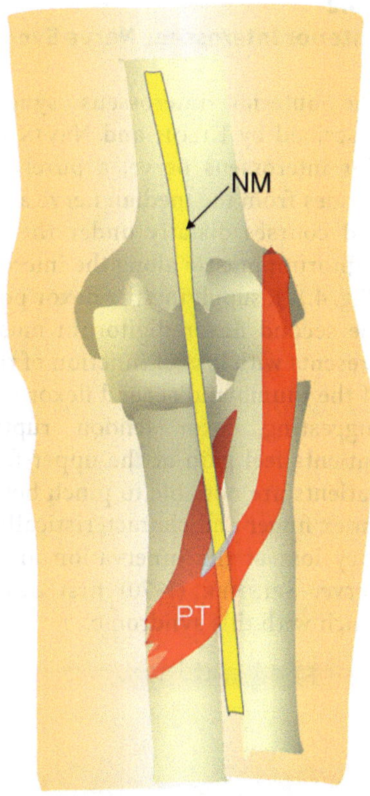

Fig. 4.10. Pronator teres syndrome. The course of the median nerve (*MN*) running between the two heads of the pronator teres muscle (*PT*) is shown

Treatment is primarily conservative, including avoidance of aggravating physical activity, and an arm sling or splint is usually beneficial initially, especially in those cases where only mild symptoms are present. Cortisone injection is reported to be beneficial. In severe cases, and in those where conservative or minimally invasive treatment fails, a surgical approach is advocated. Surgical treatment includes exploration of the median nerve in the proximal forearm, with incision of the fibrotendinous fascial layers.

Although sonography has the potential to assess nerve changes and abnormal muscles in the elbow area, only one report has been published in the literature so far (Martinoli et al. 2004). Flattening of the median nerve between the pronator muscle area suggests this mononeuropathy; comparison with the contralateral side is mandatory.

4.5.2 Anterior Interosseus Nerve Syndrome

The anterior interosseus syndrome was first described by Kiloh and Nevin (1952). The anterior interosseus nerve, a purely motoric branch, divides from the median nerve at the cubital fossa, and courses distally under the superficial flexor digitorum muscle along the interosseus membrane (Fig. 4.11), supplying the flexor pollicis longus and the second flexor digitorum muscle. Clinically it presents with loss of function of the distal phalanx of the thumb and second flexor tendon, frequently suggesting flexor tendon rupture. Sometimes patients feel pain at the upper forearm. Typically patients are not able to pinch between thumb and index finger and characteristically there is no sensory loss at the innervation area of the median nerve. Spinner (1970) first described the weak pinch with this syndrome.

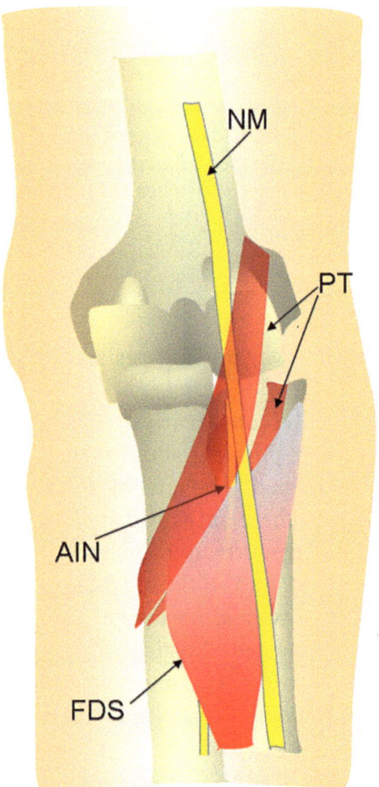

Fig. 4.11. Anterior interosseus nerve. The anterior interossseus nerve (*AIN*) branches at the cubital fossa, running distally, across the flexor digitorum superficialis muscle (*FDS*) underneath the pronator teres muscle (*PT*)

The nerve may by compressed by fibrous bands from the pronator teres muscle (Hausmann and Patel 1996). The etiology in most cases is unclear. Different causes for nerve compression have been described in cases of fracture, fascicular compression (Haussmann and Patel 1996) or anomalous muscles (Gantzer muscle = accessory head of the flexor pollicis muscle) (Degreef and De Smet 2004). Differential diagnosis of this type of syndrome is extremely important since the most commonly misdiagnosed problem is that of a tendon rupture.

Electrophysiologic studies are much more useful in anterior interosseous nerve syndrome than in the pronator syndrome. Electromyography has a high positive diagnostic rate in localizing the affected muscles and therefore in confirming the diagnosis of anterior interosseus syndrome.

Sonographic findings are limited to indirect signs such as increase of muscle echogenicity due to loss of innervation and loss of muscle volume of the affected muscles. Sonography also shows lack of active contraction of the affected muscle (Hide et al. 1999; Martinoli et al. 2004). According to our experience in most of the cases the nerve does not show any abnormalities on sonographic scans; the value of sonography lies in the assessment of the integrity of the nerve and exclusion of compressing masses along the anterior interosseus nerve.

Treatment is usually conservative; only in selected cases, when re-innervation does not occur within 2–6 months, nerve exploration and tendon or band release is advised (Lubahn and Cermak 1998).

4.5.3 Carpal Tunnel Syndrome

4.5.3.1 Epidemiology and Clinical Presentation

Compression of the median nerve at the carpal tunnel due to a healed radial fracture was first described by Paget in 1854. Marie and Foix (1913) were the first to describe the median nerve compression beneath the transverse carpal ligament. Learmonth (1933) first performed carpal tunnel release to treat median nerve compression.

Carpal tunnel syndrome (CTS) is the most common entrapment syndrome of the upper extremities with an estimated incidence in the general community of 125 per 100,000 per year. Typically, the dominant hand is affected first. The clinical hallmark and usual presenting feature of CTS is a pain syndrome called brachialgia paresthetica nocturna (MUMENTHALER et al. 1998). Patients, usually women in their fourth and fifth decade, are awakened from sleep in the early morning hours with pain radiating from the wrist proximally into the forearm and arm, and report numbness and tingling in the hand, stiffness of the fingers, and characteristic swelling sensations. All complaints rapidly resolve after repeated hand movements such as shaking. Episodes of pain in the night may be exacerbated by prolonged strenuous manual work. In the early stage no gross abnormalities can be observed within the nerve. With more severe nerve compression the patient experiences permanent paresthesias or sensory loss over the palmar thumb and digits innervated by the median nerve (Fig. 4.12), and in advanced disease weakness and wasting of part of the thenar muscles. In this stage swelling and deformation of the nerve is found, leading to sclerotic and fibrotic changes. Significant vasomotor disturbances are comparatively rare. Sensory disturbance usually appears before motoric deficiency since sensory fibers are more pressure sensitive than motoric fibers .According to NORA et al. (2005) paresthesia is the most characteristic feature followed by pain and cramps. Early diagnosis of CTS is essential to avoid late sequelae such as permanent muscle waisting and persistent pain, both of which can greatly affect quality of life.

4.5.3.2
Etiology

CTS arises from compression of the median nerve in the canal formed by the transverse carpal ligament and carpal bones (Fig. 4.13). Under pathological circumstances tissue pressure in the carpal tunnel reaches 30 mmHg, i.e. four times the normal level (SZABO and CHIDGEY 1989). Chronic or recurrent compression of the median nerve causes focal demyelination and eventually axon degeneration as the pathological counterpart to the emerging clinical deficits. Temporary ischemia due to compression of the vasa nervorum accounts for the reversible pain manifesting during the night. Factors contributing to the development of CTS are numerous and often coexist in individuals: (1) congenital smallness of the tunnel or anatomical peculiarities (persistent median artery, abnormal course or insertion of finger flexor and palmaris muscles); (2) susceptibility of the nerve to pressure (diabetic or other neuropathies, etc.); (3) systemic and endocrine disorders (pregnancy, hypothyroidism, acromegaly, amyloidosis, etc.), and (4) reduced space in the carpal tunnel due to space-occupying lesions (osteophytes, exostosis, ganglia, hematoma, tenosynovitis, articular deformities in rheumatoid arthritis, etc.) (ROSENBAUM and OCHOA 1993). The application of sonography has expanded our knowledge of the diversity of the pathological conditions underlying CTS (BEEKMAN and VISSER 2003; TAGLIAFICO et al. 2007).

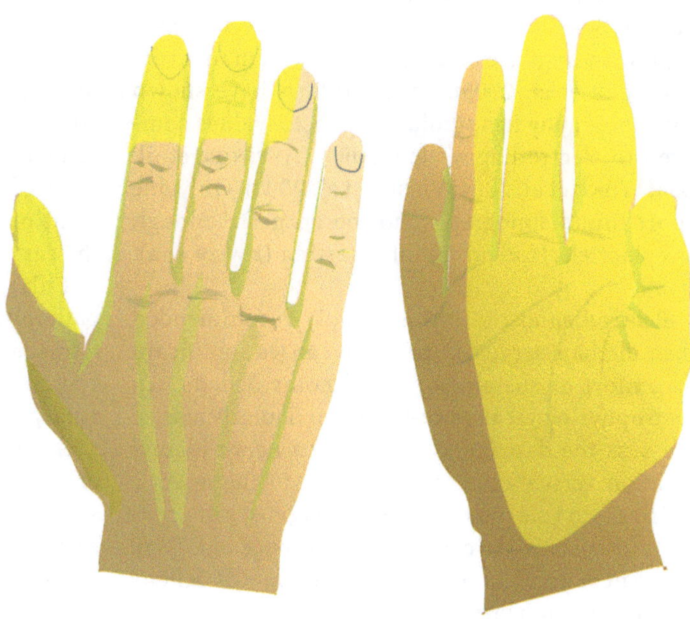

Fig. 4.12. The sensory innervation at of the median nerve at the volar and palmar aspect at the right hand

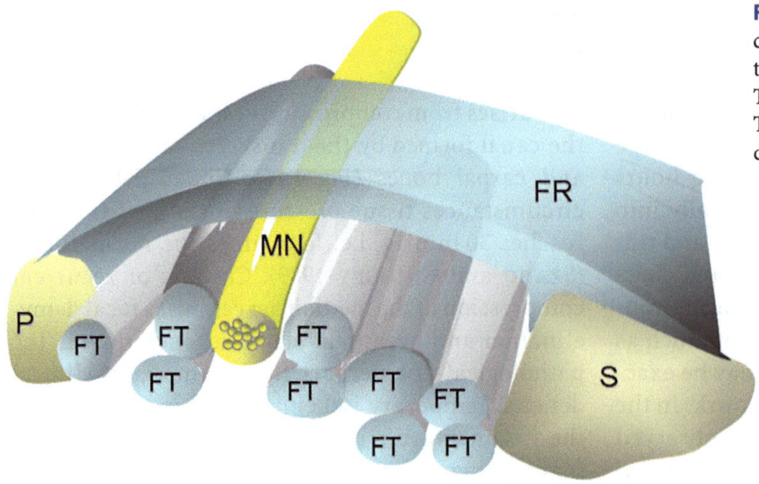

Fig. 4.13. The proximal carpal tunnel. The carpal tunnel on the lateral sides is formed by the pisiforme (*P*) and the scaphoid (*S*) bones. The flexor retinaculum (*FR*) forms the roof. The carpal tunnel contains nine flexor tendons and the median nerve

4.5.3.3 Diagnosis

In most instances, the diagnosis of CTS is reliably settled by an experienced clinician based on a review of the patient's history and complaints and a careful neurological examination. Clinical assessment should include Phalen's maneuver (emergence of paresthesias in the median territory elicited by maximal passive wrist flexion for 1 min or more (Kuschner et al. 1992; Phalen 1966) and testing for Tinel's sign (paresthesias provoked by tapping with the finger over the carpal tunnel).

Recent reports suggest that sonography should be performed as a first-line investigation after clinical examinations since the diagnostic value of sonographic findings are better then physical maneuvers (Ziswiler et al. 2005). Other authors have shown that sonography has similar diagnostic values compared to electrodiagnostic studies (Altinok et al. 2004; Wong et al. 2004; Visser et al. 2008). Only one report found sonography not be accurate enough to replace electroneurographic testing (Kwon et al. 2008).

Electrodiagnostic testing is only recommended when median nerve compression causes significant discomfort or sustained sensorimotor deficits. An electrophysiological work-up is particularly useful to assess the damage to the median nerve (demyelination versus axon loss) relevant to therapeutic decisions, to rule out differential diagnoses or coexistent disease and to confirm the presence of CTS in the event of atypical complaints, pure motor deficits and prominent neuropathy.

4.5.3.4 Sonography

The value of sonography for the detection of median nerve entrapment inside the carpal tunnel has been recognized since 1991 when the first systematic approach to the sonographic diagnosis of CTS was reported based on data derived at our institution (Buchberger et al. 1991). Since then several reports in the literature have focused on the value of different sonographic criteria for CTS diagnosis (Duncan et al. 1999; Lee et al. 1999; Nakamichi and Tachibana 2007; Sarria et al. 2000; Dilley et al. 2001; Jamadar et al. 2001). All of these studies focused mainly on three sonographic techniques: measurement of median nerve diameter or cross-sectional area at distinct locations along the carpal tunnel, structural analysis of the median nerve and bowing of the flexor retinaculum. If these reports are compared, one of the reliable findings for the diagnosis of CTS found by different authors is enlargement of the median nerve at the proximal level of the carpal tunnel (Fig. 4.14).

Enlargement of a nerve seems to be a common pathophysiological pathway to peripheral nerve damage and relates to vascular congestion and edema. While there is now general agreement that enlargement of the median nerve is a sign of CTS, there is some disagreement as to the amount of enlargement considered to be pathological. In the study by Buchberger et al. (1991, 1992) a cross-sectional area of the median nerve of 10 mm^2 measured in the proximal or middle carpal tunnel coincided with CTS. This was confirmed in a study by

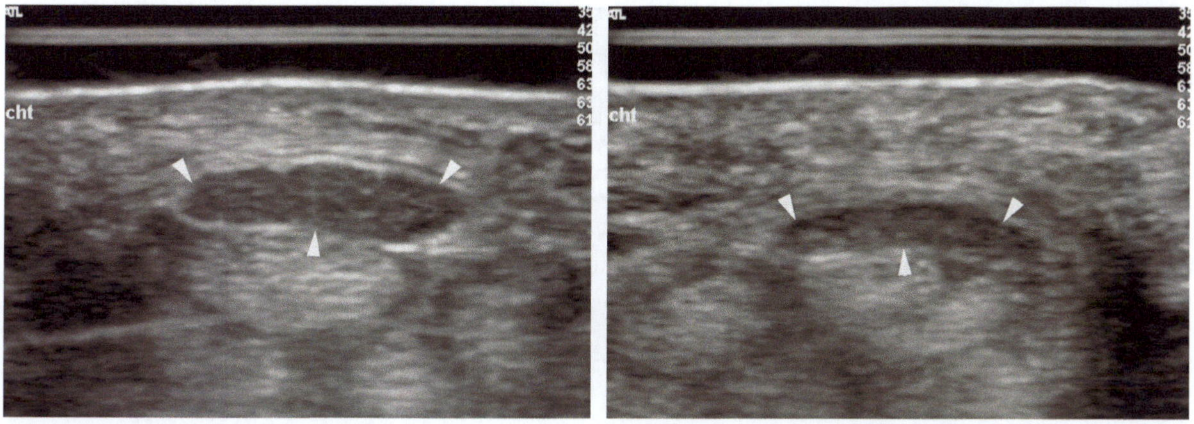

a b

Fig. 4.14a,b. Transverse sonograms through the median nerve in a patient with CTS acquired at the proximal (**a**) and distal (**b**) carpal tunnel. Marked swelling of the median nerve (*arrowheads*) is noted in the proximal carpal tunnel with loss of fascicular discrimination, whereas the nerve is somewhat flattened in the distal carpal tunnel

Nakamichi and Tachibana (2007), while in an EMG controlled study by Lee et al. (1999) a cut-off value of 15 mm^2 was considered to be pathological in patients with severe nerve damage. Altinok (2004) reported a higher sensitivity of sonographic assessment of moderate versus mild CTS, suggesting a cross sectional area of >9 mm^2 as a cut-off value. Koyuncuoglu et al. (2005) reported a cross sectional area of 8.8 mm^2 to be diagnostic in patients with positive clinical findings but negative electrodiagnostic testing.

A further sonographic sign for CTS, which relates to median nerve enlargement and has been confirmed by various studies, is palmar bowing and thickening of the flexor retinaculum (Fig. 4.15). A reliable documentation of this finding, however, will only be achieved with the application of high-frequency sonographic transducers, which allow exact discrimination of the retinaculum flexorum. A cut-off value of >4 mm between the most anterior part of the carpal ligament and the base line between the hamatum and trapezium has been reported to be significant for CTS (Buchberger et al. 1991).

In addition to median nerve enlargement, a distal flattening ratio above 3 has been defined as a cut-off value above which CTS has to be suspected (Buchberger et al. 1991, 1992). Patients with CTS included in their study had a mean distal flattening ratio of 4.6, whereas normal healthy subjects had a ratio of only 3.2. While the value of sonographic measurement of median nerve enlargement for CTS diagnosis was confirmed by other authors, the increased median nerve flattening ratio at the hook of the hamate was not confirmed in later studies to be suggestive of CTS (Nakamichi and Tachibana 2007; Sarria et al. 2000). Nevertheless, several reports agree on the finding of median nerve flattening in the distal carpal tunnel, or abrupt contour changes seen in patients with CTS (Lee et al. 1999; Nakamichi and Tachibana 2007). Based on our own experience with sonography in a large series of CTS patients, we are cautious with the interpretation of median nerve caliber changes. A considerable amount of distal median nerve flattening occurs in healthy asymptomatic volunteers. From a technical point of view this median nerve flattening is best demonstrated with longitudinal panoramic sonograms (Fig. 4.16).

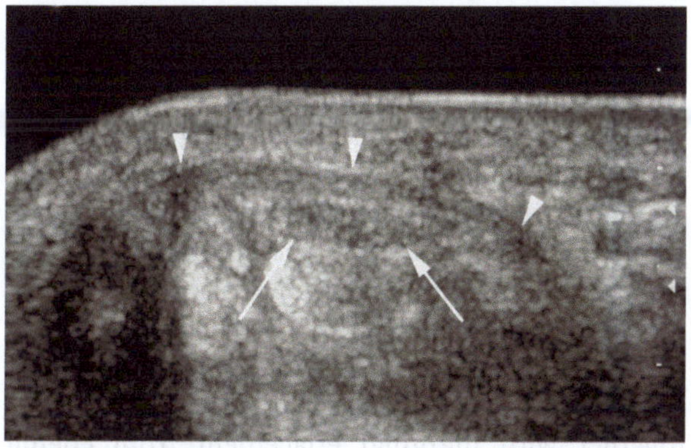

Fig. 4.15. Transverse sonogram through the carpal tunnel in a patient with CTS. Note the thickening and palmar bowing of the flexor retinaculum (*arrowheads*) and median nerve (*arrows*) with somewhat reduced fascicular discrimination

Similar results are known from the MRI literature, where the value of median nerve flattening in

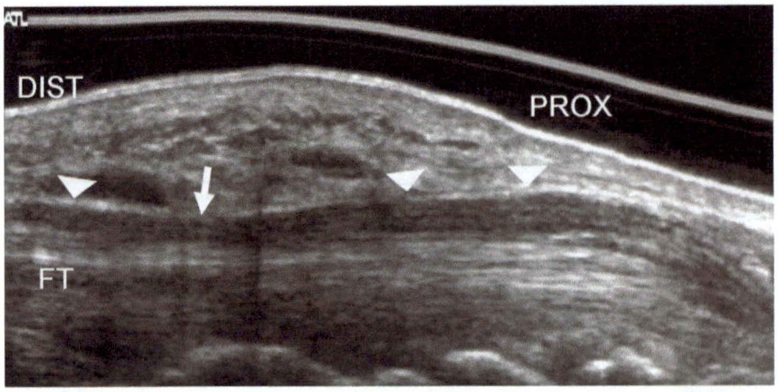

Fig. 4.16. Longitudinal extended view using a 17-MHz probe along the carpal tunnel in a volunteer without any clinical signs of CTS. A flattening of the median nerve (*arrowhead*) is seen at the proximal part of the flexor retinaculum with normal nerve caliber (*arrowheads*) proximal to the flexor retinaculum (*PROX*) and smaller caliber size distally to the flexor retinaculum (*DIST*). *FT*, flexor tendons

CTS diagnosis is disputed (Kleindienst et al. 1998; Monagle et al. 1999). Nevertheless an abrupt caliber change of the enlarged median nerve (a notch sign) at the entrance of the carpal tunnel showed a good correlation with EMG results in the study by Lee et al. (1999) (Fig. 4.17). In some cases the nerve swelling can also be seen at the distal side of the compression (Fig. 4.18a,b). We recently encountered CTS with isolated distal nerve swelling (Fig. 4.19).

An important sonographic technique for CTS diagnosis, which we consider even more reliable, is the evaluation of changes in median nerve echotexture. Several studies have shown a loss of fascicular discrimination in the enlarged median nerve (Lee et al. 1999; Nakamichi and Tachibana 2007; Martinoli et al. 2000; Mallouhi et al. 2006) together with marginal effacement from edema (Fig. 4.20a,b).

With the advent of high-frequency transducers (up to 15 MHz) and more sensitive Doppler software in the early 2000s the detection of nerve vasculature has become feasible and, according to Martinoli et al. (2000) and Mallouhi et al. (2006), an increase in internal and perineural vascularization may further aid patients with neuropathy caused by median nerve compression (Fig. 4.21a,b). However, further recent development of ultrasound equipment with higher frequency probes (up to 17 MHz) allows the visualization of small vessels in asymptomatic volunteers; therefore, sonographic detection of increased nerve blood flow should be judged cautiously and not used as a singular positive finding for CTS. Detection of vessels within the median nerve should not be mistaken for a persistent median artery (PMA). A PMA with various combinations of median nerve shape is a special condition known at the carpal tunnel which can only be assessed with color Doppler sonography. The median artery provides blood supply to the forearm and the hand during embryonic development.

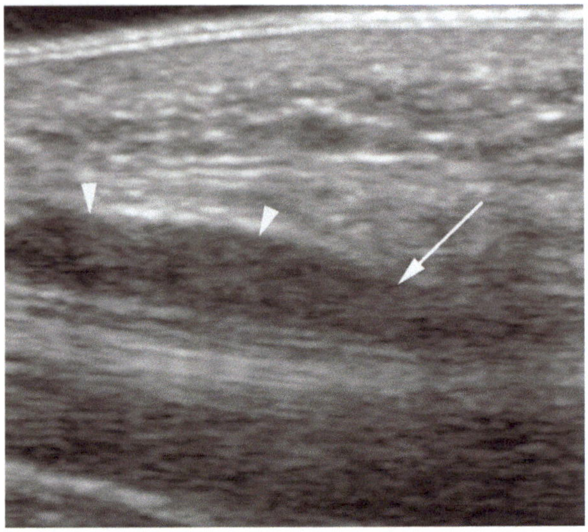

Fig. 4.17. Longitudinal sonogram through the median nerve (*arrowheads*) in a patient with CTS reveals abrupt narrowing (*arrow*) of the median nerve at its entrance into the carpal tunnel

As the radial and ulnar arteries develop, the median artery atrophies to a small vessel accompanying the median nerve in the forearm. When extending into the carpal tunnel, a PMA may join the superficial volar arch, supply the radial digits with an absent arch, or end as a thrombosed thread. An enlarged, thrombosed or calcified PMA and a PMA aneurysm in the carpal tunnel were considered causes of CTS (Eversmann 1988). In addition, a vascular anomaly inside the carpal tunnel may be of importance in the case of carpal tunnel release, as an inadvertent transection of the vessel may result in severe bleeding. Furthermore, surgical transection of the median artery is not feasible without previous knowledge concerning the contribution of the vessel to the supply of the hand. According to the literature a PMA is found in 26% of asymptomatic

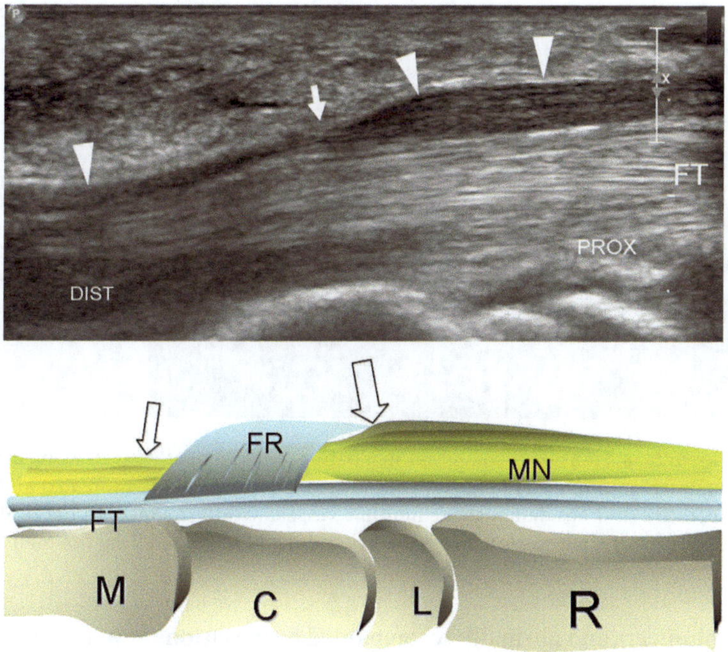

a

b

Fig. 4.18a,b. Idiopathic carpal tunnel syndrome. **a** Longitudinal extended view using a 17-MHz probe along the carpal tunnel in a patient with idiopathic CTS. A marked caliber change noted at the median nerve (*arrowhead*) is seen at the proximal part of the flexor retinaculum with marked nerve swelling (*arrowheads*) proximal to the flexor retinaculum and mild nerve swelling distally of the flexor retinaculum. **b** Corresponding schematic drawing demonstrates the "notch sign" (*large arrow*) with marked proximal nerve swelling and distal mild nerve swelling (*small arrow*). The nerve flattening is most prominent at the proximal flexor retinaculum. *FT*, flexor tendons, *M*, metacarpal bone; *C*, capitate bone; *L*, lunate bone; *R*, radial bone

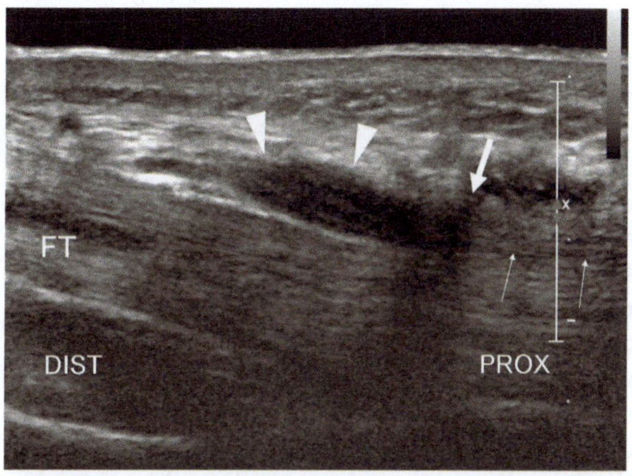

Fig. 4.19. Longitudinal extended view of the carpal tunnel in a patient with idiopathic CTS. Clinically the patient complaint of pain along the 3rd and 4th fingers, sparing the 2nd and first fingers. Marked nerve swelling (*arrowheads*) was found distally to the flexor retinaculum (*white arrow*), the nerve shows a normal caliber proximally to the flexor retinaculum (*small arrows*). Findings were confirmed by surgical nerve inspection

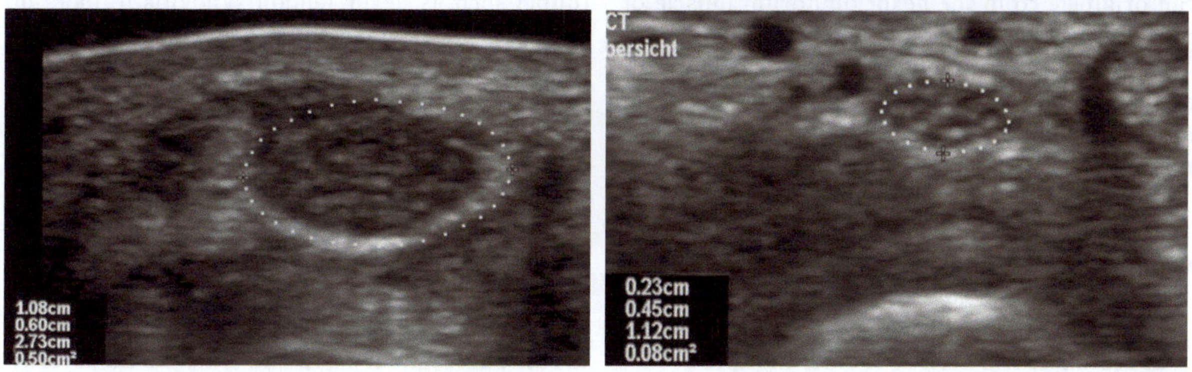

a

b

Fig. 4.20. a Transverse sonogram in a patient with idiopathic CTS showing enlargement of the median nerve with a cross sectional area of 5 mm^2 (*dotted line*) and loss of fascicular discrimination and reduced echogenicity. **b** In comparison transverse sonogram of a normal median nerve in a healthy volunteers demonstrates the typical *dotted* pattern, resembling the nerve fascicles (cross-sectional diameter is 0.8 mm^2)

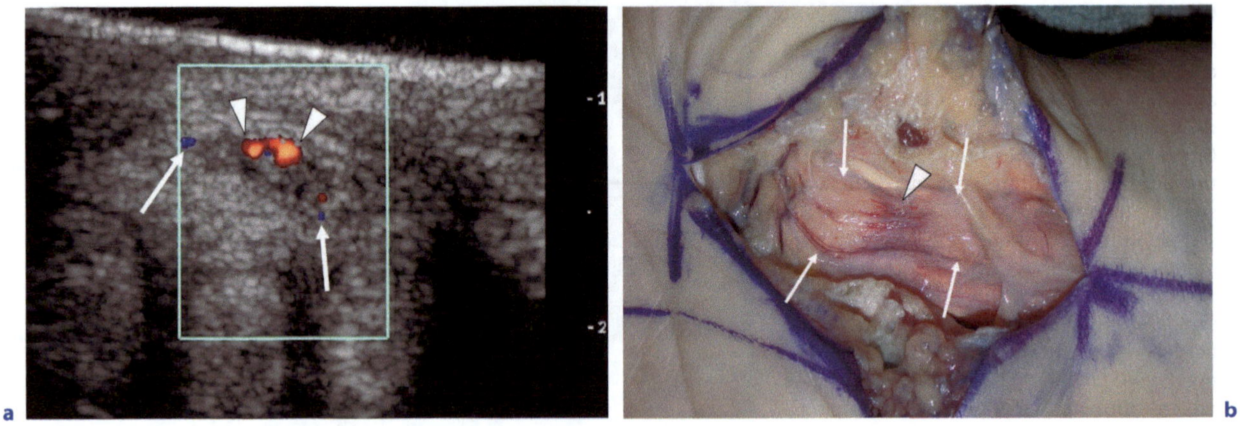

Fig. 4.21. a Transverse sonogram in a patient with idiopathic CTS using a 15-MHz transducer. Color Doppler image demonstrates multiple color signals within the median nerve (*arrowheads*) and within the perineural space (*arrows*). **b** Intraoperative findings demonstrate multiple vessels within the median nerve at the compression area and (*arrowhead*) within the perineural sheet. Note the proximal and distal nerve swelling (*arrows*)

volunteers and normally accompanied by variations in median nerve branching (high division or bifid median nerve) (Gassner et al. 2002) (Fig. 4.22a,b). In a small series of patients with clinical evidence of CTS, this anomaly was detected sonographically and postoperative patient outcome after carpal tunnel release was excellent (Gassner et al. 2002). In one of those cases we found a hypertrophic PMA with a diameter of 3 mm, with associated findings of a hypoplastic radial artery (Fig. 4.23). Dynamic sonographic imaging in a transverse and longitudinal plane during repetitive flexion and extension of the wrist and fingers enables assessment of transverse nerve gliding which has been reported to be reduced in patients with CTS. Dynamic sonography can also identify fluid collections within the tendon sheets and accessory muscle bellies; these muscles can originate from the flexor digitorum muscle or they exist as true accessory muscle (Fig. 4.24a–d).

In summary, the sonographic diagnosis of CTS may be achieved based on the following signs (in order of reliability):

- Enlargement of the median nerve at the proximal carpal tunnel with an increased cross-sectional area over 12 mm^2.
- Changes in median nerve echotexture consistent with edema, i.e. loss of fascicular discrimination with more or less homogeneous hypoechoic appearance, and indistinct outer margins.
- Abrupt caliber change (notch sign) at the proximal margin of the flexor retinaculum.
- Detection of a large PMA or increased intraneural and perineural vascularity.
- Dynamic scanning for detection of additional fluid or accessory muscle bellies

Depending on the diagnostic possibilities available at a given institution the work-up of a patient with CTS may vary. Conventionally, after obtaining a patient's history and physical examination, an electrodiagnostic study is ordered for evaluation of the median nerve. However, as stated above, we propose a different algorithm, which favors the performance of a sonographic examination early in the work-up (Fig. 4.25) (Ziswiler et al. 2005; Altinok et al. 2004; Wong et al. 2004; Visser et al. 2008).

Sonography is able to reliably diagnose idiopathic CTS in a high percentage of patients and rule out secondary CTS due to abnormalities inside the carpal tunnel such as flexor tendon synovitis, tumors or ganglia. If no abnormalities are found within the carpal tunnel, sonographic nerve inspection should be extended proximally upwards to the brachial plexus to exclude other rare and unusual abnormalities (Fig. 4.26a,b).

According to this algorithm two distinct scenarios may result after taking a patient's history and carrying out a neurological examination: (1) clear signs and symptoms of CTS, and (2) indistinct findings. In the first scenario sonography should be performed to rule out secondary CTS and to define the severity of the disease. Either conservative management or surgery may be instituted based on the sonographic findings. In the case of surgery for idiopathic CTS an electrodiagnostic study should be performed as this

Fig. 4.22. a Transverse sonogram using a 15-MHz transducer in a healthy volunteer with a bifid median nerve and a persistent median artery. Sonographic image shows two distinct fascicular groups (*dotted lines*) divided by a persistent median artery (*large arrow*), accompanied by two veins (*small arrows*). **b** Corresponding schematic drawing reveals a persistent median artery with two veins and with two distinct fascicle nerve groups surrounded by the nerve sheet

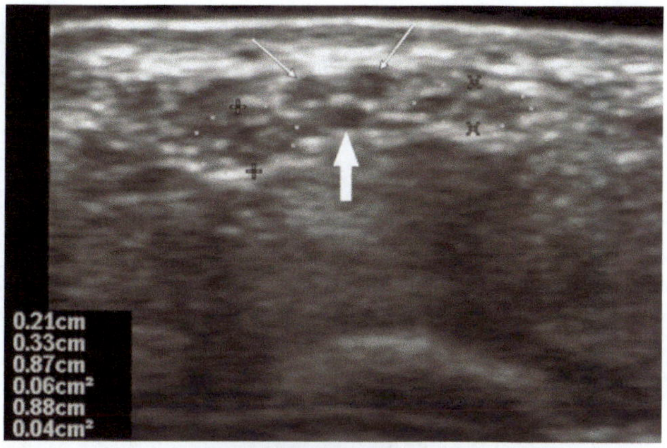

a

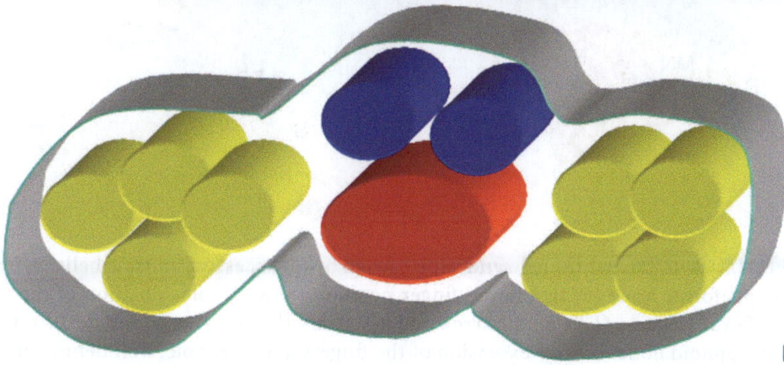

b

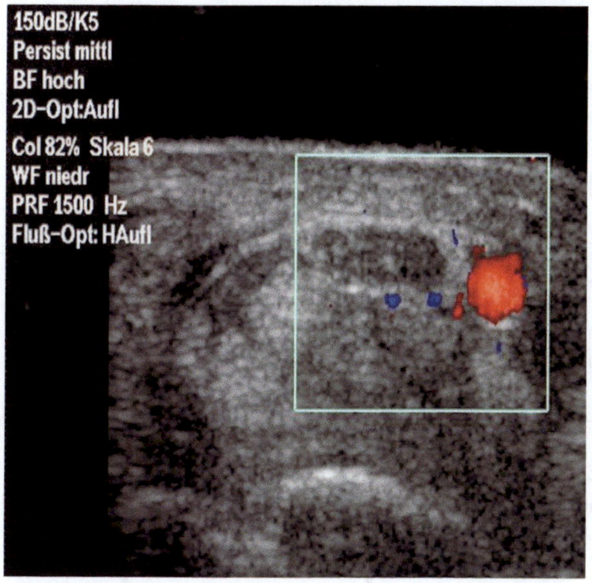

Fig. 4.23. Carpal tunnel syndrome caused by a hypertrophic persistent median artery. Transverse 15-MHz sonography with color Doppler demonstrates a hypertrophic persistent median artery adjacent to the median nerve; the nerve shows loss of fascicular discrimination. Careful surgical flexor retinaculum release was successful

may be the best way to check for functional recovery during follow-up examinations, besides clinical improvement. In the second scenario again sonography may be the first diagnostic study to be carried out. In patients with a normal sonogram or inconclusive sonographic findings an electrodiagnostic study should be performed to exclude an intrinsic pathology of the median nerve.

4.5.3.5
Therapy

The mainstays of treatment are the avoidance of wrist overuse, withdrawal of provoking factors, placement of neutral wrist splints during sleep, local corticosteroid injections adjacent to the carpal tunnel (Green 1984) and – if nonsurgical interventions fail or neurological deficits emerge – surgical sectioning of the volar carpal ligament. Pain and paresthesias bring most patients to medical attention before irreversible axonal loss has developed. Accordingly, overall prognosis of CTS is good to excellent in up to 80%–90% of patients given adequate management.

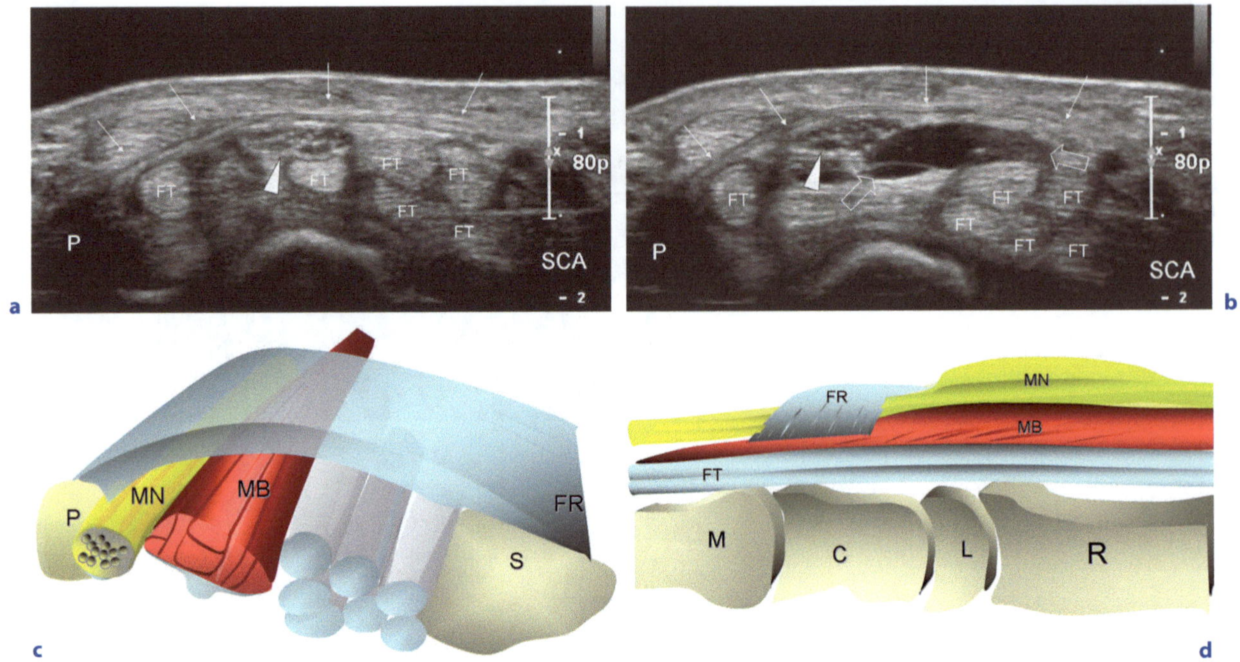

Fig. 4.24a–d. Carpal tunnel syndrome caused by an accessory muscle belly. **a** Transverse 17-MHz sonogram at the level of the pisiforme bone (*P*) in a flexed finger position shows a volar position of the median nerve (*arrowhead*) surrounded by the flexor tendons (*FT*). *Small arrows* demonstrate the crossing of the flexor retinaculum (*FR*) from the pisiforme bone to the scaphoid bone. **b** After extension of the fingers a hypoechoic, well defined muscle belly (*large arrows*) appears adjacent to the median nerve displacing the nerve to the volar side while part of the flexor tendons are displaced radially. **c** Corresponding schematic drawing of the carpal tunnel in a transverse plane shows the muscle belly (*MB*) entering the carpal tunnel beneath the flexor retinaculum and displacing the median nerve (*MN*) sideways. **d** Schematic drawing of the carpal tunnel in a longitudinal plane demonstrates the extension of the accessory muscle belly beneath the flexor retinaculum displacing the median nerve volarly

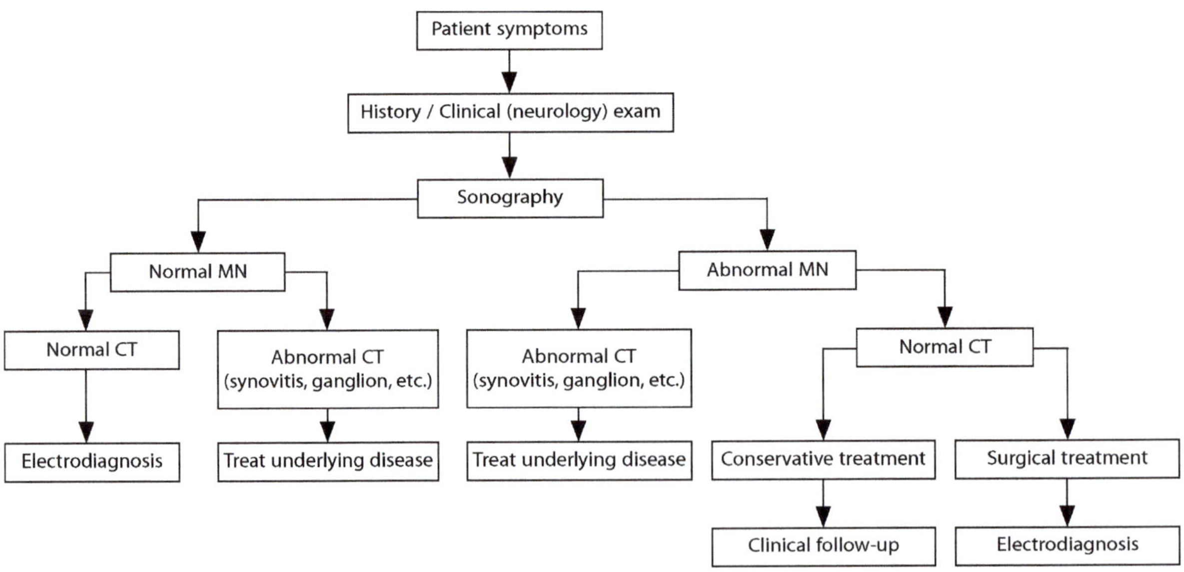

Fig. 4.25. Algorithm for diagnostic work-up of patients with suspected CTS

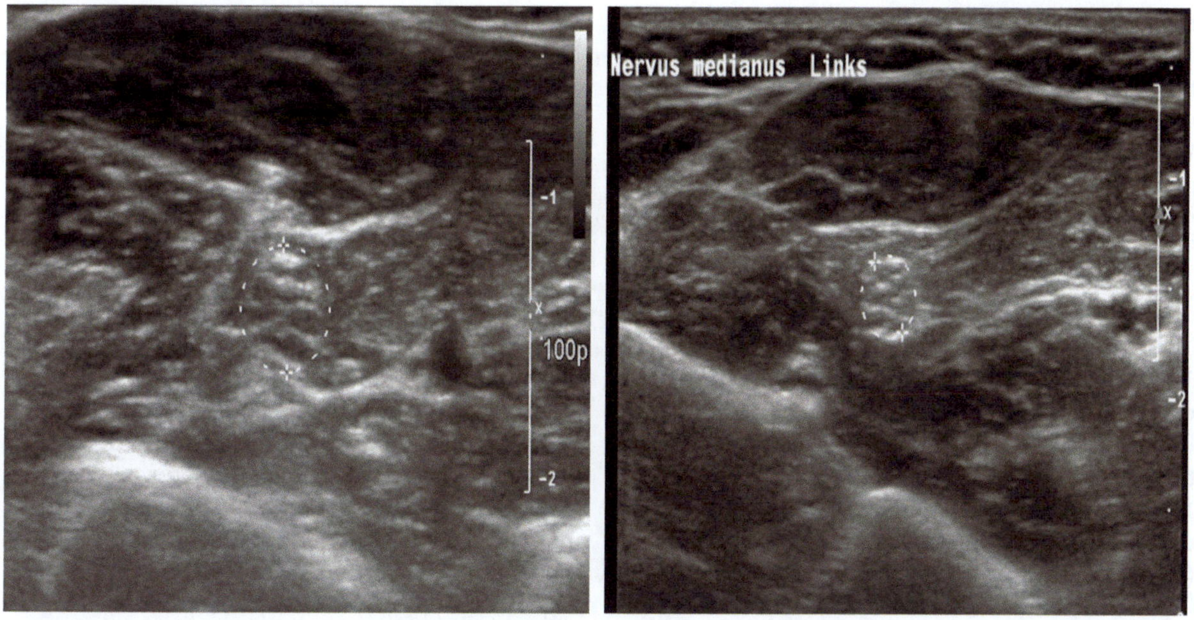

Fig. 4.26a,b. Median neuropathy with negative sonographic findings in the carpal tunnel. The patient had flu-like symptoms with fever and myalgia. After 2 weeks she developed severe pain and paresthesia in her right lower forearm and hand. **a** Transverse 17-MHz sonographic image at the proximal forearm showing enlarged median nerve (*dotted line*) with a cross-sectional diameter of 0.16 cm^2 and thickened fascicles. **b** The contralateral unaffected side shows a cross-sectional diameter of 0.11 cm^2. The affected nerve also showed increased Doppler signals (not shown). The patient showed a slow recovery after 6 months

4.6 Ulnar Nerve Compression

Ulnar nerve entrapment occurs at two distinct sites: at the elbow where the nerves courses around the medial humeral epicondyle (within or associated with the so-called cubital tunnel) and at the wrist (in Guyon's canal). Other rather rare compression areas are the arcade of Struthers and where the nerve pierces the aponeurotic fascia of the pronator teres. The cubital tunnel is the most frequent site of ulnar nerve compression and, in relation to entrapment neuropathies of other nerves, second in frequency only to median nerve compression in the carpal tunnel. In contrast to this ulnar nerve entrapment in Guyon's canal is rare.

4.6.1 Cubital Tunnel Syndrome

The ulnar nerve arises from the medial cord of the brachial plexus containing elements from C8 and T1. At the upper arm the nerve runs distally adjacent to the brachial artery and vein. At the upper third of the arm, the ulnar nerve pierces the medial intermuscular septum entering the posterior compartment of the arm lying anteriorly to the medial head of the triceps. The medial intermuscular septum extends from the coracobrachialis muscle to the medial humeral epicondyle. The nerve then reaches the arcade of Struthers, which is a potential area of rare nerve compression. The arcade of Struthers is formed by the attachments of the internal brachial ligament, the fascia and superficial muscular fibers of the medial head of the triceps, and the medial intermuscular septum. The arcade is found approximately 6–8 cm above the medial epicondyle; it should not be confused with the ligament of Struthers which also can cause median nerve entrapment.

Cubital tunnel syndrome was first described by Feindel and Stratford (1958). The cubital tunnel is an osteofibrous tunnel at the medial side of the elbow. Its roof is formed by a fibrous band called the cubital tunnel retinaculum (also called the Osborne fascia), which traverses from the medial epicondyle to the tip of the olecranon. In this region the ulnar nerve, in its course from the medial aspect of the upper arm to the palmar aspect of the forearm, bends around the medial epicondyle in direct contact with the bone (condylar groove). When entering the cubital tunnel, the ulnar nerve gives off a branch to the elbow joint (Fig. 4.27). The nerve then runs between the ulnar and humeral head of the flexor carpi ulnaris muscle. The two muscle bellies are connected by an extension of the cubital tunnel retinaculum, the so-called arcuate ligament (true cubital tunnel) (Mazurek and Shin 2001). A certain amount of motion with stretching of the nerve and decrease of ulnar tunnel diameter is an anatomical feature of this site, which occurs in the normal, asymptomatic individual (Bozentka 1998). Certain additional conditions lead to decompensation with development of neuropathy (Bozentka 1998).

After exiting the cubital tunnel the ulnar nerve pierces the flexor pronator aponeurosis, the fibrous common origin of the flexor and pronator muscles. This flexor-pronator aponeurosis is another area of possible compression of the ulnar nerve.

The blood supply for the ulnar nerve is fed by three arteries, the superior and inferior collateral artery and the posterior ulnar recurrent artery. The inferior ulnar collateral artery supplies the nerve at the area of the medial epicondyle. Because of a lack of anastomosis between the vessels, anterior transposition imposes the risk of poor blood supply to the nerve.

4.6.1.1
Epidemiology and Clinical Presentation

Ulnar nerve compression at the elbow is the second most common mononeuropathy of the upper extremities, affecting more men then women (6:1).

As the initial clinical feature patients typically note numbness in the 5th and medial half of the 4th fingers, sometimes spreading to the medial hand (Fig. 4.27). Typically sensory disturbances do not extend much beyond the wrist. Pain and tenderness occur at the medial epicondyle and radiate along the ulnar forearm to the hand. Complaints may be provoked or enhanced by trigger situations such

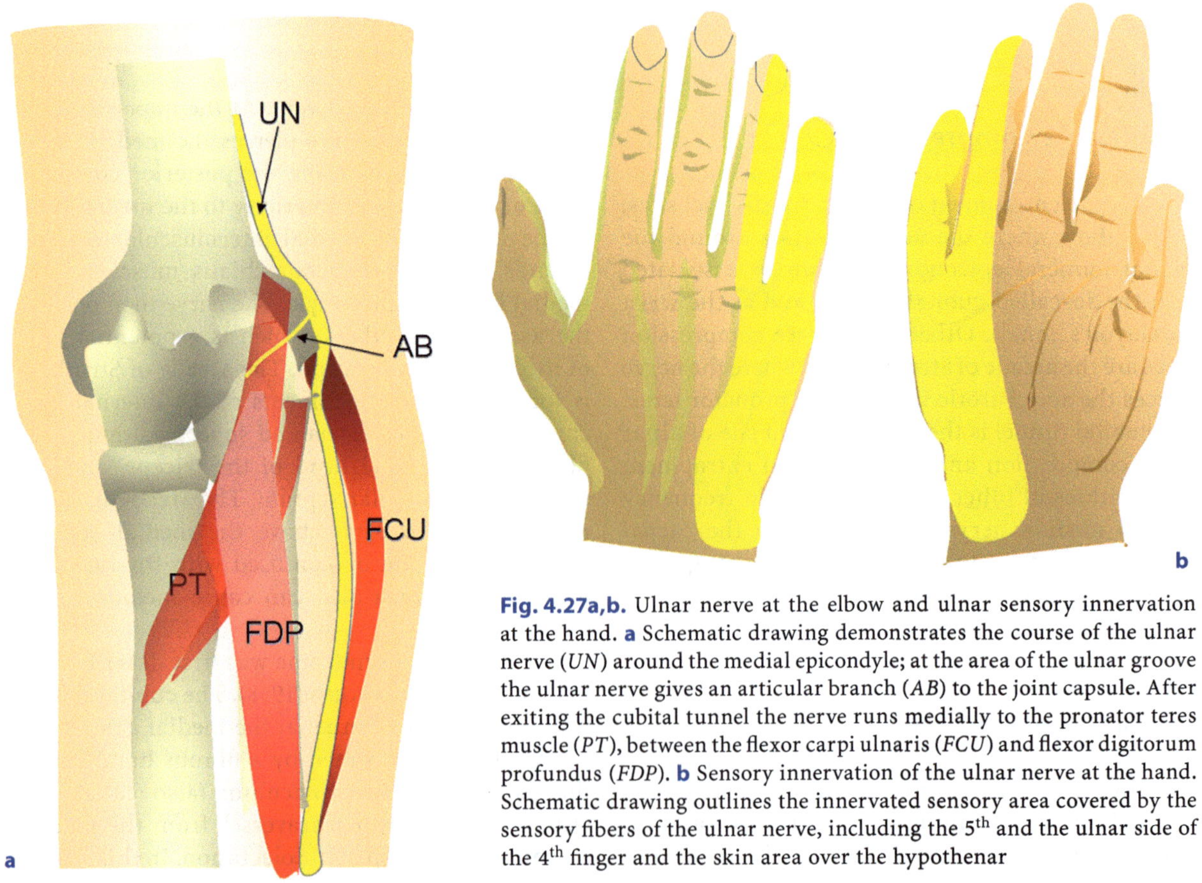

Fig. 4.27a,b. Ulnar nerve at the elbow and ulnar sensory innervation at the hand. **a** Schematic drawing demonstrates the course of the ulnar nerve (*UN*) around the medial epicondyle; at the area of the ulnar groove the ulnar nerve gives an articular branch (*AB*) to the joint capsule. After exiting the cubital tunnel the nerve runs medially to the pronator teres muscle (*PT*), between the flexor carpi ulnaris (*FCU*) and flexor digitorum profundus (*FDP*). **b** Sensory innervation of the ulnar nerve at the hand. Schematic drawing outlines the innervated sensory area covered by the sensory fibers of the ulnar nerve, including the 5th and the ulnar side of the 4th finger and the skin area over the hypothenar

as resting of the elbow on a hard surface, applying external pressure to the groove, maximal flexion of the elbow or repetitive flexion and extension movements.

In the common case of progressive nerve damage weakness of ulnar innervated hand muscles (Fig. 4.28) manifests and causes an abnormal posture of the hand ("ulnar clawing") and significant disability in the performance and fine control of finger movements. Abduction of the little finger due to paresis of the 4th interosseus muscle is recognized as the Wartenberg's sign (MUMENTHALER et al. 1998). Forearm flexors (flexor carpi ulnaris and digitorum profundus muscles) are less prominently involved or exceptionally even spared. Muscle wasting is best seen at the first interosseus space and hypothenar eminence. In some patients motor deficits develop insidiously without sensory symptoms.

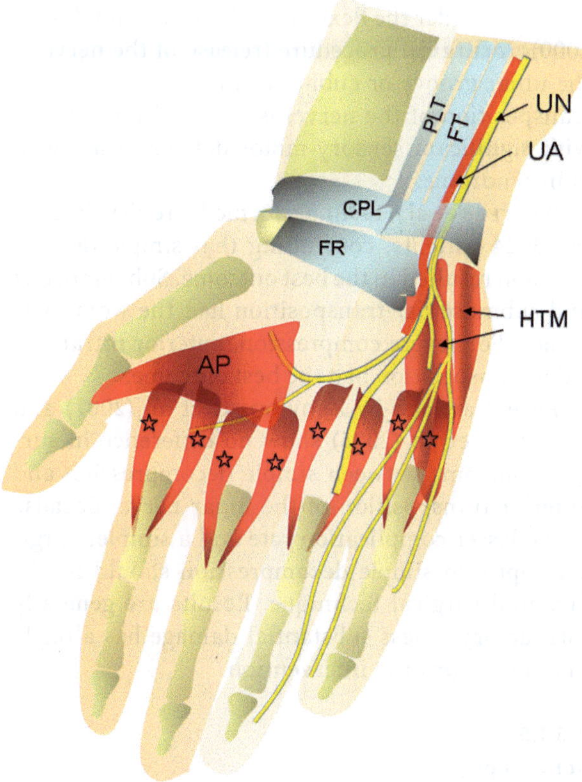

Fig. 4.28. Motoric innervation by the ulnar nerve within the hand. The course of the ulnar nerve (*UN*) running through the Guyon tunnel, adjacent to the ulnar artery, is shown. The roof of the Guyon tunnel is covered by the carpal palmar ligament. The ulnar nerve then gives branches to the hypothenar muscles, the adductor pollicis muscle (*AP*), the interosseus muscles (*asterisks*) and the lumbrical muscle (not shown)

4.6.1.2 Etiology

On passing through the ulnar groove at the elbow the nerve is susceptible to compression injury (MILLER 1991). The precise mechanisms of nerve damage and the nature of the compressive pathology are highly heterogeneous: (1) External compression is the most common cause and derives from repeated or sustained leaning on the elbow. It may cause substantial (cumulative) nerve injury, particularly in the case of a predisposing shallow condylar groove, subluxated nerve or sustained pressure in coma or anaesthetised patients (MILLER and CAMP 1979). (2) Real entrapment occurs in the ulnar sulcus if the nerve is constricted by scare tissue, in the cubital tunnel ("cubital tunnel syndrome") (MILLER and HUMMEL 1980) where the ulnar nerve passes under the aponeurotic origin of the flexor carpi ulnaris muscle (1–3 cm distal to the epicondylus) or in the flexor pronator aponeurosis (more than 4 cm distal to the epicondylus). (3) Tardy ulnar nerve palsy typically develops years after fracture or luxation of the elbow based on bone exostosis, cubitus varus or valgus abnormalities. Other causative bone abnormalities are advanced arthrosis, osteoarthritis or hyperostosis in Paget's disease, to name just a few. (4) Recurrent prominent luxation of the ulnar nerve over the medial condyle can directly damage the nerve or predispose it to repetitive trauma. (5) Soft tissue masses in the condylar groove or cubital tunnel such as organized haematoma, scarring, accessory muscles (anconeus epitrochlearis) or intraneural ganglia are further potential sources of ulnar nerve compression (O'DRISCOLL et al. 1992; PUIG et al. 1999). CONTRERAS et al. (1998) found that women have a greater amount of fat at the medial aspect of the elbow, protecting the nerve from acute trauma; furthermore, he found that the coronoid process in men is much larger then in women, also increasing the risk for ulnar nerve compression.

4.6.1.3 Diagnosis

The diagnosis of ulnar neuropathy is – in most cases – reliably established by an experienced clinician after reviewing the patient's history (with emphasis on trigger situations) and performing a thorough neurological examination. A sensitive and highly characteristic clinical test is the Froment's maneuver (Fig. 4.29). When attempting to pinch a piece

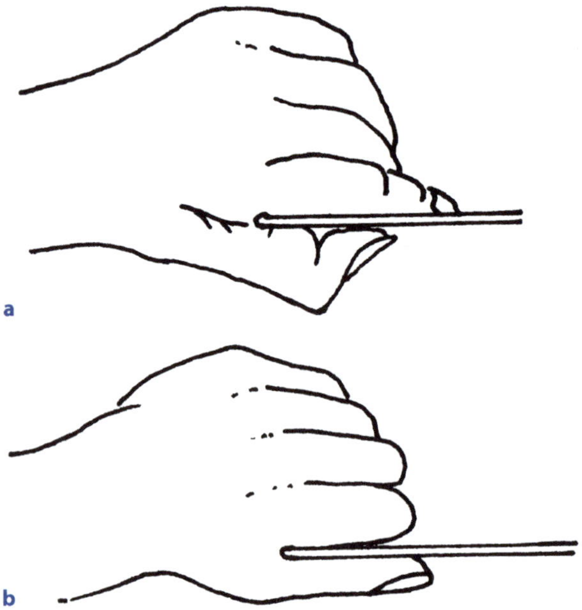

Fig. 4.29a,b. Froment's maneuver. **a** In the case of ulnar nerve palsy a typical flexed thumb posture emerges when the patient attempts to pinch a piece of paper between the thumb and index finger. **b** Maneuver in a normal subject

of paper between the thumb and index finger, the patient primarily utilises the median innervated long flexor of the thumb as compensation for the ulnar hand weakness, and a typical flexed-thumb posture emerges.

Other diagnoses mimicking ulnar neuropathy, such as lower trunk or medial cord brachial plexus palsy, combined C8 and Th1 radiculopathy or distal ulnar nerve entrapment, can be differentiated based on the pattern of sensory and motor deficits. Diagnostic work-up of patients with ulnar compression at or adjacent to the elbow should include a palpation examination of the ulnar nerve at the ulnar groove for an abnormal thickening, tenderness, decreased mobility or luxability. Further on, provocation tests (maximal elbow flexion for the cubital tunnel syndrome and assessment of the Tinel's sign), X-ray of the elbow and sonography or magnetic resonance imaging of the nerve and neighbouring tissues should be performed.

Electrodiagnostic studies play a central role in evaluating suspected ulnar nerve lesions. Standard nerve conduction studies performed in a flexed elbow position are sometimes sufficient for demonstrating segmental slowing of sensory and motor fibres (focal demyelination) across the elbow difference compared to forearm nerve conduction.

4.6.1.4 Therapy

Careful exploration for relevant trigger events and behaviour causing external nerve compression are crucial to successful therapy. In such cases strict avoidance strategies are often sufficient for a reversal of symptoms and prevention of progressive nerve damage (Dellon et al. 1993).

Conservative treatment includes avoiding occupationally-induced micro trauma, using cushions or pads and strengthening of the extensor and flexor muscles.

Steroid injection and oral anti-inflammatory drugs are usually not useful.

Surgical treatment of cubital tunnel syndrome either consists of complete decompression of the nerve (releasing the nerve from compressive adhesions and bands), decompression with epicondylectomy or of decompression with transposition of the nerve under the flexor muscle (Arle and Zager 2000). A surgical procedure (release of the nerve at the ulnar groove or cubital tunnel or submuscular transposition of the nerve) is reserved for patients with significant sensory-motor deficits or a severe pain syndrome.

Bartels et al. (1998) performed a review including 3024 patients, concluding that simple decompression resulted in the best outcome. Subcutaneous and submuscular transposition had the worst outcomes. For severe compression, anterior intramuscular transposition had the best outcome.

Recent articles by Zlowodzki et al. (2007) and Gervasio et al. (2005) show no difference in surgical outcome between simple decompression and anterior transposition of the ulnar nerve. Because of the lesser complication rate and a simpler surgical approach simple decompression should be the favoured surgical technique. Results are generally satisfactory unless substantial damage has already manifested prior to intervention.

4.6.1.5 Sonography

From a technical point of view sonography of the cubital tunnel is best performed with a high resolution linear scan head of 12–17 MHz. A standoff pad may also be used to improve image quality; this allows better contact to the angulated course of the elbow. There is standard documentation of findings in transverse and longitudinal planes at the medial aspect of the upper arm, medial epicondyle and at the forearm just distal to the cubital tunnel.

The best sonographic access to the ulnar nerve is gained with the patient lying supine on the examination table, with the arm to be examined close to the sonographer. We normally use an additional small pillow to position the fully stretched arm in about 45 degrees of abduction with forced supination (Fig. 4.30).

This maneuver results in a stable position, which is easily held by the patient for longer times and permits access to the ulnar nerve along its complete course at the upper arm and forearm. Forced supination and external rotation of the outstretched arm positions the nerve in an almost straight course from above the elbow to the proximal forearm, which facilitates the acquisition of longitudinal sonograms inside the cubital tunnel. The latter is of considerable importance if panoramic images are taken, as the sweep of the scan head along the nerve is much more easily accomplished with the nerve in an elongated position (Fig. 4.31).

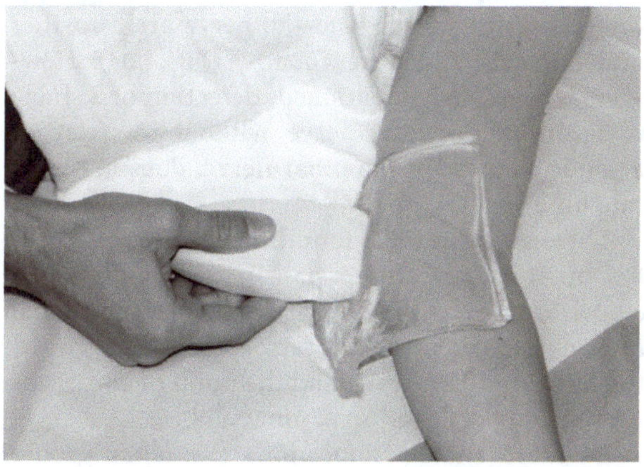

Fig. 4.30. Position of transducer for identification of the ulnar nerve at the level of the upper arm. With positioning of the transducer posterior to the medial epicondyle, the superficially coursing nerve is easily identified

Tension on the nerve is minimal in this position, as the outstretched arm limits tractional forces (Bozentka 1998), which is why we recommend this position for the measurement of nerve diameters. With elbow flexion the nerve gets flattened even in healthy individuals, which must not be mistaken for compression (Okamoto et al. 2001). After documentation of the nerve's shape and echotexture in this basic position, functional sonograms are acquired with passive flexion and/or rotation of the elbow. With these maneuvers we aim to detect reduced longitudinal nerve motion or subluxation, as well as changing nerve diameter in certain positions of the elbow.

We usually start the examination by identifying the ulnar nerve in a transverse plane at the inner side of the upper arm, where it courses in a superficial position alongside the dorsal margin of the biceps muscle. From here we follow the nerve down to the ulnar groove and onward to the proximal forearm. During this first sweep we record any changes in nerve diameter, with standard measurements acquired about 3 cm above and below, as well as inside the cubital tunnel. While the nerve has a more oval shape at the level of the upper arm and forearm it typically appears to be round inside the cubital tunnel. In a study by Chiou et al. (1998) on ten healthy volunteers short and long axis diameters of the ulnar nerve, as well as cross section areas, were measured at the level of the epicondyle and 5 cm above and below the elbow. Measurements in volunteers were as follow: mean values of the short axis (cm) x long axis (cm) at the arm, epicondyle, and forearm levels were 0.057+/−0.01, 0.068+/−0.019 and 0.062+/−0.01 Their measurements show an increase in cross-sectional area at the level of the epicondyle, where the nerve has a more rounded shape. Similar

Fig. 4.31. Longitudinal panoramic sonogram in a patient with cubital tunnel syndrome. The ulnar nerve (*arrowheads*) shows mildly edematous, hypoechoic fascicles along its course inside the sulcus, with a smooth transition to a more normal appearing echotexture at the level of the upper arm (at the right hand margin of image)

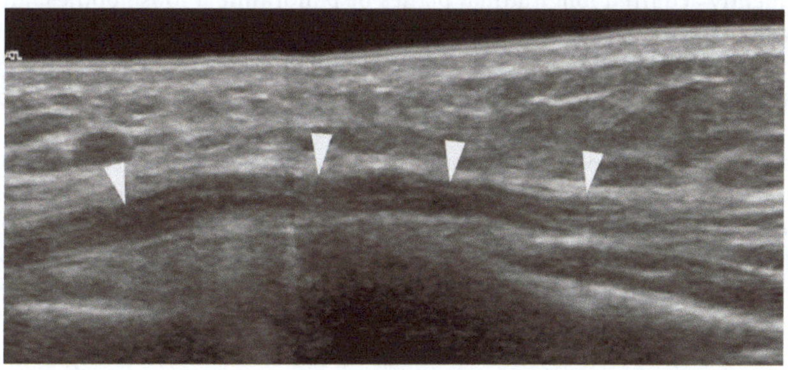

measurements in healthy volunteers were reported by Cartwright et al. (2007); he further described that women have a slightly smaller nerve size then men. Jacob et al. (2004) found that the ulnar nerve has a mean cross-sectional area at the elbow of 7.9+/–3.1 mm^2; he also found lower values in women compared to men, especially in the age group between 40 and 60. In addition he found an ulnar nerve division to be a normal variant

The sonographer has to be aware of this typical increase in ulnar nerve size inside the cubital tunnel and avoid mistaking it for cubital tunnel disease. On the contrary, we believe this fact to represent a reaction of the nerve to a normal amount of traction and stretching inside the narrow osteofibrous canal, without any implication of disease. Changes in nerve diameter have traditionally been used for the diagnosis of carpal tunnel disease (Buchberger et al. 1991; Lee et al. 1999; Martinoli et al. 2000), and the same has been advocated for the cubital tunnel. In contrast to healthy asymptomatic subjects, patients with cubital tunnel syndrome show an enlarged ulnar nerve at the level of the epicondyle, while measurements at the upper arm and forearm do not differ significantly (Chiou et al. 1998). Chiou (1998) described that an increase in cross-sectional diameter > 7.5 mm^2 is suggestive for ulnar neuropathy whereas Jacob (2004) reported 7.9 mm^2 to be the threshold for ulnar neuropathy. Increased cross-sectional diameter in ulnar neuropathy has also been reported by Wiesler et al. (2006) and Yoon et al. (2007). Park et al. (2004) measured the length of the swollen ulnar nerve and found that the longitudinal nerve swelling in retrocondylar compression syndrome is significantly longer than in the cubital tunnel syndrome (2.58 cm versus 1.64 cm).

While the sonographic features of the ulnar neuropathy are more easily seen in the transverse plane with diminished fascicular discrimination and indistinct outline of the nerve (Fig. 4.32), subsequently acquired longitudinal planes or panoramic views are better suited for evaluation of abrupt changes in nerve diameter at the level of compression (Fig. 4.33).

Color Doppler and/or power Doppler scans are acquired in nerves with B-mode findings suggestive for neuropathy. Increase of epi- and perineural vessels may be detected representing a hypervascular inflammatory state. The investigator, however, needs to be aware that, due to improvements in software and ultrasound equipment, small vessels are constantly found within and adjacent to normal nerves. Currently no published data are available to support the positive value of color Doppler sonography; however, according to our experience multiple vessels within and around the nerve are a further indication for ulnar neuropathy (Fig. 4.34). However, as previously mentioned, detection of a single vessel inside the ulnar nerve, without any relevant B-mode changes of the ulnar nerve, does not indicate ulnar neuropathy.

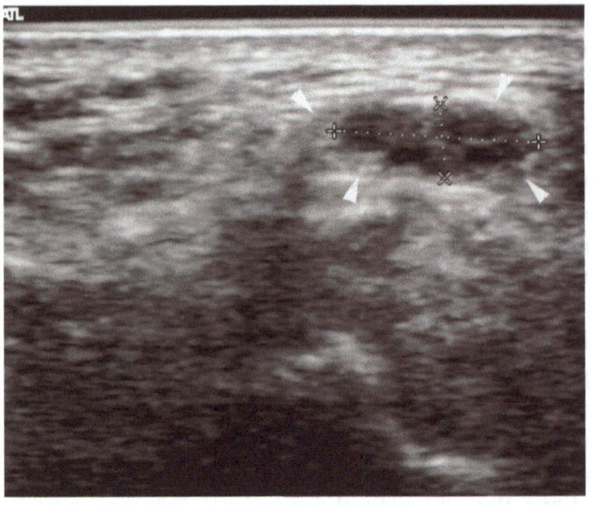

Fig. 4.32. Transverse sonogram

There are essentially four different sites of potential ulnar nerve compression in the region of the elbow. From proximal to distal they are: the medial intermuscular septum, the retroepicondylar groove, the humeroulnar arcade and the point of exit of the nerve from the flexor carpi ulnaris.

Of these anatomic locations the ulnar groove is the site most frequently responsible for entrapment, while compression at the other sites is rare. Pathological conditions such as arthrotic bone spurs in the condylar groove, extrinsic or intrinsic ganglia (Fig. 4.35), heterotopic ossifications or loose bodies, an accessory anconeus epitrochlearis muscle (Fig. 4.36) or a hypertrophic crossing aberrant ulnar artery (Fig. 4.37) may promote development of entrapment neuropathy (O'Driscoll et al. 1992; Puig et al. 1999).

In contrast to the carpal tunnel retinaculum the normal cubital tunnel retinaculum is only infrequently visualized with sonography. In cases of cubital tunnel syndrome, however, a thickened retinaculum may occasionally be detected. In the case of compression the ulnar nerve presents with abrupt narrowing at the site of compression and marked

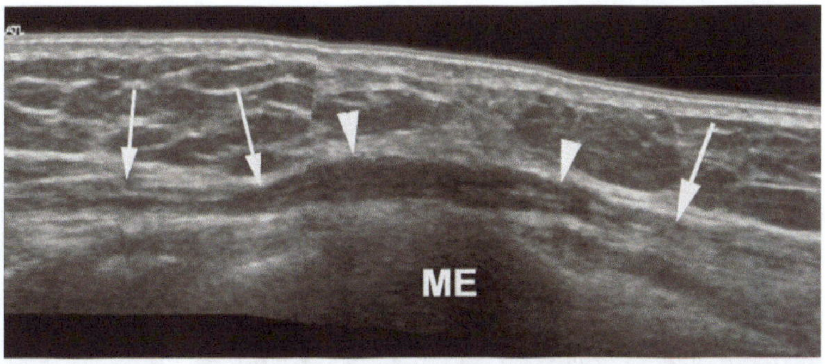

Fig. 4.33. Longitudinal panoramic sonogram through ulnar nerve at the elbow in a patient with cubital tunnel disease. Marked swelling of the nerve on its course through the cubital tunnel is seen (*arrowheads*) with normal caliber and echotexture proximally and distally (*arrows*). *ME*, medial epicondyle

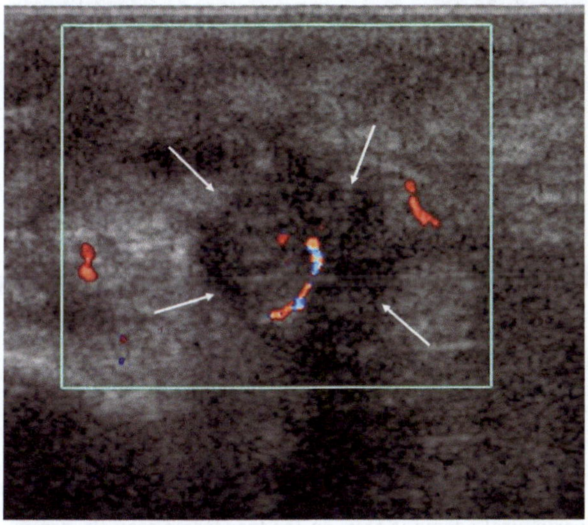

Fig. 4.34. Occupation-related cubital tunnel syndrome. Transverse 15-MHz sonogram of the cubital tunnel in a patient with marked sensory and motoric ulnar neuropathy shows an enlarged ulnar nerve (*arrows*) with poor discrimination of the epineural boarders, lack of fascicular discrimination. Color Doppler sonography demonstrates multiple intra- and perineural Doppler signals. Surgical findings confirmed severe ulnar neuropathy

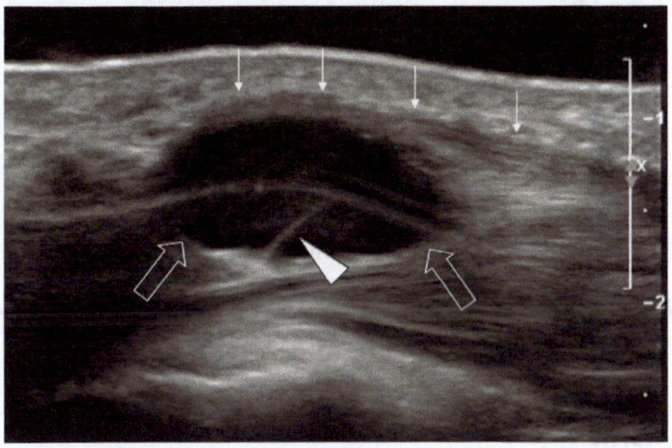

Fig. 4.35. Cubital tunnel syndrome caused by a ganglion. Longitudinal 17-MHz scan along the ulnar nerve demonstrates a well defined anechoic mass (*large arrows*) displacing and thinning out the ulnar nerve (*small arrows*). The septated mass was arising from the joint (not shown)

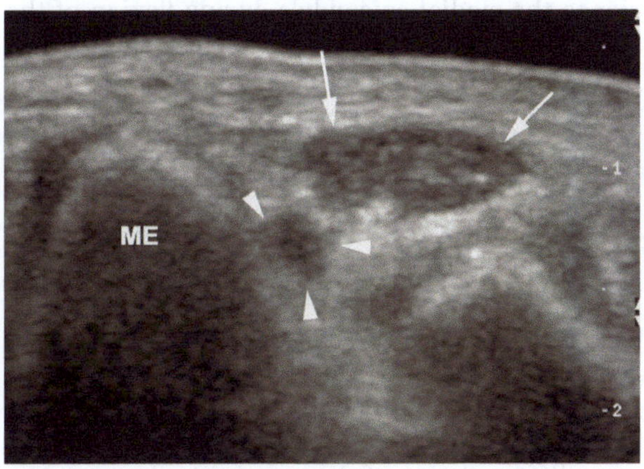

Fig. 4.36. Transverse sonogram at the medial side of the elbow in a patient with a palpable mass and associated evidence of ulnar nerve compression. A large accessory muscle belly (*arrows*) overlying the ulnar nerve is demonstrated consistent with anconeus epitrochlearis muscle. Note loss of fascicular discrimination in the ulnar nerve with epineural edema (*arrowheads*). *ME*, medial epicondyle

swelling with loss of fascicular texture proximal to this level (Fig. 4.38a). Marked edema in the epineurium and surrounding soft tissues are characteristic findings (Fig. 4.38b).

In summary the typical features of cubital tunnel syndrome are:

- Abrupt narrowing of the ulnar nerve at the site of compression
- Swelling of the nerve above the level of compression
- Loss of fascicular texture
- Indistinct outer surface of the nerve
- Edema in surrounding soft tissue

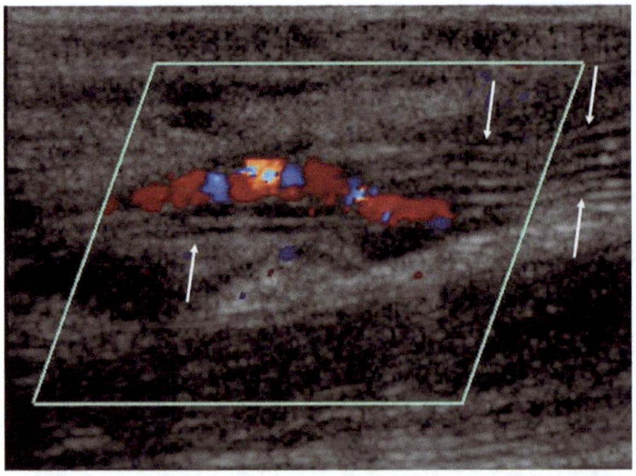

Fig. 4.37. Cubital tunnel syndrome caused by a hypertrophic aberrant ulnar artery. Longitudinal 15-MHz sonogram demonstrates an enlarged aberrant ulnar artery crossing over the ulnar artery at the cubital tunnel. The ulnar nerve did not show any caliber changes (*arrows*) but electroneurographic testing was highly positive for ulnar neuropathy. Surgical inspection confirmed the aberrant ulnar artery and release of he ulnar ligament improved clinical signs

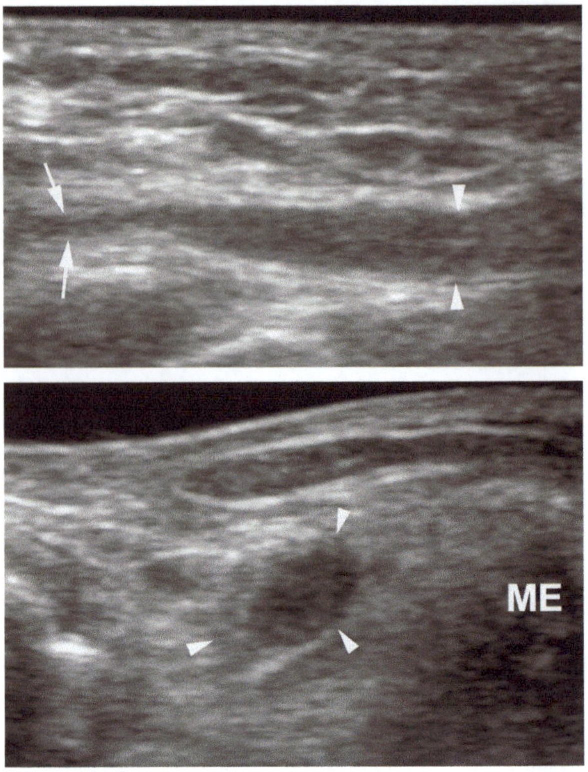

a

b

Fig. 4.38a,b. Longitudinal (**a**) and transverse (**b**) sonograms in a patient with cubital tunnel disease. Marked swelling of the ulnar nerve above the level of compression (**a**, *arrowheads*) with return to normal size distal to the medial epicondyle (**a**, *arrows*). Loss of fascicular discrimination and perineural edema is seen on the transverse scan (**b**, *arrowheads*). *ME*, medial epicondyle

4.6.1.6
Snapping Ulnar Nerve

A special condition, which may be present in asymptomatic individuals but also account for ulnar neuropathy at the elbow is ulnar nerve dislocation. The latter represents an abnormal movement of the ulnar nerve out of the cubital tunnel and anterior to the medial epicondyle during flexion of the elbow (Childress 1975), which is caused by absence of the cubital tunnel retinaculum. Neuropathy is induced by abnormal friction and tear to the nerve during recurrent dislocation. Ulnar nerve dislocation shares a common clinical feature – a transient snapping sensation during flexion of the elbow – with snapping triceps syndrome, which represents medial dislocation of the medial head of the triceps muscle. Both syndromes may exist side by side or in isolation. Because of the overlap in clinical findings they are not easily distinguished during physical examination (Spinner and Goldner 1998). However, differentiation of the two entities is necessary since the approach for surgical treatment will differ. Dynamic sonography is helpful in this regard, as it permits direct visualization of ulnar nerve and/or triceps muscle dislocation during active flexion and extension of the elbow (Jacobson et al. 2001; Okamoto et al. 2000). However, the diagnosis of ulnar nerve dislocation may be missed if excessive transducer pressure is applied, which can prevent the nerve from dislocating. Sonography typically shows abnormal movement of the nerve and/or muscle at the level of the medial epicondyle (Fig. 4.39).

In addition, the characteristic snap may be felt with the transducer. In symptomatic individuals enlarged cross section of the nerve and edema are signs of neuropathy, just as in the traditional cubital tunnel syndrome (Jacobson et al. 2001).

4.6.2
Guyon's Canal

Proximal to the wrist the ulnar nerve runs superficial to the flexor retinaculum and lies under the tendon of the flexor carpi ulnaris. The nerve turns radially to the pisiform bone entering a fibrous

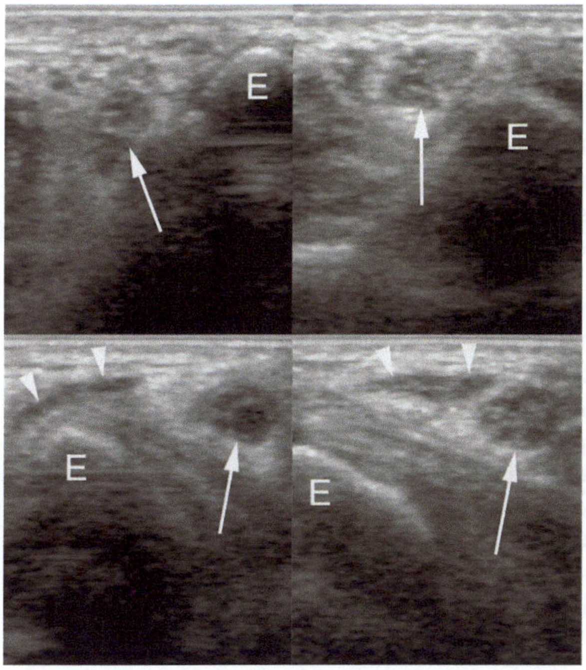

Fig. 4.39. Series of transverse sonograms acquired during flexion of the elbow (*left* to *right* extension to maximum flexion). The ulnar nerve (*arrow*) dislocates ventrally to the epicondyle during elbow flexion and is followed by the medial head of the triceps muscle (*arrowheads*) later in the movement. *E*, epicondyle

tunnel called Guyon's canal. The roof of this canal consists of the palmar carpal ligament and the palmaris brevis muscle; the floor is formed mostly by the flexor retinaculum with contributions of the flexor digitorum profundus, the piso-hamate and piso-metacarpal ligaments and the opponens digiti minimi. It is bordered by the pisiform the hook of the hamate (Mazurek and Shin 2001). On its course through the canal the ulnar nerve is accompanied by the ulnar artery and vein. In the distal portion of the tunnel the nerve bifurcates into a deep motor branch and superficial sensory branch (Fig. 4.28). Compared with cubital tunnel syndrome, entrapment of the ulnar nerve inside Guyon's canal is rare.

4.6.2.1
Clinical Considerations

The ulnar nerve may be compressed anywhere along its course through Guyon's canal resulting in sensory, motor or sensorimotor symptoms. According to the level of compression three distinct neurological syndromes are discerned. More proximal compression at the entrance of the nerve into the canal results in weakness of intrinsic hand muscles innervated by the ulnar nerve (all interossei, lumbricalis II and IV, hypothenar muscles), plus a sensory deficit in the hypothenar and ulnar half of the ring finger, both on the palmar surface only. Compression along the deep branch results only in motor deficits, whereas compression in the distal canal results in sensory deficits only.

There is a variety of reasons for ulnar neuropathy at the level of Guyon's canal: reduction of the canal's diameter by space-occupying lesions such as ganglia (Shea and McClain 1969), lipoma (Bui-Mansfield et al. 2002), or pseudoaneurysms (Lorea and Schuind 2000); posttraumatic nerve irritation, for example by the hook of the hamate fractures or Galeazzi fracture-dislocation (Pecina et al. 2001); occupationally related external compression, vascular disturbances and hypertrophy of the flexor carpi ulnaris muscle or anomalous abductor digiti minimi muscle (Harvie et al. 2003) are further reasons, among others.

A trial of conservative treatment is usually instituted in patients with neuropathy, which will take up to 6 months to work. If no improvement is achieved within this time the lesion should be treated surgically with decompression of the nerve.

4.6.2.2
Sonography

With the patient sitting the hand is positioned on a pillow with the palm facing up; a standoff pad is always used. After identification of the nerve at the distal forearm in a transverse plane, it is followed to the canal, where it is easily visualized and consists of a tiny ovoid structure with a hyperechoic epineurium and only two or three small fascicles. With high-resolution equipment the bifurcation of the nerve and its branches can be visualized and followed to its distal branches. While the sensory branch tends to follow the ulnar artery, the motor branch runs more deeply. As already mentioned above, ulnar neuropathy at Guyon's canal is rare and in many cases due to additional pathologies, such as tiny ulnar artery aneurysms, ganglia related to the pisotriquetral joint or malaligned fractures. These space-occupying lesions are easily assessed with sonography. In all of these situations the nerve additionally shows the findings characteristic of peripheral nerve compression mentioned above: swelling, edema, etc. (Fig. 4.40).

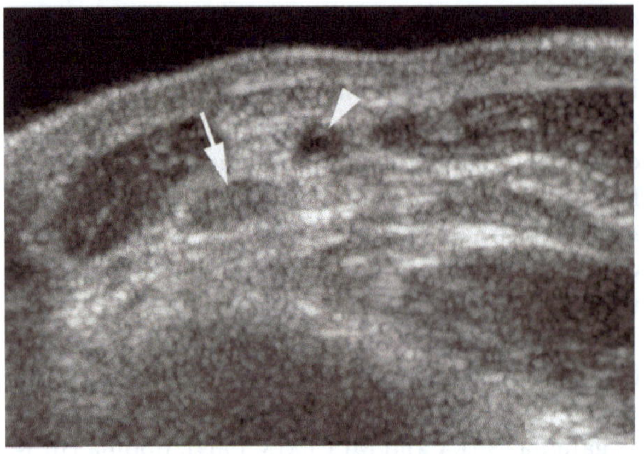

Fig. 4.40. Transverse sonogram in a patient with numbness and paresthesias in the fifth finger. Swelling of the ulnar nerve (*arrow*) with loss of fascicular discrimination is shown on its course through Guyon's canal (*arrowhead*, ulnar artery)

4.7 Iliohypogastric Syndrome

Iliohypogastric syndrome is a rare syndrome presenting with weakness of the abdominal muscle and sensory disturbance at the gluteal and/or inguinal area.

The iliohypogastric nerve arises from the ventral fascicles of L1 and sometimes receives fibers from L2. The nerve runs across the psoas muscle, then along the posterior side of the abdominal wall and motoric branches (Fig. 4.41a). One sensory branch pierces and innervates the oblique muscles, one branch innervates the skin over the gluteal area and one branch innervates the skin in the area of the symphysis and groin (Fig. 4.41b).

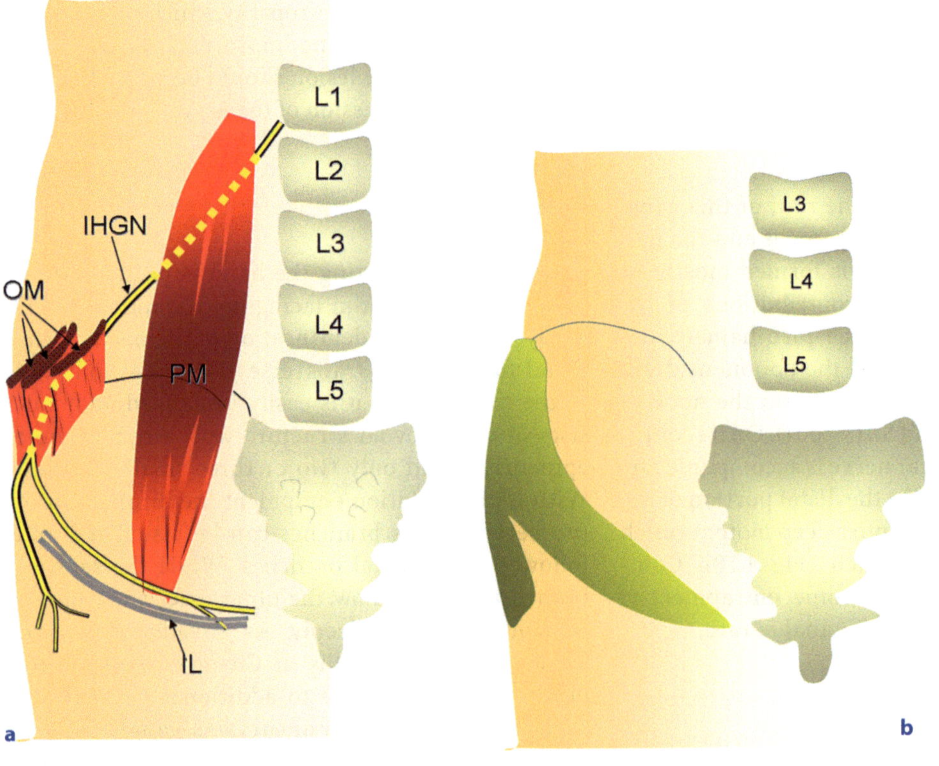

Fig. 4.41a,b. Iliohypogastric nerve. **a** The course of the iliohypogastric nerve (*IHGN*) running beneath the psoas muscle (*PM*) is shown. After piercing the aponeurotic fascia of the oblique muscle (*OM*) the nerve runs between the oblique muscles to reach the iliac crest area. The nerve gives a branch to the skin overlying the gluteal area and the area over the tensor fascia latae. One branch runs along the inguinal canal towards the symphysis. *L1–5*, lumbar vertebrae. **b** The sensory area covered by the sensory filaments of the iliohypogastric nerve is outlined

4.7.1
Etiology

Particularly at the iliac crest, where the nerve runs very superficially, the iliohypogastric nerve is prone to trauma which can cause nerve injury. Reports in the literature show that the nerve is at risk from a variety of surgical procedures such as hernia repair, bone grafting and even appendectomy (STULZ and PFEIFFER 1982; STARK et al. 1999; GROSZ 1981). Sports-related injuries such as direct trauma or muscle tears of the lower abdominal muscles may also cause traction or contusional injury to the nerve. This syndrome may also be seen in pregnancy, especially when the abdomen is rapidly expanding during the final months (CARTER and RACZ 1994).

4.7.2
Clinical Signs

Clinical signs depend on the area of compression. If motoric and sensory deficiency is present then the compression is localized more proximally. Clinical signs include burning and sharp pain over the gluteal area and/or within the groin. Loss of sensation is usually absent or only minimal.

Gradual onset induces a bent-body posture in order to prevent stretching of the nerve. If only sensory deficiency exists then the compression is more distal.

No reliable electrodiagnostic tests are currently available to define the integrity of this nerve; therefore, accurate clinical investigation (look out for previous surgery) is essential to diagnose this rare compression syndrome.

4.7.3
Sonography

Sonography may be of potential aid to diagnose this nerve palsy. We encountered three cases where a thickened sensory branch was riding over the edge of the iliac crest (Fig. 4.42). Sonography-guided injection of local anaesthetic proved to be very helpful in confirming the diagnosis.

4.7.4
Treatment

Conservative treatment includes anti-inflammatory medication and physiotherapy to correct abnormal body posture. If conservative treatment fails, sonography-guided cortisone injection should be performed next. Surgical treatment, as a last option, includes nerve resection or neurolysis.

4.8
Meralgia Paresthetica

Meralgia paresthetica is an uncommon, but not rare, painful condition mainly caused by the entrapment of the lateral femoral cutaneous nerve(LFCN) at the site where the nerve pierces the inguinal ligament. This syndrome was first described by Hager in 1885 (WILSON 1955), then reported more accurately by BERNHARDT (1878, 1895). ROTH (1878) gave the syndrome its name, merging the Greek words "meros", for thigh, and "algos", for pain, to meralgia. Men are more affected then women; approximately

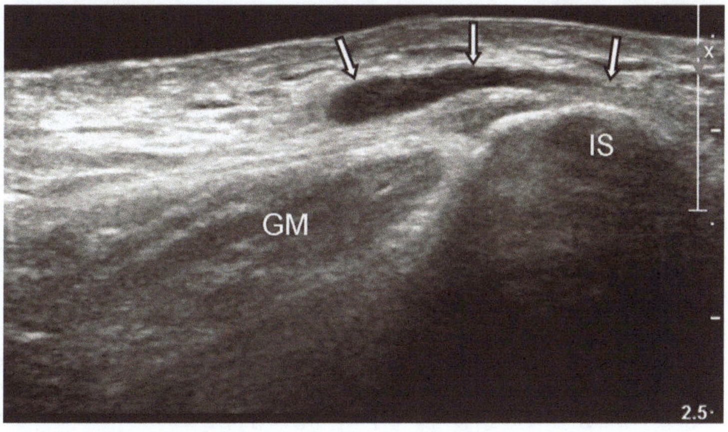

Fig. 4.42. Idiopathic iliohypogastric syndrome. Transverse 17-MHz sonogram across the iliac crest (*IC*) in a patient with severe pain at the right flank of 1 year's standing. At the level of the most acute pain a hypoechoic tubular structure can be appreciated (*arrows*) riding over the edge of the iliac crest, reaching towards the gluteal area. GM, gluteal muscle

three cases per 10,000 are to be expected. It occurs mainly in the 4th to 6th decade. Interestingly, Freud and his son suffered from this syndrome (Freud 1895).

The LFCN is a small, purely sensory nerve that arises from the lumbar plexus. By crossing underneath the psoas muscle and piercing the inguinal canal in a sharp change of its course, the nerve reaches the left thigh (Fig. 43a), innervating the skin of the lateral thigh, down to the knee (Fig. 4.43b). According to the literature there is a large variability regarding the area where the nerve pierces the inguinal ligament, and this may be of potential risk for iatrogenic injury during any type of surgery in the groin (Grothaus et al. 1997; Mirovsky and Neuwirth 2000; Yang et al. 2005). The nerve may also be compressed at the area where it pierces the inguinal ligament. The area where the nerve pierces the ligament can vary with several reports showing a wide anatomic variation. Bujrlin et al. (2007) found the LFCN medially to the anterior superior iliac spine (ASIS) ranging from 0.3 to 6.5 cm.

Various hypotheses have been postulated for the cause of this condition. The nerve may be angulated or compressed against a sharp edge of fascia as it pierces the iliac fascia prior to exiting the pelvis beneath the inguinal ligament. The nerve may be subjected to friction where it is wedged between the attachment of the inguinal ligament with the ASIS. Tight clothing and obesity predispose to compression of the nerve at the inguinal ligament. Meralgia paresthetica is more common in diabetics than in the general population. Strenuous exercise may also trigger the symptoms (Kho et al. 2005). Although rare, impingement of the LFCN by masses (e.g. neoplasms; contained iliopsoas haemorrhages) in the retroperitoneal space before it reaches the inguinal ligament can cause the same symptoms. LFCN injury has been reported in the surgical procedures such as iliac crest bone grafting, inguinal lymph node dissection or appendectomy (Harney and Patijn 2007).

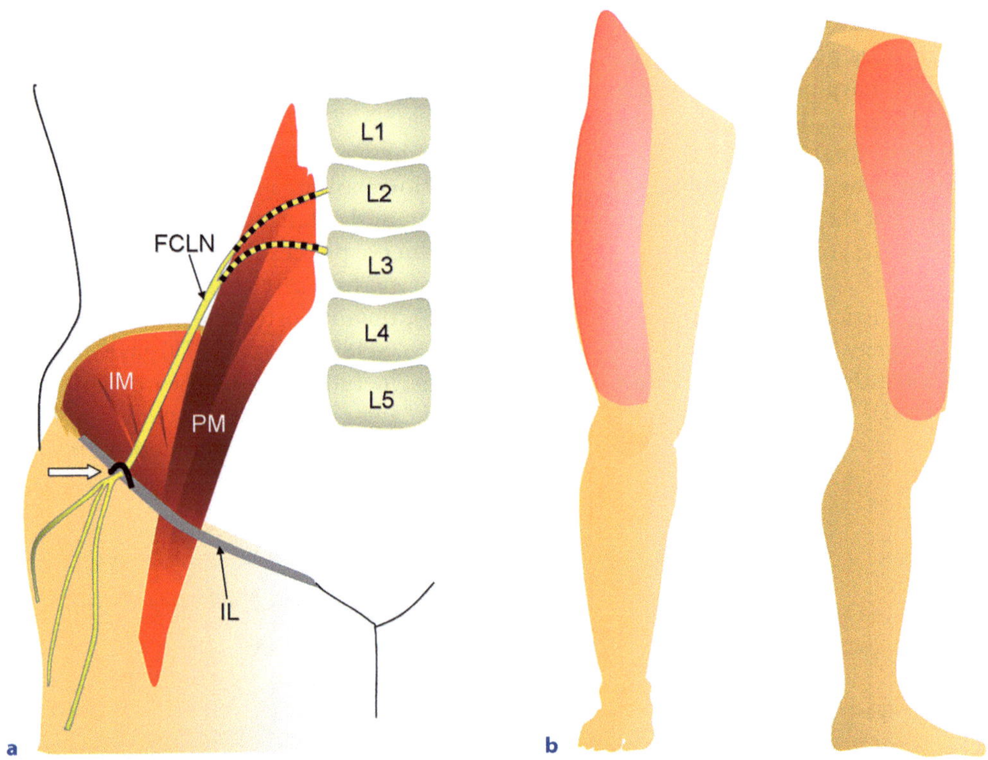

Fig. 4.43a,b. Femoral cutaneous lateral nerve. **a** The drawing demonstrates the formation of the femoral lateral cutaneus nerve (*FCLN*) arising from the nerve fibers at the level L2–L3. The nerve runs beneath the psoas muscle (*PM*), crosses the iliac muscle (*IM*) and pierces the inguinal ligament (*IL*), and by changing its course by almost 90 degrees (*large arrow*) reaches the skin of the anterolateral thigh. **b** The area covered by the sensory innervation of the FCLN extending to the anterior and lateral thigh, reaching from the anterior superior iliac spine down the knee is shown

4.8.1
Clinical Signs

Characteristic signs are burning sensation at the anterior-lateral thigh. Patients also describe a tingling sensation, coldness and local hair loss. In severe cases the slightest touch of clothing triggers the pain. Tinel sign over the iliac crest is frequently positive.

Patients describe burning, coldness, lightning pain, deep muscle ache, frank anesthesia or local hair loss in the anterolateral thigh. The symptoms can be minimal and/or severely limit the patients in there daily life. Patients may first present with hip, knee and calf pain as they try to modify their activities to minimize the symptoms. Some patients already undergo a large number of investigations for presumed lumbar, hip or groin pain before final diagnosis is made.

Electroneurographic testing has shown to be inconclusive and the diagnosis of meralgia paresthetica has to be made mainly on clinical findings. Seror (1999) reported that sensory nerve conduction is a reliable method for meralgia paresthetica electrodiagnosis.

4.8.2
Sonography

Recent reports show the feasibility of sonography to visualize the LCFN in patients with meralgia paresthetica (Hurdle et al. 2007; Tumber et al. 2008). The normal LCFN appears as a small hypoechoic tubular structure in a transversal scan and as a hypoechoic linear structure in a longitudinal plane (Fig. 4.44a–c). Currently the strength of sonography is less in diagnosing and visualizing nerve changes than in assessing the course of the nerve and assist in needle guidance for diagnostic and therapeutic injection, considering the vast variability of the nerve when passing the inguinal ligament. However, we recently encountered a few cases were sonography showed distinct changes along the affected nerve (Fig.4.45).

Initial treatment is usually conservative, by advising the patient to wear looser clothing, avoid tight belts or lose weight in the case of obesity. Medication includes nonsteroidal antiinflammatory drugs.

Patients who fail to respond to conservative therapy should be considered for sonography-guided injection of local anesthetic and a small amount of

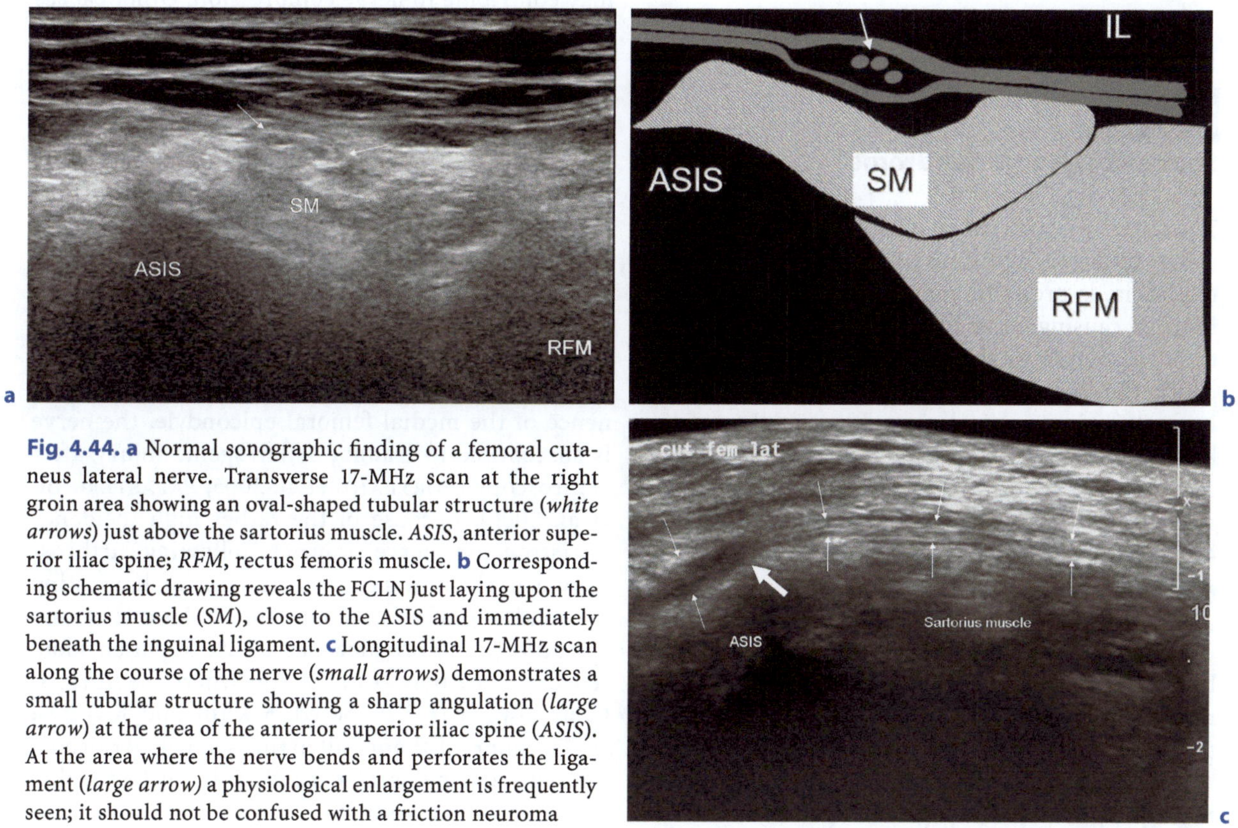

Fig. 4.44. a Normal sonographic finding of a femoral cutaneus lateral nerve. Transverse 17-MHz scan at the right groin area showing an oval-shaped tubular structure (*white arrows*) just above the sartorius muscle. *ASIS*, anterior superior iliac spine; *RFM*, rectus femoris muscle. **b** Corresponding schematic drawing reveals the FCLN just laying upon the sartorius muscle (*SM*), close to the ASIS and immediately beneath the inguinal ligament. **c** Longitudinal 17-MHz scan along the course of the nerve (*small arrows*) demonstrates a small tubular structure showing a sharp angulation (*large arrow*) at the area of the anterior superior iliac spine (*ASIS*). At the area where the nerve bends and perforates the ligament (*large arrow*) a physiological enlargement is frequently seen; it should not be confused with a friction neuroma

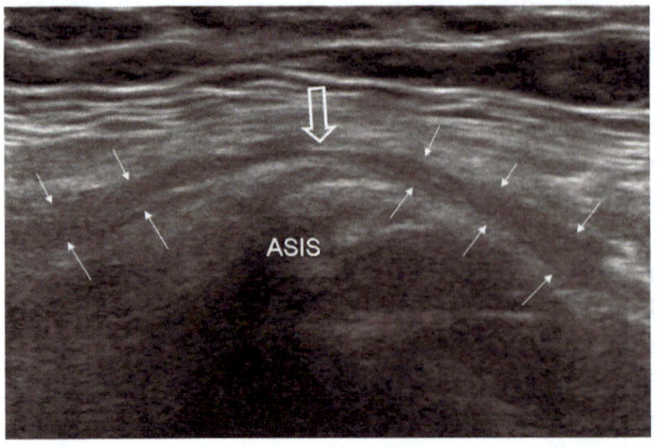

Fig. 4.45. Idiopathic meralgia paresthetica. Longitudinal 17-MHz sonographic image demonstrates an FCLN stretched and thinned out over the anterior superior iliac spine (*ASIS*) (*large arrow*). Nerve swelling (*small arrows*) is seen proximally and distally to the ASIS

cortisone. Surgical treatment should be reserved for resistant cases and for those where sonography clearly shows the course of the nerve being in close relationship with the ASIS. Surgical therapy includes nerve decompression, nerve transposition and nerve dissection.

4.9 Saphenous Nerve Syndrome

The saphenus nerve, when passing through Hunter's canal (adductor canal) and when piercing the adductor fascia, is prone to compression and stretching injuries causing knee pain and paresthesia along the distribution of the affected dermatome. Especially the infrapatellar branches are frequently injured during surgical procedures at the medial knee area.

4.9.1 Anatomy

The saphenous nerve is the longest and the terminal branch of the femoral nerve. It is a pure sensory nerve that is made up of fibers from the L3 and L4 spinal segments.

The saphenous nerve branches from the femoral nerve just distal to the inguinal ligament and runs together with the superficial femoral vein and artery within Hunter's canal into the distal third of the thigh. The canal is somewhat triangular in shape, the walls formed by the vastus medialis muscle laterally and the adductor magnus muscle medially, covered by the vasto-adductoria membrane. The last third segment of the nerve is covered by the sartorius muscle. After piercing the sartorius muscle the nerve becomes subcutaneous (Hunter et al. 1979), branching into the infrapatellar nerve and running distally behind the medial border of the tibia accompanied by the great saphenous vein, and then dividing into two branches: one continuing its course along the margin of the tibia, and ending at the ankle; the other passing in front of the ankle, and distributing to the skin on the medial side of the foot, and finally reaching the great toe (Fig. 4.46a,b).

4.9.1.1 Etiology

Due to its long course the nerve is prone to traumatic injuries, including stretching injuries or direct blow to the nerve, especially in contact and ball sports (Balaji and DeWeese 1981; Lippitt 1993). Dynamic forces of the muscle around Hunter's canal may contribute to nerve compression. Other causes of entrapment include meniscus ganglion and varicose vein surgery. Iatrogenic injuries following knee surgery are frequent.

The infrapatellar nerve may also become entrapped on its own. This is because it pierces the sartorius muscle tendon. House and Ahmed (1977) described entrapment of the infrapatellar nerve behind the sartorius tendon against the prominent edge of the medial femoral condyle with a sharply angulated course when passing around the sartorius muscle.

Due to its horizontal course across the prominence of the medial femoral epicondyle, the nerve is susceptible to trauma or iatrogenic injury after arthroscopy (Portland et al. 2005; Papastergiou et al. 2006). Because of the rather high incidence of iatrogenic nerve injuries following arthroscopy a horizontal surgical incision for harvesting the tendon grafts is recommended. Mochida and Kikuchi (1995) revealed that 22.2% of patients had sensory disturbances in the area where the infrapatellar branch is distributed. Mándi and Kalmár (1973) reported that of all arthroscopies performed for suspected meniscal tear 4.2% actually had saphenous nerve compression.

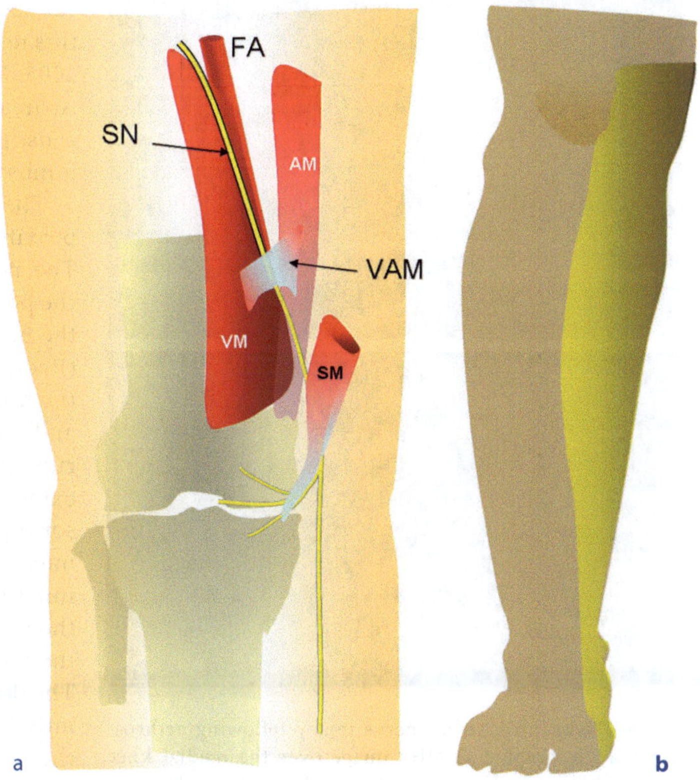

Fig. 4.46. a The anatomical course and relationship between the saphenus nerve and the muscles forming the Hunter's canal; Vastus medialis muscle (*VM*) at the lateral side, adductor muscle (*AM*) at the medial side, covered by the vasto-adductor membrane (*VAM*). The infrapatellar nerves pierces the sartorius muscle (*SM*), innervating the skin of the medial knee region. *FA*, femoral artery. Superficial cutaneous branches run distally on the medial side of the calf. **b** The right lower leg showing the skin innervation by the saphenus nerve, extending from the medial knee area, anteriorly to the tibial shin, reaching down to the medial malleolus and the medial site of the great toe

4.9.1.2 Clinical Signs

Clinical symptoms include constant pain over the medial knee region and paresthesia at the medial calf and foot. Flexion of the knee usually aggravates the symptoms. Deep palpation at the area of Hunter's canal may reinforce the pain. If only the infrapatellar nerve is affected (usually after arthroscopy) the patient can pinpoint the area of pain. Thinel's sign is strongly positive, while numbness in the medial knee area is usually associated. ENG and EMG testing are inconclusive, and should not be performed if no muscular weakness is present.

4.9.2 Sonography

On sonography the saphenus nerve and its branches appear as small tubular oval-shaped structures in a transversal scan. Between three and five fascicles can be depicted. It may take a few sweeps up and down the medial knee region to recognize the nerve. Longitudinal scan should be performed to document the extent of the lesion. Lundblad et al. (2006) successfully detected the saphenus nerve in ten of ten volunteers using a 10-MHz probe. High frequency probes working up to 17 MHz should be used to detect potential abnormalities within small nerves such as the infrapatellar nerve. According to the literature no cases of nerve palsy in Hunter's canal or iatrogenic nerve palsy after arthroscopy have been described using sonography. However, in our experience small stump neuroma are frequently visualized, appearing as a small hypoechoic round or oval-shaped mass in continuity with a small nerve. An infrapatellar nerve palsy caused by scar appears as a hypoechoic, ill-defined lesion with oedematous enlargement of the nerve compared to the contralateral side (Fig. 4.47a,b).

4.9.2.1 Treatment

Conservative treatment of the entrapment in Hunter's canal is primarily advocated. Sonography-guided injection of local anaesthetic and cortisone may aide diagnosis and treatment of this rare neuropathy. In cases of nerve dissection or scar forma-

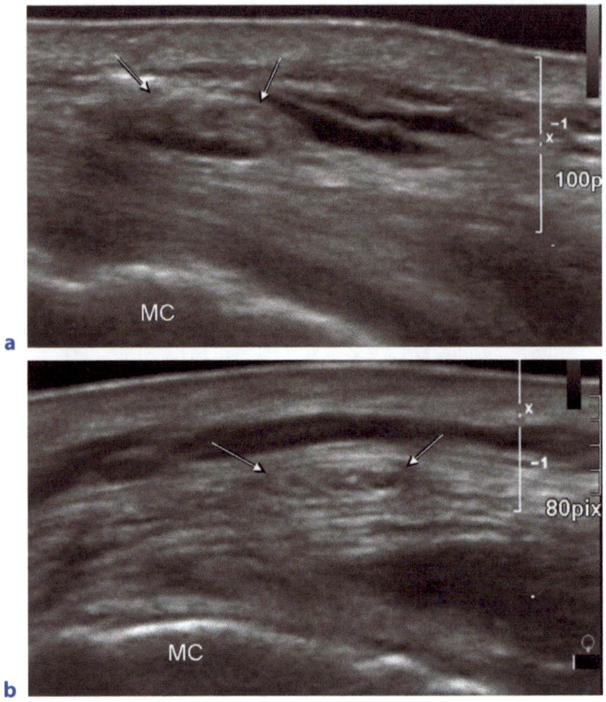

Fig. 4.47a,b. Infrapatellar nerve injury following arthroscopy. **a** Sonographic 17-MHz image over the medial knee region shows an edematous infrapatellar nerve with hypoechoic scar formation and poorly recognized fascicles (*arrows*). **b** Comparison with contralateral sonographic image shows a normal infrapatellar nerve with its typical oval shape appearance and tubular *dotted pattern* (*arrows*). *MC*, medial condyle)

tion along the infrapatellar nerve repeated sonography-guided injection of local anaesthetic, cortisone or phenol may be advised. Neurolysis or nerve resection should be considered last.

4.10 Peroneal Nerve Compression

Peroneal nerve compression is the most frequent mononeuropathy of the lower limb, affecting all age groups. Depending on the site of nerve involvement (common peroneal nerve, deep peroneal nerve and superficial peroneal nerve) various syndromes (peroneal tunnel syndrome, anterior tarsal tunnel syndrome) of peroneal nerve compression may be discerned. Foot drop is the most striking clinical finding, followed by pain and sensory disturbances. Direct trauma, ganglia, stretching injury, postsurgical sequelae or inflammatory disease may trigger this nerve palsy (Dallari et al. 2004; Gruber et al. 2005; Malghem et al. 1998; McCrory et al. 2002). Acute or chronic compartment syndrome may also cause peroneal palsy. Differential diagnosis includes lumbar discopathy.

The peroneal nerve leaves the sciatic nerve in the proximal portion of the popliteal fossa (Fig. 4.48a). The nerve passes between the superficial head of the peroneus longus muscle and the bony surface of the fibular neck, referred to as the peroneal tunnel (Pecina et al. 2001). Shortly after its course around the fibular neck the nerve divides into a superficial and a deep branch. The superficial peroneal nerve runs between the peroneus longus muscle and the extensor digitorum muscle proximally and the extensor digitorum distally, supplying the foot elevating muscles (peroneus longus and brevis muscle) and innervates the skin over the lateral calf, supplying the skin on the dorsolateral region of the foot, and the skin on the third, fourth and fifth toe (Fig. 4.48b). The deep peroneal nerve enters the peroneus longus muscle, after passing the extensor digitorum muscle the nerve reaches in front of the interosseus membrane, and adjacent to the anterior tibial artery, runs distally passing underneath the inferior extensor retinaculum (Fig. 4.48c). The nerve innervates the muscles running within the anterior tarsal tunnel and gives branches to the medial and lateral ankle joint. The distal branches of the nerve supply the skin between the first and second toe and innervate the extensor digitorum brevis (Fig. 4.48d).

4.10.1 Peroneal Tunnel Syndrome

The most common causes of compression neuropathy of the common peroneal nerve are external, such as a ganglion, tight short leg plaster casts, malaligned fibular head fractures and knee surgery (Asp and Rand 1990; Spinner et al. 2003). Stretching nerve injury following knee luxation has also been reported (Gruber et al. 2005) (see Chap. 5). Although relatively rare, an idiopathic entrapment syndrome of the common peroneal nerve is known, which typically occurs in the restricted space between the bone and the fascia of the peroneus longus muscle. In many instances these lesions may be related to functional anatomic changes: inversion and plantar flexion of the foot tenses the peroneus longus muscle and squeezes the nerve towards

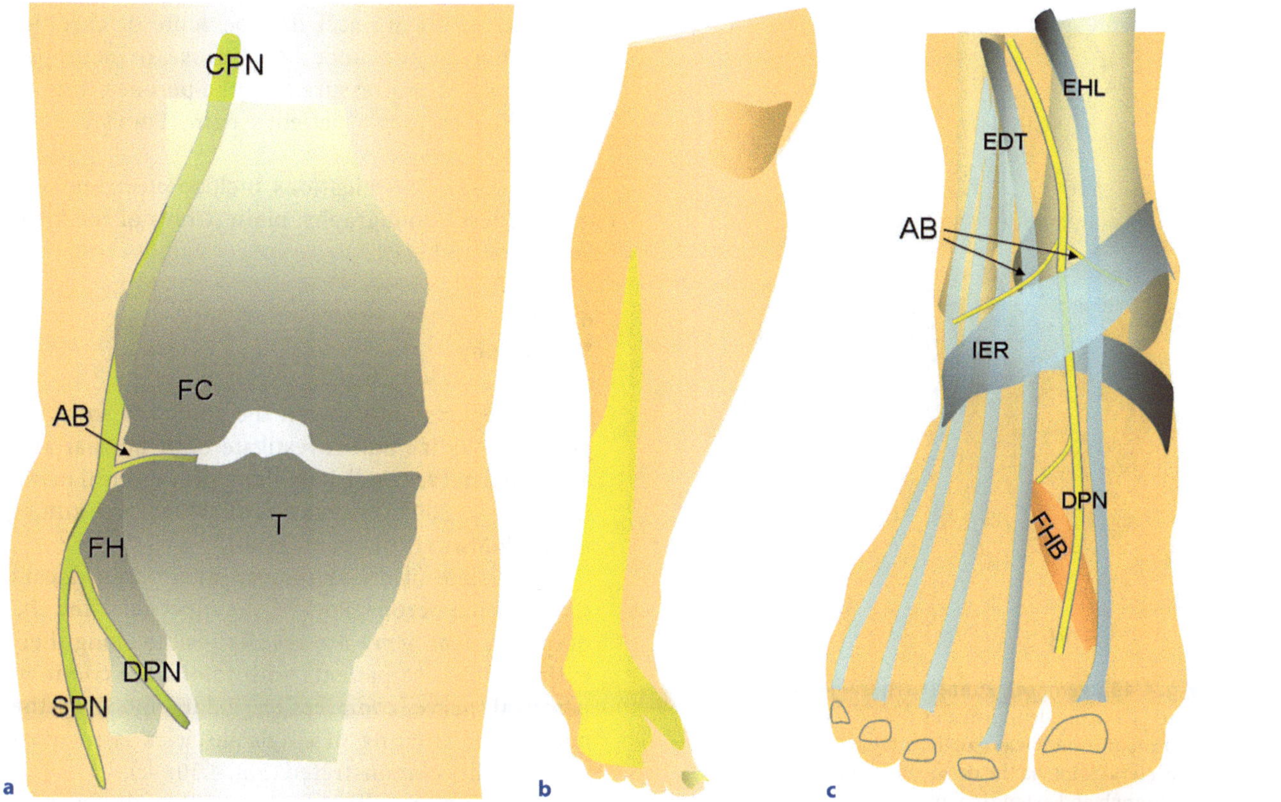

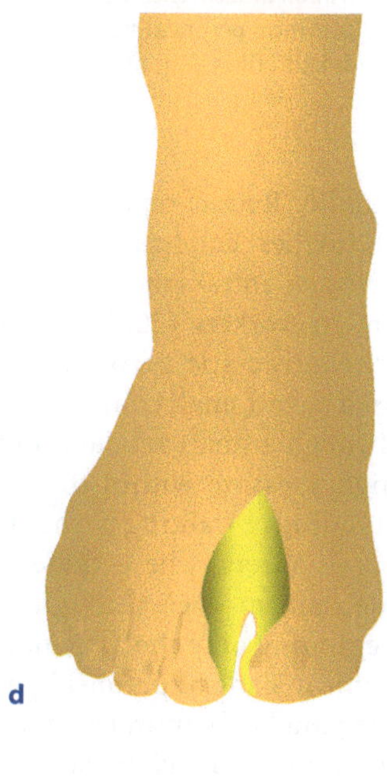

Fig. 4.48a–d. Common peroneal nerve. **a** Schematic illustration of the knee joint shows the close relationship of the common peroneal nerve (*CPN*) slinging around the fibular head (*FH*), and dividing into the superficial peroneal nerve and deep peroneal nerve (*DPN*), a small articular branch (*AB*) breach from the common peroneal nerve to innervate the knee joint. **b** The sensory innervation extending from the lateral upper leg to the skin around the lateral malleolus and covering the dorsal foot, including the skin on the 3rd, 4th and 5th toe. **c** At the lower the deep peroneal nerve (*DPN*) leg passes underneath the inferior extensor retinaculum (*IER*), giving articular branches to the medial and lateral ankle, then innervates the flexor hallucis brevis muscle (*FHB*). **d** The terminal branch innervates the skin between the first and second toe. *T*, tibia; *FC*, femoral condyle

the fibular neck. Repetitive actions with inversion and pronation (long distance running, operating machines with pedals), habitual overuse (sleeping position, wheel chair sitting, sitting with crossed legs) are therefore known to predispose the nerve to development of neuropathy (Hamdan et al. 2008; Kopell and Thompson 1960; Kumak 1987; Legeyt and Ambrose 1998; Sidey 1969; Kaminsky 1947).

A ganglion arising from the tibiofibular joint is one of the most frequent causes for peroneal tunnel syndrome. In most cases the ganglion arising from the joint tibiofibular joint, displaces the common peroneal nerve and causes cumulative nerve palsy (Fig. 4.49). Buckwalter et al. (1979) and Malghem et al. (1998) postulated that cysts arising from the joint have communication to the neurovascular

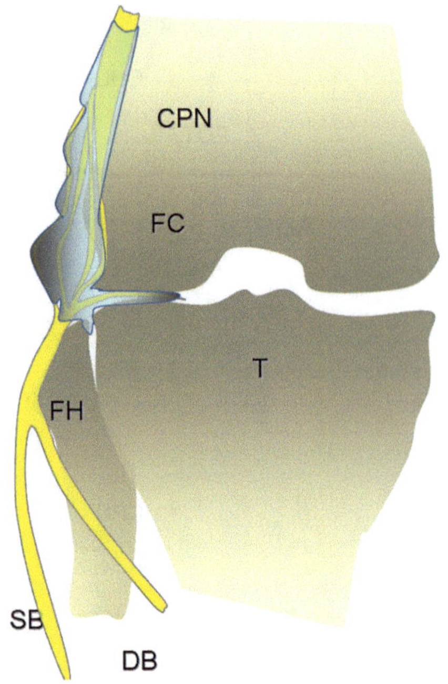

Fig. 4.49. Peroneal tunnel syndrome. Schematic drawing demonstrates the genesis of the intraneural peroneal ganglion by arising from the lateral joint via the nerve sheet of the articular branch and extending into the nerve sheet of the common peroneal nerve (*CPN*). *FC*, femoral condyle; *T*, tibia; *FH*, fibular head

bundle. Recent reports by Spinner (2003, 2006a–c) further emphasize the distinct differentiation between intra- and extraneural ganglia. Spinner and coworkers (2003, 2006a–c)have shown nicely that intracystic peroneal ganglia around the knee area have a small connection to the tibiofibular joint through a small articular branch (see Chap. 5). The high pressure within the tibiofibular joint during standing or walking pushes the joint fluid into small nerve sheets, where there is less resistance. This mechanism goes through different stages: at the beginning only the articular branch is affected (no clinical signs of peroneal palsy), as the build up of the ganglion continues, following the peroneal and finally also the sciatic nerve is affected.

4.10.1.1 Clinical Signs

Common peroneal nerve compression results in burning pain in the sensory regions mentioned above, motor weakness and atrophy with a gradual transition to a dropping foot in complete peroneal paralysis. Clinical onset may be acute or chronic, depending on the underlying cause of neuropathy. Palpation or pressure over the peroneal tunnel typically increases a patient's pain (Pecina et al. 2001).

Diagnostic investigations include electroneurographic tests, sonography, plain X-rays of the knee and ankle and MRI.

4.10.1.2 Sonography

Recent reports have shown the ability of sonography to visualize and investigate both normal and abnormal nerve conditions along the peroneal nerve (Peer et al. 2002; Peeters et al. 2004; Créteur et al. 2007; Martinoli et al. 2000).

With state-of-the-art linear array transducers the common peroneal nerve, the superficial and the deep peroneal nerve are readily visible along their entire course. In patients with idiopathic common peroneal nerve compression enlargement of the nerve with swelling of single fascicles is in most cases readily demonstrated (Fig. 4.50a–c).

A frequent associated finding of chronic peroneal palsy is the increase in echogenicity of the affected anterior tibial and extensor muscles of the foot.

The detection of coexisting abnormalities with external compression is straightforward, such as ganglia, tumors, bony ridges, etc. which are easily visualized with sonography (Fig. 4.51) (Pedrazzini et al. 2002; Visser et al. 2006; Dallari et al. 2004). An attempt should be made to differentiate extra- and intraneural ganglia with sonography by demonstrating any subtile connection between the intraneural cystic and the tibio-fibular joint. Extraneural ganglia usually displace the entire peroneal nerve without spreading the fascicles because they are still contained by the nerve sheet, whereas intraneural ganglia show intraneural displacement of the fascicles in a fan-like matter with proximal thickening of the nerve fascicles (Fig. 4.49).

4.10.1.3 Therapy

Therapeutic management of peroneal nerve palsy can be either straightforward or very challenging, depending on the type of nerve injury. Mild forms of nerve palsy may resolve by eliminating the compressing agent such as plasters or tight dressings. Surgical management of peroneal nerve lesions should be

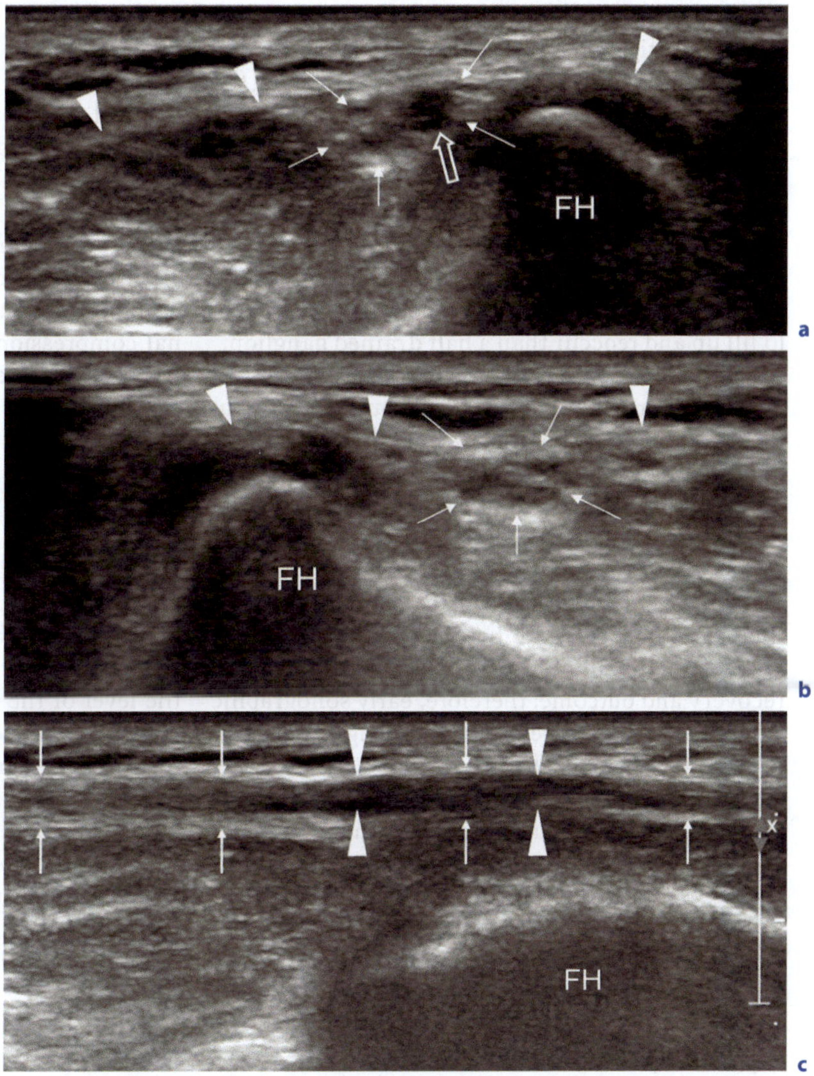

Fig. 4.50a–c. Idiopathic peroneal tunnel syndrome. **a** Transverse 17-MHz scan at the level of the fibular head (*FH*) shows a hypoechoic slightly enlarged common peroneal nerve in close relationship to the fibular head and the fibrous part of the peroneus longus muscle (*arrowheads*). One of the fascicles which is closest to the bone appears to be even thicker (*large arrow*) than the other remaining fascicles. **b** Comparative transverse scan on the contralateral healthy side demonstrates that there is more space between the common peroneal nerve and the fibular head and the fascicles are better discernible. **c** Longitudinal 17-MHZ scan along the affected common peroneal nerve (*small arrows*). Note the change of echotexture at the level above and proximally (*arrowheads*) to the fibular head (*FH*)

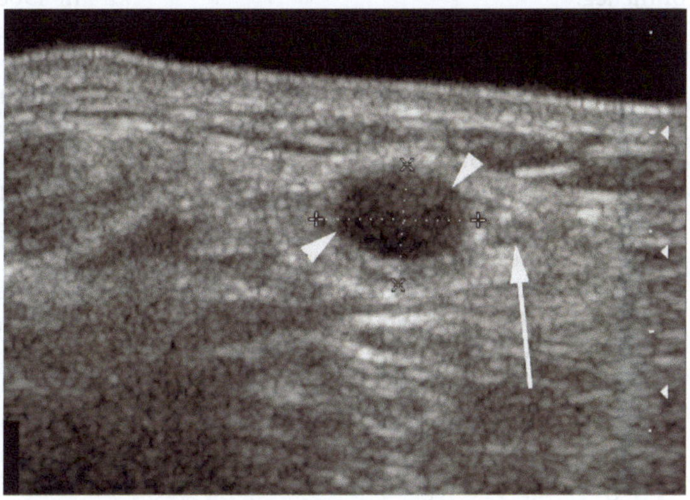

Fig. 4.51. Peroneal tunnel syndrome caused by intraneural ganglion. Transverse 12-MHz scan at the level of the fibular head reveals a well defined intraneural cyst (*arrowheads*) with lateral displacement of the fascicles (*large arrow*)

immediate in the case of direct laceration or if diagnostic investigations show a compromising mass.

If a ganglion cyst is compressing or displacing the peroneal nerve sonography-guided aspiration with a large needle (14-gauge) is advised. We use a large needle because the ganglion cyst has a very viscous consistence. It is further helpful to put pressure on the ganglion with one finger to guarantee complete drainage in order to achieve complete collapse of the ganglion. The collapsed ganglion is much less likely to fill up and reoccur than a half drained ganglion.

In idiopathic peroneal tunnel syndrome the nerve is released proximally from its fibrous enclosure at the fibular neck. The attachment of the peroneus longus at the fibular neck also is released.

Stretching injury after knee luxation frequently shows a long segment of damaged nerve, sometimes exceeding 10 cm; this per se is already an indicator for a poor outcome. It is worth mentioning again that the time interval between symptom onset and decompression or nerve implant is crucial for recovery and outcome; therefore, early sonographic assessment of the extent of the damaged peroneal nerve is very beneficial.

Failing sufficient recovery from nerve decompression, nerve grafting or repair tendon transfer procedures may be considered after 12 months.

4.10.2 Superficial Peroneal Nerve Syndrome

Superficial peroneal nerve syndrome is a rare compression syndrome first described by Henry in 1945. The nerve can be compressed at the level where the nerve penetrates crural fascia, within the lower third of the leg.

4.10.2.1 Etiology

Common causes for superficial peroneal palsy are direct trauma or fibrous processes involving the superficial peroneal nerve after inversion ankle injury. Compression of the superficial peroneal nerve at the level where the nerve pierces the fascia cruris with and without muscle herniation have been reported in a variety of sports activities (Daghino et al. 1997; Yang et al. 2006; Lorei and Hershman 1993). The nerve is continuously stretched during repetitive flexion and extension of the foot, as occurs in long-distant running.

4.10.2.2 Clinical Signs

Clinical symptoms include pain and dysesthesia or paresthesia at the dorsum of the foot; nocturnal leg pain is sometimes reported. Tinel sign is frequently positive, weak dorsiflexion is sometimes noted. Symptoms increase during specific leg exercise.

In cases of muscular hernia a palpable bulging lesion is found at the level of the anterior leg. External compression by tight socks and fracture callus has been reported.

4.10.2.2.1 Sonography

As stated above, sonography permits investigation of the superficial peroneal nerve along its entire course, also showing the penetrating of the nerve at the crural fascia. Sonography demonstrates a fusiform swelling of the superficial nerve palsy at the level of the crural piercing; comparison to the contralateral in exactly the same plane is mandatory for correct diagnosis (Fig. 4.52a,b). Diagnostic confirmation of this nerve palsy includes sonography-guided local anesthetic injection; cortisone injection is usually not beneficial since the fibrosing process at the level of the nerve passage is pronounced and therefore surgical release of the fascia is advocated (De Fijter et al. 2006).

4.10.3 Anterior Tarsal Tunnel Syndrome

This syndrome was first described by Marinacci in 1968. The deep peroneal nerve, when reaching the dorsum of the foot, passes beneath the inferior retinaculum extensorum (Fig. 4.48c), where it can be compressed, causing pain, dysesthesia and paresthesia at the dorsum of the foot.

4.10.3.1 Anatomy

The deep peroneal nerve originates from the common peroneal nerve at the fibular neck. After passing the extensor digitorum muscle it reaches in front of the interosseus membrane, and adjacent to the anterior tibial artery the nerve runs distally passing underneath the inferior retinaculum extensorum. The inferior retinaculum extensorum runs from the

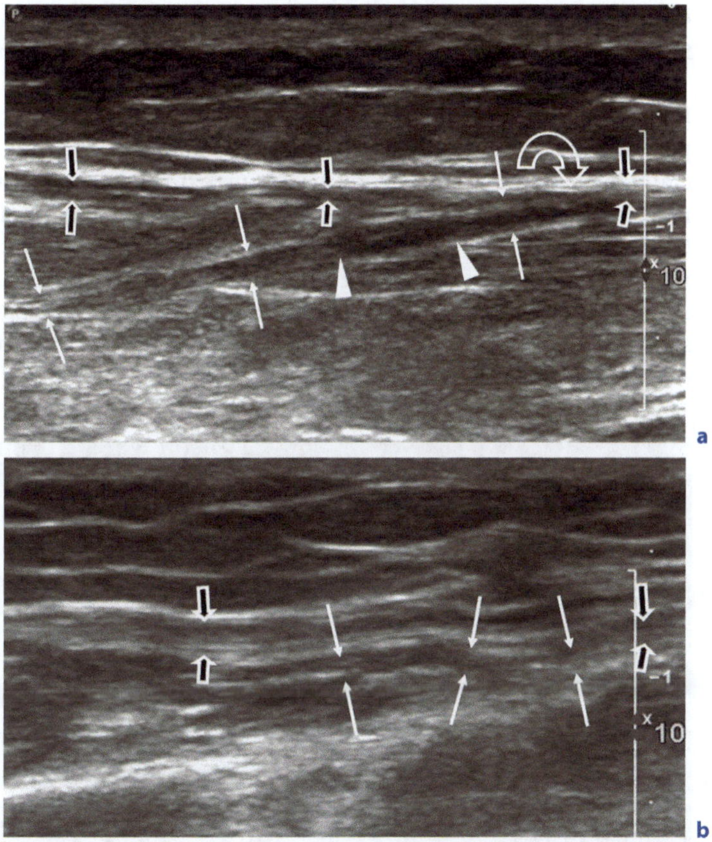

Fig. 4.52. a Superficial peroneal nerve syndrome. Longitudinal 17-MHZ scan along the superficial peroneal nerve (*small arrows*). The nerve shows a fusiform swelling (*arrowheads*) starting from where the nerve pierces (*rounded arrow*) the crural fascia (*large arrows*). **b** Comparison with the contralateral scan of the non-injured leg shows a normal superficial peroneal nerve with a wave-like course (*arrows*), suggesting that the nerve has a better range of motion during extension and flexion of the foot. There is no caliber change at the area where the nerve penetrates the crural fascia (*large arrows*)

medial to the lateral malleolus in a y-shaped form, building the roof for the anterior tarsal tunnel. The floor is built by the overlaying fascia of the talar and navicular bone. The nerve within the tunnel is accompanied by four extensor tendons (anterior tibial, extensor hallucis, extensor digitorum longus, peroneus tertius), the anterior tibial artery and anterior tibial veins. The nerve innervates the muscles running within the anterior tarsal tunnel and gives branches to the medial and lateral ankle joint. The distal branches of the nerve supply the skin between the first and second toe and innervate the extensor digitorum brevis (Fig. 4.48d).

4.10.3.2
Etiology and Clinical Findings

The anterior tarsal tunnel is a rare compression syndrome presenting with pain and paresthesia when only sensory fascicles are compressed; when motoric fascicles are affected extension of the first toe is weakened. Anterior tarsal tunnel syndrome is mostly caused by compression of the deep peroneal nerve due to repetitive mechanical irritation of the deep peroneal nerve at the region beneath the inferior extensor retinaculum.

Other etiologies of anterior tarsal tunnel include chronic ankle sprains, fractures, dislocations, posttraumatic fibrosis, ganglions, tendon sheath tumors, penetrating injuries and chronic overuse from a variety of endurance sports activities. Sensory deficits involves the area between the first and second toes as well as paresis and atrophy of the extensor digitorum brevis.

4.10.3.3
Diagnosis

Electroneurographic testing of anterior tarsal tunnel is helpful in the differential diagnosis of radiculopathy. The distal latency of the deep peroneal nerve is increased; in cases where only the motoric fascicles are affected, the EMG shows active and chronic denervation of the extensor digitorum brevis. In cases with partial anterior tarsal tunnel syndrome only the sensory branch of the deep peroneal nerve after the division under the inferior extensor retinaculum is compressed.

4.10.3.4 Sonography

High frequency probes are used to detect the deep peroneal nerve since the nerve runs very superficially beneath the inferior retinaculum extensorum. The nerve can be recognized more easily when lymph edema is present at the dorsum of the foot. An inflammation process involving the extensor tendon shows hyperemic changes on color Doppler ultrasound. Soft tissue masses that compromise the nerve can be depicted; most of the masses are ganglions, typically they are lobulated, septated and they displace the nerve. A connection between the ganglion and the joint can be visualized. Ultrasound can also differentiate intraneural ganglia from extraarticular ganglia. As previously described intraneural ganglia have a typical appearance, showing cystic changes within the nerve with marginal displacing of the fascicles, careful investigation may show the joint communication via the articular branch (Fig. 4.53a–c) (see also Chap. 6). Ultrasound may also well depict complete disruption of the nerve after a penetrating injury (Fig. 4.54).

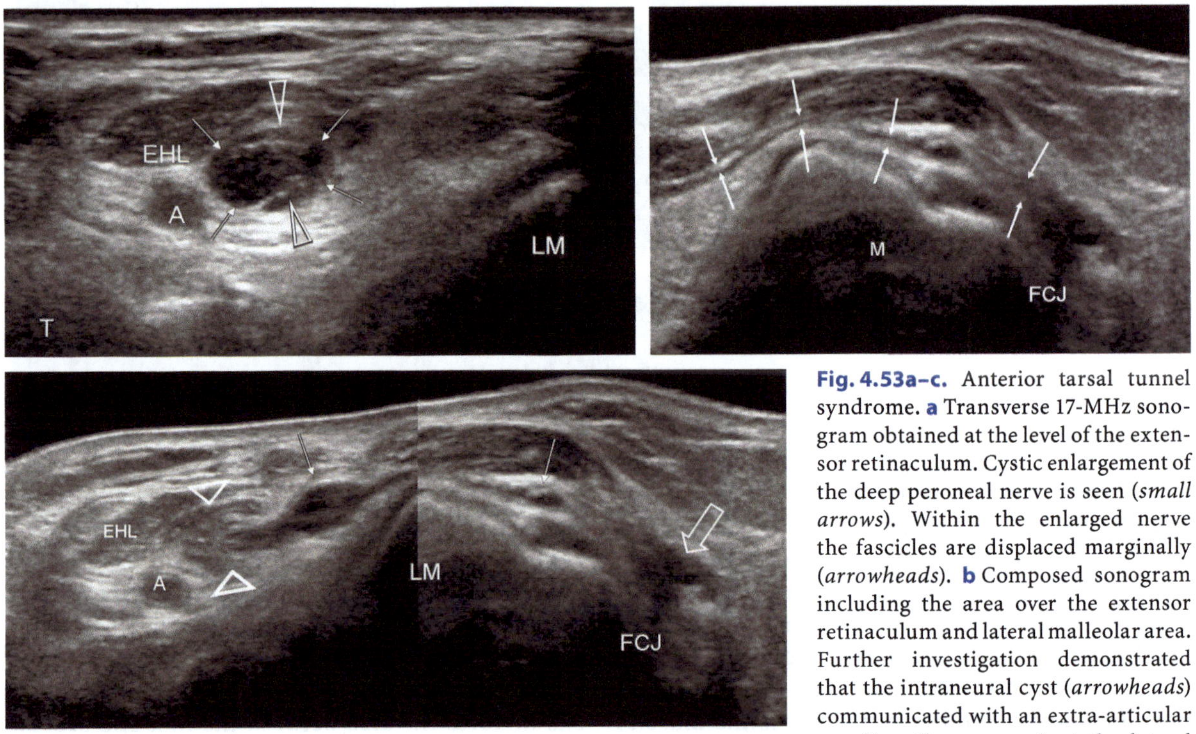

Fig. 4.53a–c. Anterior tarsal tunnel syndrome. **a** Transverse 17-MHz sonogram obtained at the level of the extensor retinaculum. Cystic enlargement of the deep peroneal nerve is seen (*small arrows*). Within the enlarged nerve the fascicles are displaced marginally (*arrowheads*). **b** Composed sonogram including the area over the extensor retinaculum and lateral malleolar area. Further investigation demonstrated that the intraneural cyst (*arrowheads*) communicated with an extra-articular ganglion (*large arrow*) at the lateral fibulo-calcaneal joint (*FCJ*). *EHL*, extensor hallucis longus muscle; *A*, anterior tibial artery; *LM*, lateral malleolus; *T*, tibia. Along the communication between the deep peroneal nerve and the FCJ multiple small cystic bulges are noted. Sonography-guided aspiration confirmed viscous fluid within the cyst. **c** Zoomed sonographic image demonstrated a small articular branch arising from the deep peroneal nerve and arching over the malleolus (*M*) to reach the fibulo-calcaneal joint

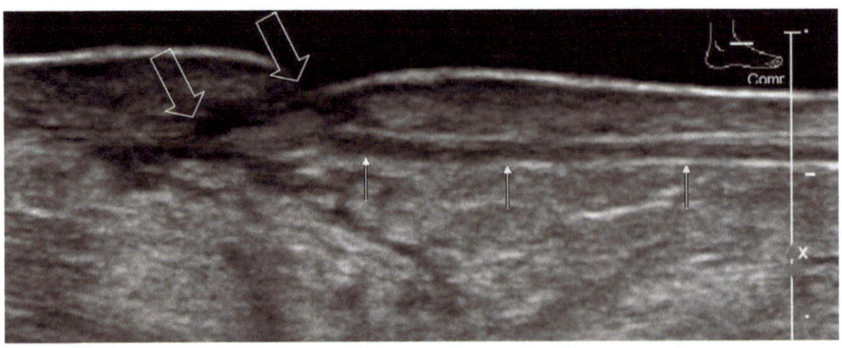

Fig. 4.54. Complete dissection of the deep peroneal nerve at the dorsum of the foot after a glass cut injury. Longitudinal 17-MHz scan was performed along the course of the terminal branch of the deep peroneal nerve (*small arrows*). Complete dissection of the deep peroneal nerve is depicted at the level of the penetrating cutting injury (*large arrows*)

4.10.3.5
Treatment

Conservative management should be used first and is suggested prior to surgical decompression. Avoiding any chronic overuse such as jogging may ease the neurological symptoms; tight shoes should also not be worn. In case of a compressing ganglion, ultrasound-guided aspiration should be attempted; in the case of synovial thickening along the tendons ultrasound-guided cortisone injection is advised.

4.11 Tibial Nerve Compression

From the sciatic nerve bifurcation the tibial nerve enters the calf between the two gastrocnemius heads and continues, lying between the posterior tibial muscle and the flexor hallucis muscle, in a relatively straight course down to the medial ankle accompanied by the tibial artery and vein. On its passage around the medial malleolus the nerve enters a fibro-osseous canal, referred to as the posterior tarsal tunnel. The tibial nerve sends a calcaneal and lateral plantar branch that supplies the area around the heel (Fig. 4.55a). On its passage through the tarsal canal, the nerve may be compressed resulting in posterior tarsal tunnel syndrome, a recognized clinical entity first described in the early 1960s by Kopell and Thompson (1960). Within the posterior tarsal tunnel the nerve splits into a medial and plantar nerve. Compression syndromes can occur to the medial plantar nerve (Jogger's foot) and to the lateral plantar nerve (Fig. 4.55b). The tibial nerve can be compressed anywhere from the popliteal fossa down to the ankle (Fig. 4.56).

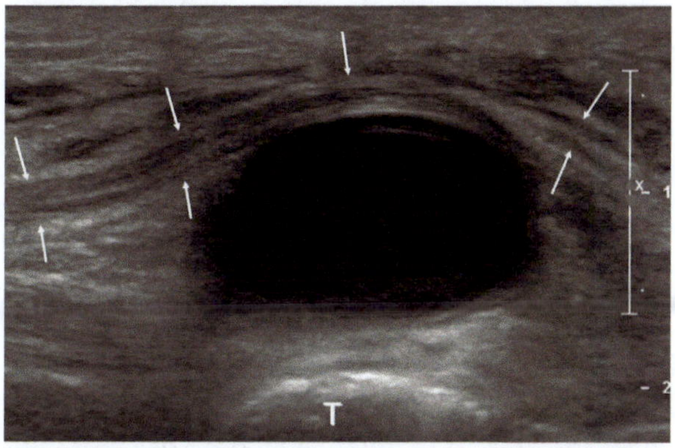

Fig. 4.56. Tibial nerve compression at the popliteal fossa. Longitudinal 17-MHz scan along the tibial nerve (*arrows*) shows bowing displacement of the nerve caused by an extra-articular ganglion. *T*, tibia)

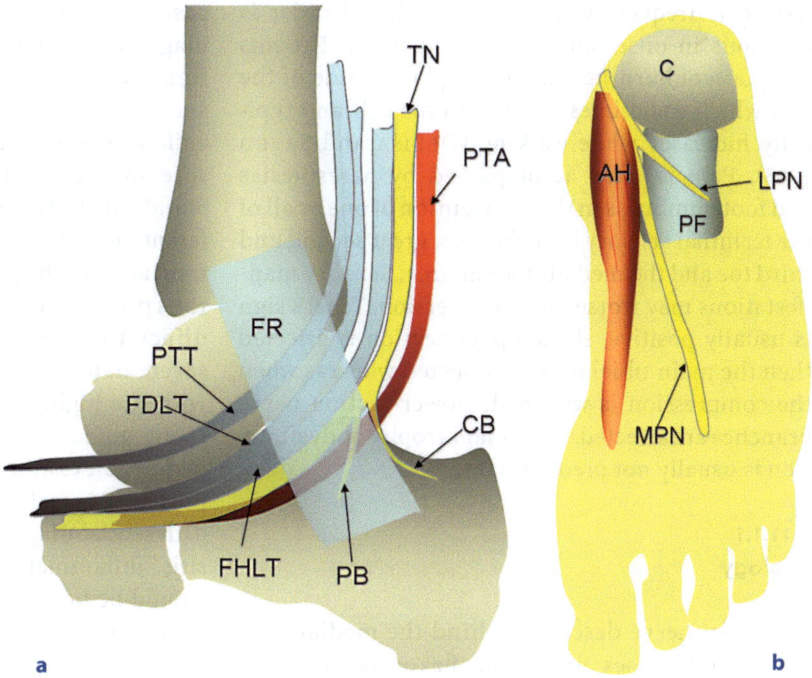

Fig. 4.55a,b. Tibial nerve at the tarsal tunnel. The posterior tarsal tunnel and the branching into the medial and lateral plantar nerve are shown. **a** The tibial nerve (*TN*) runs between the posterior tibial artery (PTA) and the flexor hallucis longus tendon (FHLT), flexor digitorum longus tendon (*FDLT*), anteriorly the posterior tibial tendon (*PTT*) covered by the retinaculum flexorum (*RF*). The tibial nerve gives a branch to the calcaneal area (*CB*) and a branch to the lateral plantar area (*PB*). **b** Schematic drawing of the plantar foot demonstrates the bifurcation of the tibial nerve into the medial plantar nerve (*MPL*) and lateral plantar nerve (*LPN*). Compression of the plantar nerve (jogger's syndrome) can occur due to the tight anatomical relationship between the calcaneus and the adductor hallucis muscle (*AH*)

4.11.1 Posterior Tarsal Tunnel Syndrome

The tarsal tunnel is a fibro-osseous canal consisting of a bony sulcus on the medial side of the calcaneus, the posterior talar process and the medial malleolus. According to Pecina et al. (2001) the upper section of the tarsal tunnel is narrower then the lower section, therefore the medial plantar nerve is at higher risk for compression.

The roof of the canal consists of the flexor retinaculum, which covers the tendons of the tibialis posterior, flexor digitorum and flexor hallucis longus muscles. The tibial artery and veins run together with these three tendons and the tibial nerve and the tarsal tunnel may in fact be considered the hilum of the planta pedis, as it houses virtually all of its neurovascular supply (Fig. 4.55a). Before entering the tarsal tunnel the tibial nerve sends a small sensory branch towards the heel and at the upper margin of the retinaculum or after a short distance in the canal divides into its terminal branches, the medial and lateral plantar nerve. The distal branches innervate the skin of the heel, the medial plantar area, including the great, second and third toe.

The posterior tarsal tunnel syndrome (Keck 1962; Mumenthaler et al. 1998) is clearly less frequent than the aforementioned entrapment syndromes of upper extremities, but is the most frequent entrapment in the foot. Clinical and electroneurographic testing is frequently inconclusive; the disorder is insidious in onset and mostly unilateral. Patients complain of burning pain at the plantar side of the foot which sometimes radiates to the calf and typically increases while walking (DeLisa and Saeed 1983). Pain is often accompanied by paresthesias and foot numbness in the distribution of one or all of the terminal sensory branches, i.e. great second and third toe and the medial-plantar area. Sensory manifestations may worsen by foot eversion. Tinel's sign is usually positive. If the upper section is affected then the main tibial nerve is affected whereas when the compression is within the lower section nerve branches are affected. Muscular atrophy or dysfunction is usually not predominant.

4.11.1.1 Etiology

The tibial nerve descends behind the medial malleolus and passes under the flexor retinaculum ("laciniate ligament") to the plantar side of the foot, where it divides into the calcaneal, medial and lateral plantar branches. In the tarsal tunnel, roofed by the flexor retinaculum, the nerve is prone to compression injury (Goodgold et al. 1965, Oh and Meyer 1999). In the majority of patients tarsal tunnel syndrome is idiopathic with no clear precipitating factors detectable. The second most common cause is entrapment due to scare tissue or articular deformities originating from previous trauma (distortion or fracture of the ankle). Similar to the carpal tunnel, inflammatory, autoimmune (McGuigan et al. 1983) or hormonal changes (Oloff et al. 1983) can further decrease the lumen of the tunnel. Other sources of compression are an accessory flexor digitorum longus muscle (Kinoshita et al. 2003) and space occupying lesions within the tunnel such as lipoma, varicose veins, ganglia (Nagaoka and Satou 1999), intraneural ganglia (Spinner et al. 2007), non-traumatic exostosis or schwannoma. When predisposing physical factors are present strenuous sporting activities may aggravate the neurological symptoms (Kinoshita et al. 2006).

4.11.1.2 Diagnosis

If fully expressed (characteristic sensory and motor deficits), the posterior tarsal tunnel syndrome can easily be diagnosed on clinical grounds only. In the case of a pure pain syndrome, however, a correct diagnosis may be much more demanding and sometimes requires ancillary, e.g. radiological testing. In such patients a positive compression test (provocation of typical complaints by 30 s manual pressure applied on the tarsal tunnel) may be helpful. Standard electrodiagnostic testing may help to differentiate; however, normal results are not contraindicative to the presence of posterior tarsal tunnel. Interpretability of electrodiagnostic testing may be difficult in the events of coexisting neuropathy or severe damage of the nerve root S1. The procedure with the highest diagnostic sensitivity is a sonography-guided anaesthetic nerve block. Finally, an orthopedic examination is mandatory to distinguish posterior tarsal tunnel syndrome from numerous differential diagnoses such as stress fractures, bursitis, inflammatory arthritis or plantar fasciitis. It should be borne in mind that some of these conditions may affect tibial nerve function in terms of a (non-compressive) local irritation.

4.11.1.3 Sonography

Technical considerations for sonography of the tibial nerve at the tarsal tunnel are similar to what has been said for peroneal tunnel evaluation. A high resolution 12- to 17-MHz transducer is certainly recommended for this region. A stand-off gel pad may by helpful to achieve better contact to the concave tarsal surface. Identification of the distal tibial nerve is easily achieved in a transverse scan plane just above the medial malleolus, if the transducer is positioned in the groove that exists between the Achilles tendon and the posterior tibial margin (Peer et al. 2002). Here the nerve lies close to the posterior tibial vessels between the flexor hallucis longus and flexor digitorum muscle. Color Doppler may be used to identify the vascular bundle, which provides a fine landmark for localization of the nerve. The nerve is larger compared to the common peroneal nerve and its fascicular texture is normally better discernible. From this position the nerve is followed downward to the tarsal tunnel with documentation of its bifurcation. The two terminal tibial nerve branches are normally easily followed a certain way along their course to the planta pedis. The flexor retinaculum may normally be identified as a distinct hypoechoic line.

Sonographic findings in patients with tarsal tunnel syndrome depend on the etiology: with the existence of extra-articular ganglia displacement and bowing of the tibial nerve can be visualized (Fig. 4.56). When cystic enlargement of the tibial nerve is detected, a connection to the near joint should be suspected (Fig. 4.57) (Spinner et al. 2007). Posttraumatic changes causing external compression are easily confirmed in the same way as in any other anatomic regions, with direct nerve compression and reactive nerve edema representing a common pathway of neuropathy (Martinoli et al. 2000; Nagaoka and Satou 1999; Peer et al. 2002). Color Doppler ultrasound can confirm venous engorgement demonstrating venous vessels surrounding the tibial nerve. After long-standing nerve compression the affected nerve shows a wave-like appearance in a longitudinal scan, similar to the median nerve in carpal tunnel syndrome (Fig. 4.58). It is important to assess and compare the cross-sectional area on both nerves especially in idiopathic posterior tarsal tunnel syndrome. Direct trauma to the nerve with partial or complete dissection can easily be assessed with sonography (see Chap. 5).

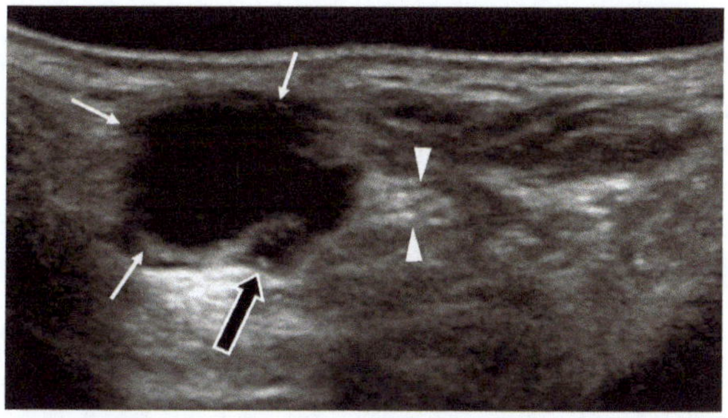

Fig. 4.57. Posterior tibial tunnel syndrome. Transverse 15-MHz scan at the level of the medial malleolus. A cystic mass (*small arrows*) is seen expanding within the medial plantar nerve, displacing the nerve fascicles marginally (*large arrow*). The lateral branch is unaffected (*arrowheads*)

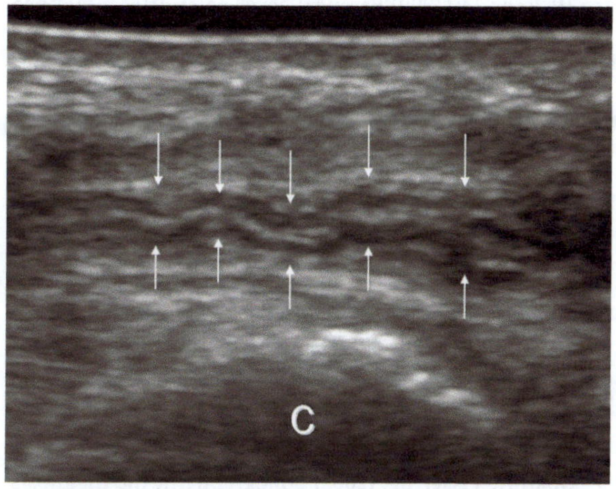

Fig. 4.58. Posterior tibial tunnel syndrome. At the level of the posterior tarsal tunnel, proximal to the compression, caused by an extra-articular cyst the tibial nerve demonstrates a wave-like appearance, typical for nerve compression of long-standing

4.11.1.4 Therapy

Potential sources of external compression, like poorly fitting shoes, should be eliminated. Sonography-guided local corticosteroid injections are sometimes helpful and sonography-guided aspiration of a ganglion may relieve pressure on the nerve. If posterior tarsal tunnel syndrome causes substantial discomfort or sensory-motor deficits and conservative treatment options fail operative release of the flexor retinaculum is the therapy of choice. Outcome after surgery is favourable in about 75% of patients (MONDELLI et al. 1998). NAGAOKA and SATOU (1999) described good surgical outcome resecting the talocalcaneal ganglion that caused posterior tarsal tunnel. A minority of patients develop chronic pain syndromes with features of reflex sympathetic dystrophy.

References

Altinok T, Baysal O, Karakas HM et al. (2004) Ultrasonographic assessment of mild and moderate idiopathic carpal tunnel syndrome. Clin Radiol 59:916–925

Arle JE, Zager EL (2000) Surgical treatment of common entrapment neuropathies in the upper limbs. Muscle Nerve 23:1160–1174

Asp JP, Rand JA (1990) Peroneal nerve palsy after total knee arthroplasty. Clin Orthop 233–237

Bahm J (2007) Critical review of pathophysiologic mechanisms in thoracic outlet syndrome (TOS). Acta Neurochir Suppl 100:137–179

Balaji MR, DeWeese JA (1981) Adductor canal outlet syndrome. JAMA 245:167–170

Balogh B, Vass A, Piza-Katzer H (1997) Ist eine Vorverlagerung des N. ulnaris beim Sulcus nervi ulnaris-Syndrom wirklich indiziert? Handchir Mikrochir Plast Chir 29:133–139

Baltopoulos P, Tsintzos C, Prionas G, Tsironi M (2008) Exercise-induced scalenus syndrome. Am J Sports Med 36:369

Bartelsls RH, Menovsky T, Van Overbeeke JJ (1998)Surgical management of ulnar nerve compression at the elbow: an analysis of the literature. J Neurosurg 89:722–727

Beekman R, Visser LH (2003) Sonography in the diagnosis of carpal tunnel syndrome: a critical review of the literature. Muscle Nerve 27:26–33

Bernhardt M (1878) Neuropathologische Beobachtungen. Deutsches Archiv für klinische Medizin, Leipzig 22:362–393

Bernhardt M (1895) Über isoliert im Gebiete d. Nervus cutaneus femoris externus vorkommende Paraesthesien. Neurologisches Zentralblatt 14:242–244

Bjurlin MA, Davis KE, Allin EF, Ibrahim DT (2007) Anatomic variations in the lateral femoral cutaneous nerve with respect to pediatric hip surgery. Am J Orthop 36:143–146

Blankstein A, Ganel A, Diamant L, Chechick A (2006) Cervical rib – preliminary data on diagnosis by ultrasound. Ultraschall Med. Aug 7 [Epub ahead of print]

Bodack MP, Tunkel RS, Marini SG, Nagler W (1998) Spinal accessory nerve palsy as a cause of pain after whiplash injury: case report. J Pain Symptom Manage 15:321–328

Bodner G, Buchberger W, Schocke M et al. (2001) Radial nerve palsy associated with humeral shaft fracture: evaluation with US – initial experience. Radiology 219:811–816

Bodner G, Harpf C, Meirer R et al. (2002) Ultrasonographic appearance of supinator syndrome. J Ultrasound Med 21:1289–1293

Bozentka DJ (1998) Cubital tunnel syndrome pathophysiology. Clin Orthop 351:90–94

Buchberger W, Schoen G, Strasser K et al. (1991) High resolution ultrasonography of the carpal tunnel. J Ultrasound Med 101:531–537

Buckwalter JA, Dryer RF, Mickelson MR (1979) Arthrography in juxta-articular cysts of the knee. Two cases diagnosed by delayed roentgenograms. J Bone Joint Surg Am 61:465

Buchberger W, Judmaier W, Birbamer G et al. (1992) Carpal tunnel syndrome: diagnosis with high resolution sonography. AJR Am J Roentgenol 159:793–798

Bui-Mansfield LT, Williamson M, Wheeler DT et al. (2002) Guyon's canal lipoma causing ulnar neuropathy. AJR Am J Roentgenol 178:1458

Carter BL, Racz GB (1994) Iliohypogastric nerve entrapment in pregnancy: diagnosis and treatment. Anesth Analg 79:1193–1194

Cartwright MS, Shin HW, Passmore LV, Walker FO (2007) Ultrasonographic findings of the normal ulnar nerve in adults. Arch Phys Med Rehabil 88:394–396

Chien AJ, Jamadar DA, Jacobson JA (2003) Sonography and MR imaging of posterior interosseous nerve syndrome with surgical correlation. AJR Am J Roentgenol 181:219–221

Childress HM (1975) Recurrent ulnar nerve dislocation at the elbow. Clin Orthop 108:168–173

Chiou HJ, Chou YH, Cheng SP et al. (1998) Cubital tunnel syndrome: diagnosis by high resolution ultrasonography. J Ultrasound Med 17:643–648

Contreras MG, Warner MA, Charboneau WJ (1998) Anatomy of the ulnar nerve at the elbow: potential relationship of acute ulnar neuropathy to gender differences. Clin Anat 11:372–378

Créteur V, Bacq C, Fumière E, Bissen L, Delcour C (2007) Sonography of peripheral nerves. Part II: lower limbs. J Radiol 88:349–360

de Fijter WM, Scheltinga MR, Luiting MG (2006) Minimally invasive fasciotomy in chronic exertional compartment syndrome and fascial hernias of the anterior lower leg: short- and long-term results. Mil Med 171:399–403

Daghino W, Pasquali M, Faletti C (1997) Superficial peroneal nerve entrapment in a young athlete: the diagnostic contribution of magnetic resonance imaging. J Foot Ankle Surg 36:170–172

Dallari D, Pellacani A, Marinelli A (2004) Deep peroneal nerve paresis in a runner caused by ganglion at capitulum peronei. Case report and review of the literature. J Sports Med Phys Fitness 44:436–440

Degreef I, De Smet L (2004) Anterior interosseous nerve paralysis due to Gantzer's muscle. Acta Orthop Belg 70:482–484

DeLisa JA, Saeed MA (1983) The tarsal tunnel syndrome. Muscle Nerve 6:664–670

Dellon AL, Hament W, Gittelshon A (1993) Nonoperative management of cubital tunnel syndrome: an 8-year prospective study. Neurology 43:1673–1677

Dilley A, Greening J, Lynn B et al. (2001) The use of cross correlation analysis between high frequency ultrasound images to measure longitudinal median nerve movement. Ultrasound Med Biol 27:1211–1218

Demondion X, Vidal C, Herbinet P (2006) Imaging assessment of thoracic outlet syndrome. Radiographics 26:1735–1750

Duncan I, Sullivan P, Lomas F (1999) Sonography in the diagnosis of carpal tunnel syndrome. AJR Am J Roentgenol 173:681–684

Eversmann W (1988) Entrapment and compression neuropathies. In: Green DP (ed) Operative hand surgery, vol 2. Churchill Livingstone, New York, pp 1430–1441

Feindel W, Stratford J (1958) The role of the cubital tunnel in tardy ulnar palsy. Can J Surg 1:287–300

Foxall GL, Skinner D, Hardman JG, Bedforth NM (2007) Ultrasound anatomy of the radial nerve in the distal upper arm. Reg Anesth Pain Med 32:217–220

Freud S (1895) Über die Bernhardsche Sensibilitätsstörung. Neurol Centralbl 14:491–492

Garfin S, Mubarak SJ, Owen CA (1977) Exertional anterolateral-compartment syndrome. Case report with fascial defect, muscle herniation, and superficial peroneal-nerve entrapment. J Bone Joint Surg Am 59:404–405

Gassner E, Schocke M, Peer S et al. (2002) Persistent median artery in the carpal tunnel – color Doppler ultrasonographic findings. J Ultrasound Med 21:455–461

Gervasio O, Gambardella G, Zaccone C, Branca D (2005) Simple decompression versus anterior submuscular transposition of the ulnar nerve in severe cubital tunnel syndrome: a prospective randomized study. Neurosurgery 56:108–1017

Goodgold J, Kopell HP, Spieholz NI (1965) The tarsal tunnel syndrome. N Engl J Med 273:742–746

Green DP (1984) Diagnostic and therapeutic value of carpal tunnel injection. J Hand Surg 9:850–854

Gillard J, Pérez-Cousin M, Hachulla E et al. (2001) Diagnosing thoracic outlet syndrome: contribution of provocative tests, ultrasonography, electrophysiology, and helical computed tomography in 48 patients. Joint Bone Spine 68:416–420

Grosz CR (1981) Iliohypogastric nerve injury. Am J Surg 142:628

Grothaus MC, Holt M, Mekhail AO et al. (1997) Lateral femoral cutaneous nerve: an anatomic study. Surg Radiol Anat 19:307

Gruber H, Peer S, Meirer R, Bodner G (2005) Peroneal nerve palsy associated with knee luxation: evaluation by sonography – initial experiences. AJR Am J Roentgenol 185:1119–1125

Hamdan FB, Jaffar AA, Ossi RG (2008) The propensity of common peroneal nerve in thigh-level injuries. J Trauma 64:300–303

Harney D, Patijn J (2007) Meralgia paresthetica: diagnosis and management strategies. Pain Med 8:669–677

Harvie P, Patel N, Ostlere SJ (2003) Ulnar nerve compression at Guyon's canal by an anomalous abductor digiti minimi muscle: the role of ultrasound in clinical diagnosis. Hand Surg 8:271–275

Haussmann P, Patel MR (1996) Intraepineurial constriction of nerve fascicles in pronator syndrome and anterior interosseous nerve syndrome. Orthop Clin North Am 27:339–344

Harpf C, Rhomberg M, Rumer A, Hussl H (1999) Iatrogenic lesion of the accessory nerve in cervical lymph node biopsy. Chirurg 70:690–693

Hide IG, Grainger AJ, Naisby GP, Campbell RS (1999) Sonographic findings in the anterior interosseous nerve syndrome. J Clin Ultrasound 27:459–464

Hurdle MF, Weingarten TN, Crisostomo RA et al. (2007) Ultrasound-guided blockade of the lateral femoral cutaneous nerve: technical description and review of 10 cases. Arch Phys Med Rehabil 88:1362–1364

House JH, Ahmed K (1977) Entrapment neuropathy of the infrapatellar branch of the saphenous nerve. Am J Sports Med 5:217–224

Hunter LY, Louis DS, Ricciardi JR, O'Connor GA (1979) The saphenous nerve: its course and importance in medial arthrotomy. Am J Sports Med 7:227–230

Jacob D, Creteur V, Courthaliac C et al. (2004) Sonoanatomy of the ulnar nerve in the cubital tunnel: a multicentre study by the GEL. Eur Radiol 14:1770–1773

Jacobson JA, Jebson PJL, Jeffers AW et al. (2001) Ulnar nerve dislocation and snapping triceps syndrome: diagnosis with dynamic sonography – report of three cases. Radiology 220:601–605

Jamadar DA, Jacobson JA, Hayes CW (2001) Sonographic evaluation of the median nerve at the wrist. J Ultrasound Med 20:1011–1014

Johnson RK, Spinner M, Shrewsbury MM (1979) Median nerve entrapment syndrome in the proximal forearm. J Hand Surg [Am] 4:48–51

Kalb K, Gruber P, Landsleitner B (1999) Die nicht traumatisch bedingte Parese des Ramus profungdus nervi radialis. Aspekte eines seltenen Krankheitsbildes. Handchir Mikrochir Plast Chir 32:26–32

Kaminsky F (1947) Peroneal palsy by crossing the legs. JAMA 134:206

Keck C (1962) The tarsal tunnel syndrome. J Bone Joint Surg 44A:180–182

Kho KH, Blijham PJ, Zwarts MJ (2005) Meralgia paresthetica after strenuous exercise. Muscle Nerve 31:761–763. KHO 2005

Kierner AC, Zelenka I, Heller S, Burian M (2000) Surgical anatomy of the spinal accessory nerve and the trapezius branches of the cervical plexus. Arch Surg 135:1428–1431

Kiloh LG, Nevin S (1952) Isolated neuritis of the anterior interosseous nerve. Br Med J 1:850–851

Kinoshita M, Okuda R, Morikawa J, Abe M (2003) Tarsal tunnel syndrome associated with an accessory muscle. Foot Ankle Int 24:132–136

Kinoshita M, Okuda R, Yasuda T, Abe M (2006) Tarsal tunnel syndrome in athletes. Am J Sports Med 34:1307–1312

Kleindienst A, Hamm B, Lanksch WR (1998) Carpal tunnel syndrome: staging of median nerve compression by MR imaging. J Magn Reson Imaging 8:1119–1125

Kopell HP, Thompson WA (1960) Peripheral entrapment neuropathies of the lower extremities. N Engl J Med 262:56–60

Kumak D (1987) The facts of Kathmandu: squatters palsy. JAMA 257:28

Kuschner SH, Ebramzadeh E, Johnson D et al. (1992) Tinel's sign and Phalen's test in carpal tunnel syndrome. Orthopedics 15:1297–1302

Koyuncuoglu HR, Kutluhan S, Yesildag A et al. (2005) The value of ultrasonographic measurement in carpal tunnel syndrome in patients with negative electrodiagnostic tests. Eur J Radiol 56:365–369

Kwon BC, Jung KI, Baek GH (2008) Comparison of sonography and electrodiagnostic testing in the diagnosis of carpal tunnel syndrome. J Hand Surg 33:65–71

Lacey SH, Soldatis JJ (1993) Bilateral pronator syndrome associated with anomalous heads of the pronator teres muscle: a case report. J Hand Surg [Am] 18:349–351

Lanzetta M, Foucher G (1995) Entrapment of the superficial branch of the radial nerve (Wartenberg's syndrome). A report of 52 cases. Plast Reconstr Surg 96:408–412

Learmonth JR (1933) The principle of decompression in the treatment of certain diseases of peripheral nerves. Surg Clin North Am 13:905–913

LeGeyt MT, Ambrose J (1998) Nontraumatic compression of the common peroneal nerve: a case report and review of the literature. Am J Orthop 27:521–523

Lee D, van Holsbeeck MT, Janevski PK, Ganos DL, Ditmars DM, Darian VB (1999) Diagnosis of carpal tunnel syndrome. Ultrasound versus electromyography. Radiol Clin North Am 37:859–872

Lippitt AB (1993) Neuropathy of the saphenous nerve as a cause of knee pain. Bull Hosp Jt Dis 52:31–33

Longley DG, Yedlicka JW, Molina EJ et al. (1992) Thoracic outlet syndrome: evaluation of the subclavian vessels by color duplex sonography. AJR Am J Roentgenol 158:623–630

Lorea P, Schuind F (2000) False aneurysm appearing as delayed ulnar nerve palsy after minor penetrating trauma in the forearm. J Trauma 51:144–145

Lorei MP, Hershman EB (1993) Peripheral nerve injuries in athletes. Treatment and prevention. Sports Med 16:130–147

Lubahn JD, Cermak MB (1998) Uncommon nerve compression syndromes of the upper extremity. J Am Acad Orthop Surg 6:378–86

Lundblad M, Kapral S, Marhofer P et al. (2006) Ultrasound-guided infrapatellar nerve block in human volunteers: description of a novel technique. Br J Anaesth 97:710–714

Malghem J, Vande berg BC, Lebon C, Lecouvet FE, Maldague BE (1998) Ganglion cysts of the knee: articular communication revealed by delayed radiography and CT after arthrography. AJR Am J Roentgenol 170:1579–1583

Mallouhi A, Pülzl P, Trieb T, Piza H, Bodner G (2006) Predictors of carpal tunnel syndrome: accuracy of gray-scale and color Doppler sonography. AJR Am J Roentgenol 186:1240–1245

Mándi A, Kalmár L (1973) Nervus saphenus syndrome. Orv Hetil 114:925–926

Marie P, Foix C (1913) Atrophie isolee de l'eminence thenar d'origine nevritique: role du ligament annulaire anterieur du carpe dans la pathogenie de la lesion. Revue Neurology (Paris) 26:647–649

Martinoli C, Serafini G, Bianchi S et al. (1996) Ultrasonography of peripheral nerves. J Peripher Nerv Syst 1:169–174

Martinoli C, Bianchi S, Gandolfo N et al. (2000) Ultrasound of nerve entrapment in osteofibrous tunnels of the upper and lower limbs. Radiographics 20:199–217

Martinoli C, Bianchi S, Dahmane MH et al. (2002) Ultrasound of tendons and nerves. Eur Radiol 12:44–55

Martinoli C, Bianchi S, Pugliese F et al. (2004) Sonography of entrapment neuropathies in the upper limb (wrist excluded). J Clin Ultrasound 32:438–450

Mazurek MT, Shin AY (2001) Upper extremity peripheral nerve anatomy: current concepts and applications. Clin Orthop 383:7–20

McCrory P, Bell S, Bradshaw C (2002) Nerve entrapments of the lower leg, ankle and foot in sport. Sports Med 32:371–91

McGuigan L, Burke D, Fleming A (1983) Tarsal tunnel syndrome and peripheral neuropathy in rheumatoid disease. Ann Rheum Dis 42:128–131

Miller RG (1991) AAEM case report #1: ulnar neuropathy at the elbow. Muscle Nerve 14:97–101

Miller RG, Camp PE (1979) Postoperative ulnar neuropathy. JAMA 242:1636–1639

Miller RG, Hummel EE (1980) The cubital tunnel syndrome: treatment with simple decompression. Ann Neurol 7:567–569

Mirovsky Y, Neuwirth M (2000) Injuries to the lateral femoral cutaneous nerve during spine surgery. Spine 25:126

Miyata K, Kitamura H (1997) Accessory nerve damages and impaired shoulder movements after neck dissections. Am J Otolaryngol 18:197–201

Machiels F, Shahabpour M, De Maeseneer M et al. (1999) Tarsal tunnel syndrome: ultrasonographic and MRI features. JBR-BTR 82:49–50

Mochida H, Kikuchi S (1995) Injury to infrapatellar branch of saphenous nerve in arthroscopic knee surgery. Clin Orthop Relat Res 320:88–94

Monagle K, Dai G, Chu A et al. (1999) Quantitative MR imaging of carpal tunnel syndrome. AJR Am J Roentgenol 172:1582–1586

Mondelli M, Giannini F, Reale F (1998) Clinical and electrophysiological findings and follow-up in tarsal tunnel syndrome. Electroencephalogr Clin Neurophysiol 109:418–425

Mumenthaler M, Schliack H, Stoehr M (1998) Läsionen peripherer Nerven und radikuläre Läsionen. Thieme, Stuttgart

Murphy JB (1905) IV. A case of cervical rib with symptoms resembling subclavian aneurism. Ann Surg 41:399

Nagaoka M, Satou K (1999) Tarsal tunnel syndrome caused by ganglia. J Bone Joint Surg Br 81:607

Naffziger HC, Grant WT (1938) Neuritis of the brachial plexus mechanical in origin: the scalenus syndrome. Surg Gynecol Obstet 67:722–730

Nakamichi K, Tachibana S (2007) Ultrasonographic findings in isolated neuritis of the posterior interosseous nerve: comparison with normal findings. J Ultrasound Med 26:683–687

Nason RW, Abdulrauf BM, Stranc MF (2000) The anatomy of the accessory nerve and cervical lymph node biopsy. Am J Surg 180:241–342

Nigst H, Dick W (1979) Syndromes of compression of the median nerve in the proximal forearm (pronator teres syndrome; anterior interosseous nerve syndrome). Arch Orthop Trauma Surg 93:307–312

Nora DB, Becker J, Ehlers JA, Gomes I (2005) What symptoms are truly caused by median nerve compression in carpal tunnel syndrome? Clin Neurophysiol 116:275–83

O'Driscoll SW, Horii E, Carmichael SW et al. (1992) The cubital tunnel and ulnar neuropathy. J Bone Joint Surg Br 74:84–94

Ogino T, Minami A, Kato H (1991) Diagnosis of radial nerve palsy caused by ganglion with use of different imaging techniques. J Hand Surg [Am] 16:230–235

Oh SH, Meyer RD (1999) Entrapment neuropathies of the tibial (posterior tibial) nerve. Neurol Clin 17:593–615

Okamoto M, Abe M, Shirai H et al. (2000) Morphology and dynamics of the ulnar nerve in the cubital tunnel: diagnosis by high resolution ultrasonography. J Hand Surg [Br] 25:85–89

Oloff LM, Jacobs AM, Jaffe S (1983) Tarsal tunnel syndrome: a manifestation of systemic disease. Foot Surg 22:302–307
Papastergiou SG, Voulgaropoulos H, Mikalef P et al. (2006) Injuries to the infrapatellar branch(es) of the saphenous nerve in anterior cruciate ligament reconstruction with four-strand hamstring tendon autograft: vertical versus horizontal incision for harvest. Knee Surg Sports Traumatol Arthrosc 14:789–793
Park GY, Kim JM, Lee SM (2004) The ultrasonographic and electrodiagnostic findings of ulnar neuropathy at the elbow. Arch Phys Med Rehabil 85:1000–1005
Paget J (1854) Lectures on surgical pathology. Lindsay and Blakiston, Philadelphia
Pecina MM, Krmpotic-Nemanic J, Markiewitz AD (eds) (2001) Tunnel syndromes. Peripheral nerve compression syndromes, 3rd edn. CRC-LLC Press, Boca Raton
Pedrazzini M, Pogliacomi F, Cusmano F et al. (2002) Bilateral ganglion cyst of the common peroneal nerve. Eur Radiol 12:2803–2806
Peer S, Kovacs P, Harpf C (2002) High resolution sonography of lower extremity peripheral nerves: anatomic correlation and spectrum of pathology. J Ultrasound Med 21:315–322
Peeters EY, Nieboer KH, Osteaux MM (2004) Sonography of the normal ulnar nerve at Guyon's canal and of the common peroneal nerve dorsal to the fibular head. J Clin Ultrasound 32:375–380
Phalen GS (1966) The carpal tunnel syndrome: seventeen years' experience in diagnosis and treatment of six hundred fifty-four hands. J Bone Joint Surg 48A:211–228
Phalen GS, Kendrick JI, Rodriguez JM (1971) Lipomas of the upper extremity. A series of fifteen tumors in the hand and wrist and six tumors causing nerve compression. Am J Surg 121:298–306
Portland GH, Martin D, Keene G, Menz T (2005) Injury to the infrapatellar branch of the saphenous nerve in anterior cruciate ligament reconstruction: comparison of horizontal versus vertical harvest site incisions. Arthroscopy 21:281–285
Prevel CD, Matloub HS, Zhong Y et al. (1993) The extrinsic blood supply of the ulnar nerve at the elbow: an anatomic study. J Hand Surg 18A:433–438
Puig S, Turkhof E, Sedivy R et al. (1999) Sonographic diagnosis of recurrent ulnar nerve compression by ganglion cysts. J Ultrasound Med 18:433–436
Ritts GD, Wood MB, Linscheid RL (1987) Radial tunnel syndrome. A ten-year surgical experience. Clin Orthop 219:201–205
Roles NC, Maudsley RH (1972) Radial tunnel syndrome. Resistant tennis elbow as a nerve entrapment. J Bone Joint Surg 54B:499–508
Roth VK (1878) Meralgia paresthetica. Karger, Berlin
Rosenbaum R (1999) Disputed radial tunnel syndrome. Muscle Nerve 22:960–967
Rosenbaum RB, Ochoa JL (1993) Carpal tunnel syndrome and other disorders of the median nerve. Butterworth-Heinemann, Boston
Rossey-Marec D (2004) Ultrasonographic appearance of idiopathic radial nerve constriction proximal to the elbow. J Ultrasound Med 23:1003-1007
Roos DB (1996) Historical perspectives and anatomic considerations. Thoracic outlet syndrome. Semin Thorac Cardiovasc Surg 8:183–189
Sanders RJ, Hammond SL, Rao NM (2007) Diagnosis of thoracic outlet syndrome. J Vasc Surg 46:601–604
Sanders RJ, Hammond SL (2002) Management of cervical ribs and anomalous first ribs causing neurogenic thoracic outlet syndrome. J Vasc Surg 36:51–56
Sarria L, Cabada T, Cozcolluela R et al. (2000) Carpal tunnel syndrome: usefulness of sonography. Eur Radiol 10:1920–1925
Seror P (1986) Anterior interosseous nerve syndrome. Electromyographic characteristics (2 cases) and review of the literature (62 cases) Rev Electroencephalogr Neurophysiol Clin 16:153–163
Seror P (1999) Lateral femoral cutaneous nerve conduction v somatosensory evoked potentials for electrodiagnosis of meralgia paresthetica. Am J Phys Med Rehabil 78:313–316
Seyffarth H (1951) Primary myoses in the M. pronator teres as cause of lesion of the N. medianus (the pronator syndrome). Acta Psychiatr Neurol Scand Suppl 74:251–254
Shea JD, McClain EJ (1969) Ulnar nerve compression syndromes at and bellow the wrist. J Bone Joint Surg 51:1095–1103
Sidey JD (1969) Weak ankles: a study of common peroneal entrapment neuropathy. BMJ 3:623–626
Spinner M (1968) The arcade of Frohse and its relationship to posterior interosseous nerve paralysis. J Bone Joint Surg 50B:809–812
Spinner M (1970) The anterior interosseous-nerve syndrome, with special attention to its variations. J Bone Joint Surg Am 52:84–94
Spinner RJ, Atkinson JLD, Tiel RL (2003) Peroneal intraneural ganglia: the importance of the articular branch. A unifying theory. J Neurosurg 99:330–333
Spinner RJ, Desy NM, Amrami KK (2006a) Cystic transverse limb of the articular branch: a pathognomonic sign for peroneal intraneural ganglia at the superior tibiofibular joint. Neurosurgery 59:157–166
Spinner RJ, Scheithauer BW, Desy NM et al. (2006b) Coexisting secondary intraneural and vascular adventitial ganglion cyst of joint origin: a causal rather than a coincidental relationship supporting an articular theory. Skeletal Radiol 35:734–744
Spinner RJ, Amrami KK, Rock MG (2006c) The use of MR arthrography to detect occult joint communication in a recurrent peroneal intraneural ganglion. Skeletal Radiol 35:172–179
Spinner RJ, Dellon AL, Rosson G et al. (2007) Tibial intraneural ganglia in the tarsal tunnel: is there a joint connection. J Foot Ankle Surg 1:27–31
Spinner RJ, Goldner RO (1998) Snapping of the medial head of the triceps and recurrent dislocation of the ulnar nerve. J Bone Joint Surg Am 80:239–247
Stapleton C, Herrington L, George K (2007) Sonographic evaluation of the subclavian artery during thoracic outlet syndrome shoulder manoeuvres. Man Ther [Epub ahead of print]
Stark E, Oestreich K, Wendl K et al. (1999) Nerve irritation after laparoscopic hernia repair. Surg Endosc 13:878–881
Stewart JD (1993) Compression and entrapment neuropathies. In: Dyck PJ, Thomas PK (eds) Peripheral neuropathy, 3rd edn. Saunders, Philadelphia, pp 1354–1379

Stoehr M, Bluthardt M (1993) Atlas der klinischen Elektromyographie und Neurographie. Kohlhammer, Stuttgart
Stulz P, Pfeiffer KM (1982) Peripheral nerve injuries resulting from common surgical procedures in the lower portion of the abdomen. Arch Surg 117:324–327
Sturzenegger M, Rutz M (1991) Radial nerve paralysis – causes, site and diagnosis. Analysis of 103 cases. Nervenarzt 62:722–729
Szabo RM, Chidgey LK (1989) Stress carpal tunnel pressures in patients with carpal tunnel syndrome and normal patients. J Hand Surg 14:624–627
Tagliafico A, Resmini E, Nizzo R et al. (2008) Ultrasound measurement of median and ulnar nerve cross-sectional area in acromegaly. J Clin Endocrinol Metab 93:905–909
Terrell JE, Welsh DE, Bradford CR, Chepeha DB, Esclamado RM, Hogikyan ND, Wolf GT (2000) Pain, quality of life, and spinal accessory nerve status after neck dissection. Laryngoscope 110:620–626
Tsai CC, Lin TM, Lai CS, Lin SD (2001) Tarsal tunnel syndrome secondary to neurilemoma – a case report. Kaohsiung J Med Sci 17:216-220
Tumber PS, Bhatia A, Chan VW (2008) Ultrasound-guided lateral femoral cutaneous nerve block for meralgia paresthetica. Anesth Analg 106:1021–1022
Urschel HC, Kourlis H (2007) Thoracic outlet syndrome: a 50-year experience at Baylor University Medical Center Proc (Bayl Univ Med Cent) 20:125–135
Vaccaro AR, Ludwig SC, Klein GR, McQuire M, Green D, Green NE (1998) Bilateral peroneal nerve palsy secondary to a knee board: report of two cases. Am J Orthop 27:746–748
Vandeweyer E, Goldschmidt D, de Fontaine S (1998) Traumatic spinal accessory nerve palsy. J Reconstr Microsurg 14:259–261
Visser LH, Smidt MH, Lee ML (2008) High-resolution sonography versus EMG in the diagnosis of carpal tunnel syndrome. J Neurol Neurosurg Psychiatry 79:63–67
Wartenberg R (1932) Cheiralgia Parestetica (Isolierte. Neuritis des Ramus superficialis nervi radialis). Z Ger Neurol Psychiatr 141:145–155
Wiater JM, Bigliani LU (1999) Spinal accessory nerve injury. Clin Orthop 368:5–16
Wiesler ER, Chloros GD, Cartwright MS et al. (2006) Ultrasound in the diagnosis of ulnar neuropathy at the cubital tunnel. J Hand Surg [Am] 31:1088–1093
Wilhelm A (1985) Das proximale Radialiskompressionssyndrom. Behandlung und Ergebnisse. Handchirurgie 17:215–224
Wong SM, Griffith JF, Hui AC et al. (2004) Carpal tunnel syndrome: diagnostic usefulness of sonography. Radiology 232:93–99
Wilson SAK (1955) Neurology, 2nd ed. Williams & Wilkins, Baltimore, p 369
Yang SH, Wu CC, Chen PQ (2005) Postoperative meralgia paresthetica after posterior spine surgery: incidence, risk factors, and clinical outcomes. Spine 30:547–550
Yang LJ, Gala VC, McGillicuddy JE (2006) Superficial peroneal nerve syndrome: an unusual nerve entrapment. Case report. J Neurosurg 104:820–823
Yoon JS, Kim BJ, Kim SJ et al. (2007) Ultrasonographic measurements in cubital tunnel syndrome. Muscle Nerve 36:853–855
Ziswiler HR, Reichenbach S, Vögelin E et al. (2005) Diagnostic value of sonography in patients with suspected carpal tunnel syndrome: a prospective study. Arthritis Rheum 52:304–311
Zlowodzki M, Chan S, Bhandari M et al. (2007) Anterior transposition compared with simple decompression for treatment of cubital tunnel syndrome. A meta-analysis of randomized, controlled trials. J Bone Joint Surg Am 89:2591–2598
Zöch G, Aigner N (1997) Wartenberg syndrome: a rare or rarely diagnosed compression syndrome of the radial nerve? Handchir Mikrochir Plast Chir 29:139–143

Traumatic Nerve Lesions

5

Siegfried Peer and Hannes Gruber

CONTENTS

5.1 General Considerations

Traumatic lesions of peripheral nerves are common. According to the literature a relevant lesion of a peripheral nerve exists in roughly 2%–3% of patients admitted to Level I trauma centers. If plexus and root injuries are included the incidence rises to about 5% (Noble et al. 1998; Robinson 2000). In general, these types of injuries are increasingly recognized in today's clinical practice, because of improved trauma services. Besides the medical impact of these lesions they constitute a major social problem, as recovery is often incomplete (especially in cases of delayed treatment), which may result in long lasting disability. This is even more troublesome, as patients with these types of injuries belong to a younger and highly productive age group within the trauma population. Institution of

S. Peer, MD
Professor, Department of Radiology, Section for Diagnostic and Interventional Sonography, Innsbruck Medical University, Anichstrasse 35, 6020 Innsbruck, Austria
H. Gruber, MD
Associate Professor, Department of Radiology, Innsbruck Medical University, Anichstrasse 35, 6020 Innsbruck, Austria

adequate and early treatment is the only chance to prevent unfavorable outcomes and therefore an exact diagnostic work-up is mandatory. Traditionally these lesions were evaluated with a combination of clinical examination and neurological function tests (nerve conduction studies and electromyography). Electrodiagnosis may precisely discern low grade lesions without axonal loss ("Neurapraxia" according to the Seddon/Sunderland classification), from higher grade lesions which consist of axon loss and some damage to one or more of the nerve sheath elements ("Axonotmesis/Neurotmesis") (Seddon 1975; Sunderland 1978). As far as localization of lesions is concerned electromyography and nerve conduction studies are affected by a variety of pitfalls, and therefore may often not yield reliable information about the precise site of nerve involvement. In the same way electrodiagnostic tests do not give concise information in making a decision for conservative or surgical therapy. Often a trial of conservative treatment is instituted, but distinct nerve lesions may show better outcome when operated within the first week after injury (Alan 2000; Birch and Raji 1991). If, in the case of conservative treatment, the nerve does not show recovery on follow-up examinations surgery is performed. Nevertheless, early surgery would be more appropriate even in purely neurapraxic lesions if the nerve is encased by scar tissue, in which case it may not recover during conservative treatment. This diagnosis, however, is beyond the scope of electrodiagnosis and may only be accomplished with direct imaging of the nerve itself and here sonography (Peer et al. 2001) and other imaging techniques may be helpful, as they allow for direct visualization of the nerve and its surroundings, thus setting the path for early institution of surgery in cases where improvement of nerve function with conservative treatment is not to be expected. The latter is true for completely or partially dissected nerves, nerves compressed by close lying hematomas or bony spurs in the case of coexisting fractures, etc.

The reasons for a traumatic peripheral nerve lesion are manifold but several large groups may be discerned in general: Firstly, direct lesions occurring during the course of trauma, which affects the nerve itself (sharp transection of the median nerve during suicide attempts, for example); secondly, indirect lesions, such as combination injuries with a fracture accompanied by a nerve lesion. In the same way we may delimit primary nerve lesions, such as transections, from secondary nerve lesions (gradually developing compression of a nerve by scar tissue formation, bony callus or an organizing hematoma, for example). Each of these subgroups may have distinct features, but from a mere pathophysiologic point of view the way a nerve reacts on external stress shows only small variations. Iatrogenic nerve lesions raise additional questions: while the first group implies mainly a medical problem, the latter constitute a medico-legal problem, due to coexisting issues of malpractice and insurance (Birch et al. 1991; Peer et al. 2001; Wilbourn 1998). Especially in the latter group exact documentation of the type and extent of a nerve lesion is necessary and the differentiation between a lesion which is truly related to bad medical practice (such as transection of the accessory nerve during neck dissection) and a lesion which is due to some type of unfavorable clinical outcome (development of scar tissue for example) is of outmost importance.

5.2 Traumatic Lesions of the Brachial Plexus

(H. Gruber)

Magnetic resonance imaging and computed tomographic myelography are currently considered the techniques of choice for imaging of the brachial plexus (Yoshikawa et al. 2006). In current clinical practice most centers favor MRI because of the inherent multiplanar capabilities and high soft tissue contrast. Several studies report on the use of these methods for the diagnosis of traumatic plexus lesions; Doi et al. (2002), for example, reported a sensitivity of 92% for combined MRI and CT myelography in the diagnosis of nerve root avulsion. With separate assessment of the two modalities an accuracy of 85% for CT myelography and 52% for MRI in the diagnosis of brachial plexus lesions was reported (Carvalho et al. 1997; Penkert et al. 1999). While most users are not aware of the limited spatial resolution of MRI, the latter studies addressed this issue, pointing out that high specificity can only be achieved with sufficient in plane resolution.

A general benefit of sonography is its unrivaled spatial resolution; however, paired with a relatively low imaging contrast (compared with MRI for example). For several years sonography was mainly used for imaging guided regional anesthesia (Sheppard et al. 1998; Yang et al. 1998) (see also Chap. 7, Sect. 7.2), but together with other research groups we could recently demonstrate the diagnostic power of sonography in the evaluation of brachial plexus injury (Haber et al. 2006; Gruber et al. 2007b).

In the subsequent paragraph an overview of possible applications of sonography to imaging of traumatic plexus lesions is given.

5.2.1 Etiology

A variety of traumatic events may result in direct injuries of the brachial plexus: shoulder trauma, head and neck trauma, direct thoracic trauma and subacute impairment by primary hematoma. Secondary causes for brachial plexus palsy are fractures of the clavicle with subsequent scaring or callus formation and iatrogenic injuries due to surgery of tumors at the thoracic apex or in the neck region. Nerve root avulsion injury occurs in accidents with severe traction on the upper extremity, most often seen in motorbike accidents. Depending on the force applied, such injuries may simultaneously affect the plexus from its cervical roots down to the supra- and even infraclavicular elements known as "chain injuries". Iatrogenic plexus lesions (traction due to bad positioning of the arm during operations) are often complex and difficult to diagnose (De Laat et al. 1994; Boardman and Cofield 1999), as they do not follow typical morphological patterns known from "true traumatic lesions". Nevertheless they have to be handled with special care because of the forensic aspects involved.

5.2.2 Clinical Diagnosis

Brachial plexus palsy shows a varying combination of sensory deficits, dysesthesia or hyperesthesia, together with muscle weakness and motor deficits, depending on the level and degree of injury. In most patients the clinical signs and symptoms are ambiguous and thus the injured part of the plexus (root, fascicle, etc.) is not easily identified. Electrophysiological testing shortly after the injury and in monthly controls can reliably assess the gross level of injury and show signs of nerve regeneration.

5.2.3 Sonography

We perform sonography with a 7–12 or a 9–3 MHz linear array transducer depending on patient size and weight. Standard post-processing such as image compounding and artifact reduction software is used. The patient is positioned supine, with the head turned slightly to the opposite side of the investigated area (if possible). Sonograms should always be acquired in a transverse and longitudinal scan, at the level of the intervertebral foramen (roots) and in the supra- and infraclavicular region (trunks and fascicles). The identification of the exact level of a cervical root is best done with use of the course of the vertebral artery and the configuration of the transverse processes of the cervical spine as anatomical landmarks (Martinoli et al. 2002). The cervical roots appear as hypoechoic rounded clearly bordered structures if scanned axially and tubular sometimes slightly bulbous structures arising from the intervertebral foramen in longitudinal scans. Especially in slender patients with a long and thin neck even the foraminal base of the nerve root can be assessed with sufficient clarity (Fig. 5.1). The cervical roots from C4–C7 can always be depicted, whereas the root C8 is often shadowed, especially in obese patients with short necks. However, visualization may be improved if the patient's shoulder is relaxed and lowered. Sometimes, with examination of the more inferior roots, better results may be achieved with the patient in a sitting position.

In the interscalene region the trunks of the plexus are formed and – if scanned axially – appear as a cluster of sharply lined hypoechoic nodules interposed between the scalenus anterior and medius muscle accompanied by the subclavian artery. The latter can easily be identified because of its typical appearance, with pulsation demonstrated in B-mode or with duplex sonography. The medial, posterior and lateral plexus fascicle – which surround the subclavian artery – are identified by scanning the peri-, the infraclavicular and the proximal axillary region. In longitudinal scans the plexus elements are depicted as hypoechoic tubular structures, with occasional thin internal hyperechoic elements which relate to various amounts of interfascicular epineural tissue. With optimal scanning technique only a short segment of the plexus traversing underneath the clavicle is routinely not accessible to sonography. The size and structure of each plexus element is routinely documented in comparison to the non-injured opposite side.

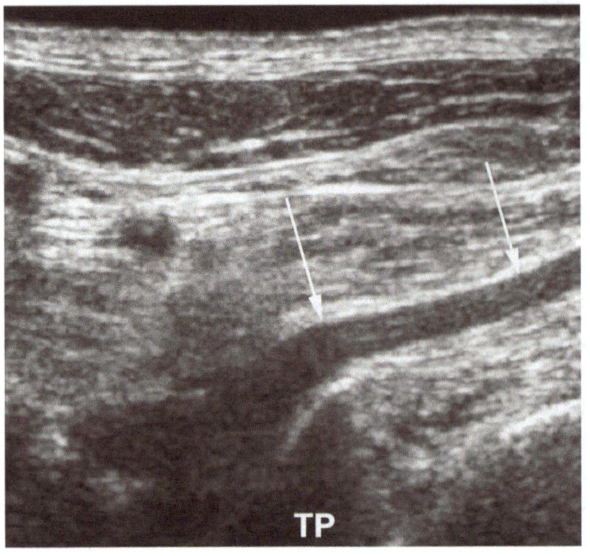

Fig. 5.1. Longitudinal sonogram through C6 nerve root (*arrows*) in a healthy asymptomatic volunteer demonstrates sonographic visualization of the entire nerve root to the neural foramen. *TP*, transverse spinal process

Traction neuroma, localized edema (Fig. 5.2) and post-traumatic scaring are the most common traumatic plexus lesions. In the plexus region traction neuromas show the same characteristic "pollywog" appearance of neuroma in a peripheral nerve, with hypoechoic enlargement of structures proximal to the level of injury (Fig. 5.3a,b). With severe traction a so-called neuroma in continuity – multiple neuromas at different levels inside a plexus segment – may develop (Fig. 5.4). If a neuroma is caused by partial avulsion it is embedded eccentrically in the partially continuous plexus element.

Dissections are demonstrated best in longitudinal scans, and in the case of an acute complete transection show a complete interruption of the fascicles with a variably sized gap between two stumps (Fig. 5.5).

These findings, however, seem to follow a temporal dynamic: when examined in the early acute setting both dissected nerve stumps may show about the same size. On subsequent controls the proximal stump changes its shape and appears bulbous and hypoechoic, which reflects proximal axonal congestion as expression of ongoing reparative mechanisms with sprouting of axons.

Even foraminal root avulsions may be demonstrated in optimal conditions, with demonstration of an empty meningeal sac at the root exit from the neural foramen (Fig. 5.6a,b) and a peripheral stump.

Especially in chronic plexus lesions hypoechoic scars may partially obstruct plexus elements and if of smaller extent may be overlooked. If they are residuals from former hematoma, internal calcifications may also be detected.

Even the first study, which compared sonographic findings in traumatic plexus lesions after motor vehicle accidents correlated with surgical findings was promising (Hayamizu et al. 1995). The authors stressed the value of sonography in the preoperative identification of patients, in whom surgery is not indicated: lesions which favor conservative treatment or lesions with avulsion of the ganglion. In a prospective controlled trial (Gruber 2007b) we were able to define the high sensitivity and specificity of sonographic plexus evaluation in traumatic injuries, establishing sonography as a first-line modality for this patient group. In this study 168 plexus elements were evaluated and minor lesions were reliably differentiated from major lesions with a positive predictive value of 100% at a negative predictive value of 92%. Sonography is therefore helpful in the assignment of patients to surgical or conservative treatment. With the application of sonography explorative surgical inspection with the risk of further plexus damage may thus be avoided in most of the patients with plexus trauma.

5.2.4 Therapy

Conservative treatment includes physiotherapy and anti-inflammatory medication, which is especially indicated and often sufficient in patients with electroneurographic evidence of spontaneous recovery.

If primary sonographic evaluation of the plexus shows an acute major lesion (incomplete or complete transection), which warrants immediate surgery, and no electrophysiological signs of recovery are seen during a trial of conservative treatment, surgical nerve inspection is presently advocated.

The treatment of dissections with nerve grafting is straight forward. In the case of scaring an internal or external neurolysis is performed depending on the extent of damage. Patients who undergo nerve inspection with neurotomy or nerve grafting within about 6 months after trauma generally have much better outcomes than patients operated later than 12 months after the injury (Penkert et al. 1999).

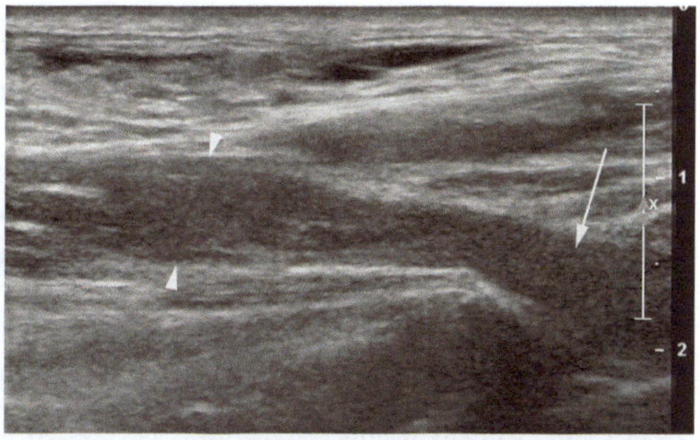

Fig. 5.2. Longitudinal sonogram through the paravertebral portion of the brachial plexus (root level) in a patient with traction injury after a humeral head fracture dislocation with demonstration of a swollen and edematous segment (*arrowheads*) but an intact root portion inside the neural foramen (*arrow*)

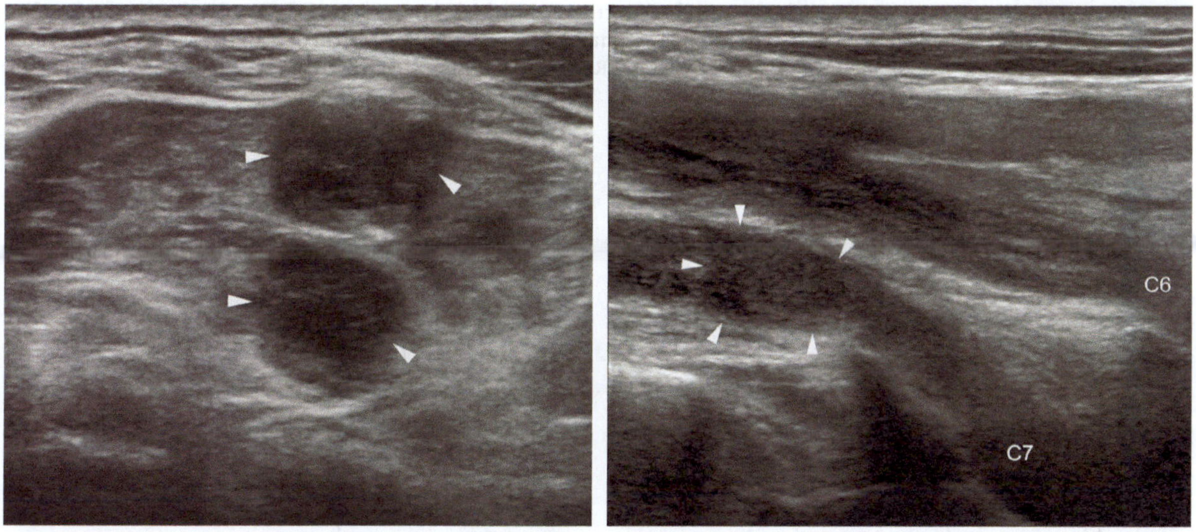

a b

Fig. 5.3. **a** Transverse sonogram through the brachial plexus (superior trunk and medial trunk/interscalene region) in a patient after a motorcycle accident shows two markedly swollen plexus trunks (*arrowheads*). **b** Longitudinal sonogram through *C6* and *C7* nerve root shows small traction neuroma of C7 (*arrowheads*)

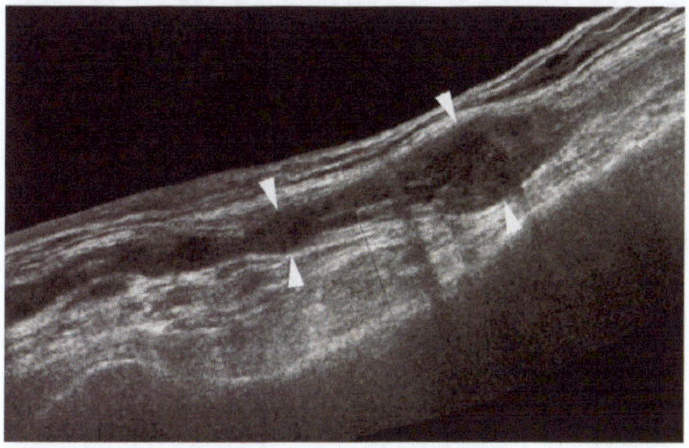

Fig. 5.4. Longitudinal panoramic sonogram in a female patient with severe traction injury of upper extremity in a motor vehicle accident. Bulbous lesions along the plexus fascicle (*arrowheads*) consistent with traction neuromas are demonstrated

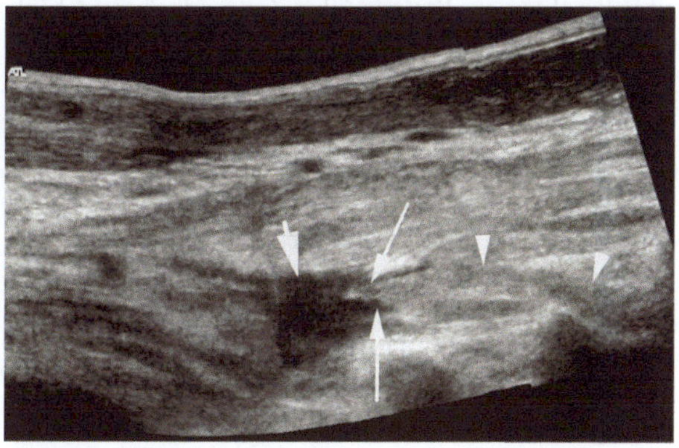

Fig. 5.5. Longitudinal sonogram in another patient with complete dissection of a nerve root (*arrowheads*) acquired on first presentation of patient to the outpatient department shows a gap with fresh hematoma (*short arrow*) and proximal stump without thickening (*arrows*)

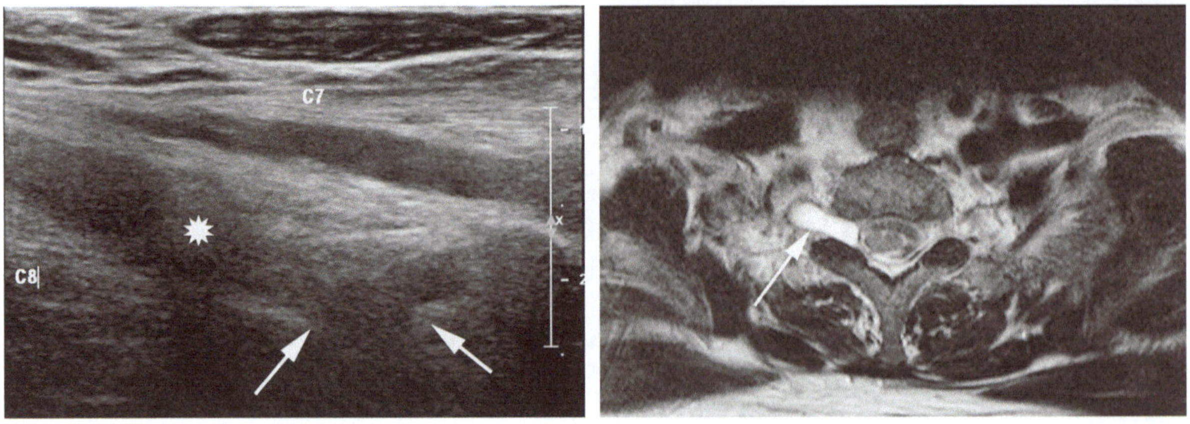

Fig. 5.6. a Longitudinal sonogram through paravertebral portion of brachial plexus (*C8* and *C7*/root level) in a patient after dislocation of the right shoulder demonstrates complete rupture of C8 nerve root with retraction of the stump (*asterisk*) and empty neural foramen (*arrows*). **b** T2 weighted transverse MR image at C8 root level confirms empty neural foramen with formation of a pseudomeningocele (*arrow*)

5.3 Traumatic Nerve Lesions in the Upper Extremity

(H. Gruber)

5.3.1 Etiology

Compared to nerves in other body regions the nerves of the upper extremity are relatively exposed to external forces. They may be injured directly during blunt or sharp trauma and indirectly by laceration, or misplaced fracture fragments which pierce or jam the nerve, or by traction over bone or bone fragments.

Especially in nerve lesions associated with fractures we have to distinguish primary lesions, which occur in the acute traumatic event from secondary lesions that appear during surgery or intervention (squeezing of the nerve or interposition between fracture fragments or implants during closed or open reposition of the fracture) or during the healing processes. Hot spots for traumatic nerve lesions are sites, where nerves are tightly connected to connective tissue or bone. Thus nerves may be impinged, partially or completely dissected, or just swollen and edematous, sometimes also due to encasing interfascicular hematoma. In secondary nerve palsy – usually developing slowly during the healing process – nerves may be surrounded or displaced by fibrous or bony callus, scar formations or even be compromised by metallic implants (Bodner et al. 2001).

5.3.1.1 Radial Nerve

The radial nerve with its close anatomic relationship to the humerus in its spiral groove is often compromised by trauma. Owing to this situation and the low mobility of the nerve at the site, where it pierces the lateral intermuscular septum, it suffers directly in many traumatic events. Fractures with radial nerve impairment are usually located at the middle or distal third of the humeral shaft and can result in various types of radial nerve lesions from simple edema (Fig. 5.7) to complete rupture (Figs. 5.8a,b and 5.9).

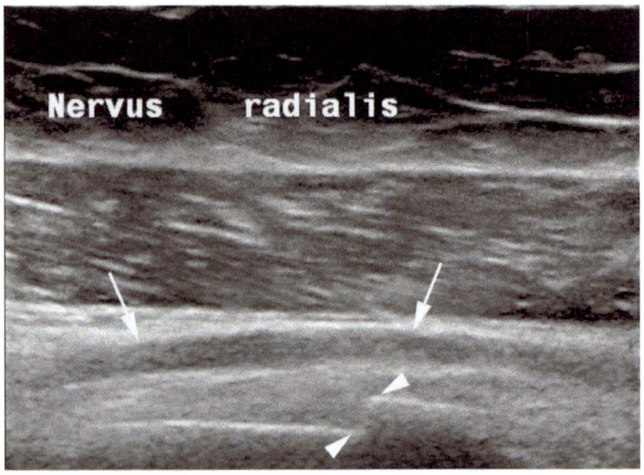

Fig. 5.7. Longitudinal sonogram through radial nerve (*arrows*) in a patient with slightly dislocated humeral shaft fracture (*arrowheads*) shows swollen edematous but continuous radial nerve

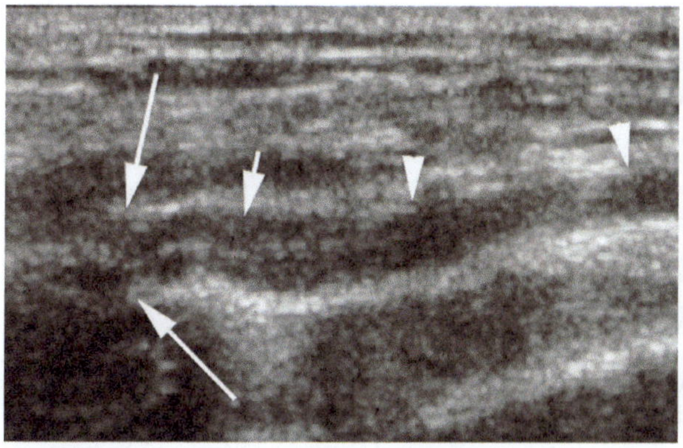
a

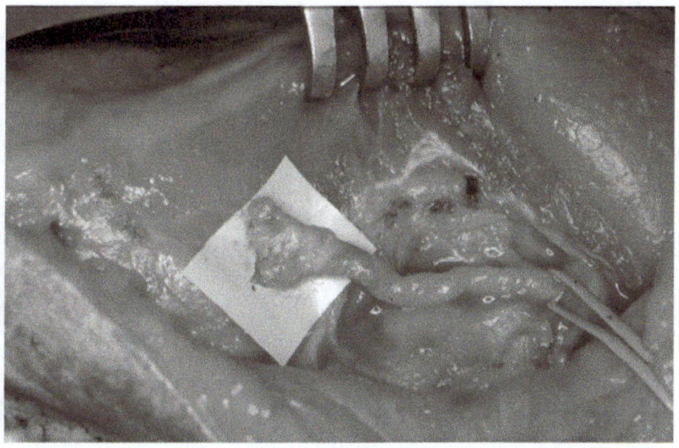
b

Fig. 5.8a,b. Longitudinal sonogram (**a**) and intraoperative photograph (**b**) of transected radial nerve (*arrowheads* in **a**) in a patient with complete radial nerve paralysis after humeral shaft fracture. The distal stump (*long arrows*) is thickened with edematous fascicles (*short arrow*), which was confirmed during surgery (**b**)

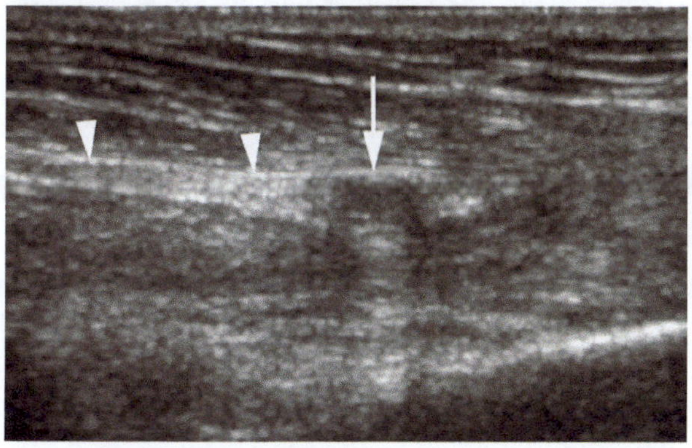

Fig. 5.9. Longitudinal sonogram of transected radial nerve in a patient with complete radial nerve paralysis after humeral shaft fracture (same patient as in Fig. 5.3). The distal stump of the radial nerve is thin (*arrow*), the nerve itself shows normal caliber (*arrowheads*)

5.3.1.2
Axillary Nerve

Along its course around the neck of the humerus heading for the lateral shoulder region, the axillary nerve pierces through a tight muscular gap. Here and at the exit out of the posterior brachial plexus fascicle it is usually injured by traction forces during dislocation of the shoulder. In the same way it may be injured by humeral head fractures or a combination of fracture and dislocation. In shoulder dislocations the spectrum of concomitant axillary nerve lesions ranges from minor strain resulting in edema or intraneural bleeding to complete avulsions (Steinmann and Moran 2001).

5.3.1.3
Accessory Nerve

True traumatic lesions of the accessory nerve – the 11th cranial nerve – with its typical course along the ventral border of the trapezoid muscle are rarely seen. However, it may be compromised by acute massive and localized external pressure during carrying of heavy loads with improper devices such as carrier belts (Bodner et al. 2002) (Fig. 5.10).

5.3.1.4
Median Nerve

In contrast to the nerves mentioned above, the median nerve and the musculocutaneous nerve – because of their relative protected course in the soft tissues of the upper extremity – have no typical segment, which is especially prone to trauma. They rather undergo direct blunt or sharp injury at various sites along their course (Jaquet et al. 2001).

5.3.1.5
Ulnar Nerve

On its course through the bony groove behind the medial humeral condyle (ulnar nerve groove) the ulnar nerve passes around one of the hardest hypomochlia in the body. While this hypomochlion may exert tensile stress on the nerve resulting in chronic nerve impairment it only rarely is a cause for direct traumatic injury (Jaquet et al. 2001). In the case of fracture dislocations of the elbow, however, a variety of ulnar nerve lesions may complicate the clinical course of a patient (Fig. 5.11a–c).

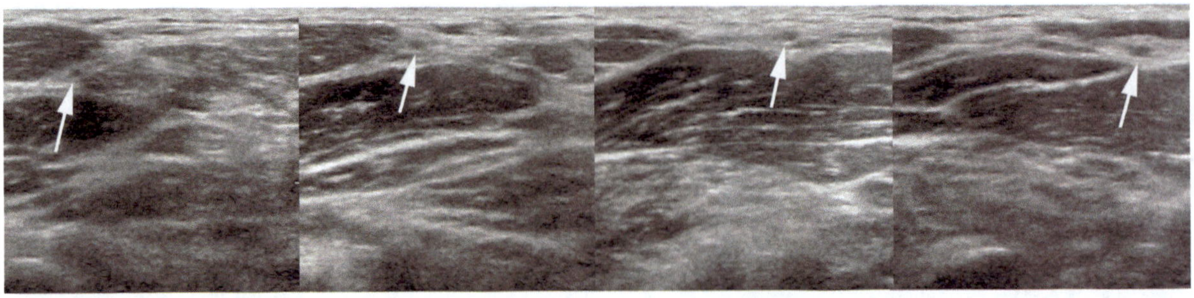

Fig. 5.10. Sequence of transverse sonograms along the course of the accessory nerve in a poacher who developed accessory nerve palsy after carrying a deer. Notice slight edematous swelling of the middle portion of the nerve (*arrows*)

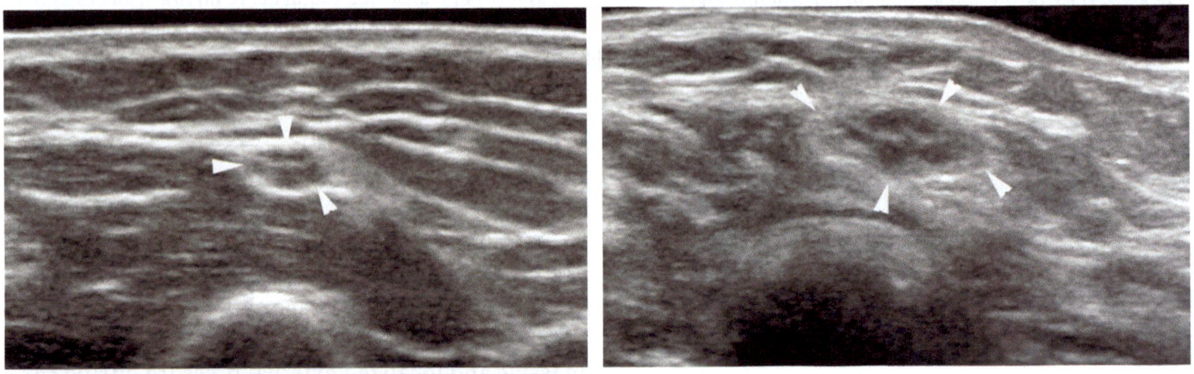

a b

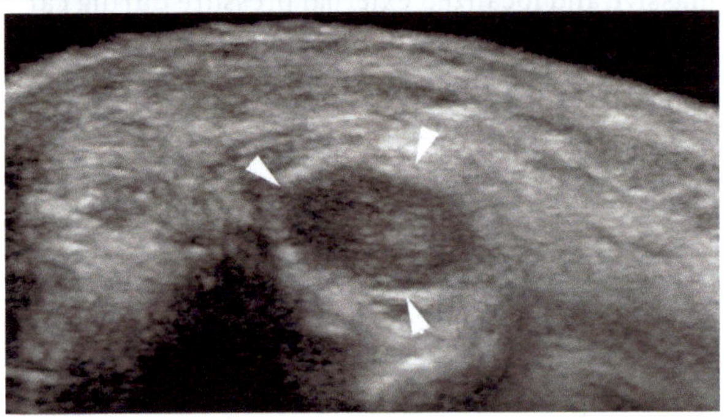

c

Fig. 5.11a–c. Series of transverse sonograms through ulnar nerve (*arrowheads*) at the elbow level in a patient after supracondylar fracture with dislocation of the elbow and ulnar nerve palsy. While the nerve shows normal caliber and texture proximal to the elbow (**a**) there is continuous enlargement (**b,c**) with marked edema and loss of the fascicular texture at the level of the medial epicondyle

5.3.2 Clinical Diagnosis

Besides a clinical neurological exam, an electrodiagnostic examination is currently the method of choice to indicate the presence and level of a nerve damage and to assess functional nerve recovery. In most cases of nerve palsy conduction studies show some amount of activity and therefore at least partial integrity of the nerve. Serial follow-up examinations can assess the amount and speed of recovery. Nerve conduction tests, however, are unable to differentiate the cause of nerve damage, for example if the nerve is partially dissected, impinged by fracture fragments (Fig. 5.12) or severely encased by callus (Fig. 5.13). In general it is important to diagnose the underlying reason of nerve impairment at an early stage and sonography proves helpful in this regard; it is able to differentiate nerve lesions that warrant early surgery from lesions that are better suited for a trial of conservative management. According to literature a nerve without signs of recovery within 3–4 months has to undergo surgical inspection. For radial nerve lesions for example spontaneous recovery is reported to occur in between 73% to 92% of cases; however, this is not to be expected in cases with direct compromise of a nerve by partial or complete rupture, by callus or scars or other stable obstructions.

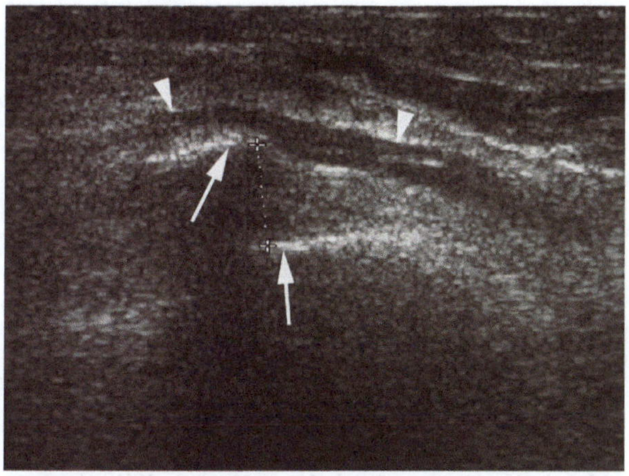

Fig. 5.12. Longitudinal sonogram through radial nerve (*arrowheads*) in a patient with radial nerve palsy after humeral shaft fracture. Sideways compression of the nerve by marked displacement of fracture fragments (*arrows*) is seen

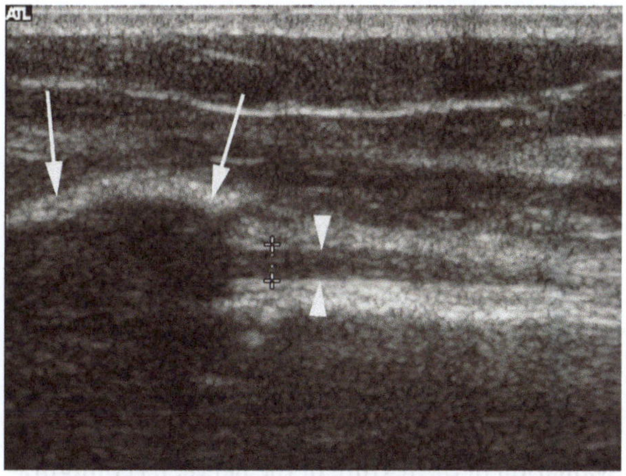

Fig. 5.13. Longitudinal sonogram through radial nerve in a different patient after humeral shaft fracture with radial nerve palsy shows nerve (*arrowheads*) traversing underneath the callus (*arrows*). The nerve could not be demonstrated beyond the callus in a transverse plane which confirmed encasement

Also for the planning of explorative surgery sonography is an easily applicable and powerful fast-forward method; if clinical diagnosis points to a nerve lesion and nerve conduction tests indicate a level, sonography can in most cases define the true extent of the lesion, the type of probably coexistent soft tissue trauma (hematoma, scar formation) and the best access route to the nerve.

5.3.3 Sonographic Findings

A 12–5 and a 17–5 MHz broad band linear array transducer is best suited for investigation of upper extremity nerves. Normally they are easily accessed in axial scans at levels with distinct anatomical and topographical features, which allow for immediate identification of the nerve. In addition color Doppler sonography allows visualization of the accompanying vessels, which may serve as a guideline for identification. Like all other peripheral nerves upper extremity nerves show the typical hypoechoic tubular structure surrounded by echoic intraneural tissues and enveloped in outer nerve sheaths. The sizes of the nerves and the number of discernible fascicles vary depending on the type of nerve, with the median nerve being the largest trunk, followed by the ulnar nerve and the terminal branches of the radial nerve. The latter are sometimes difficult to find. Here it helps to first identify the main trunk of the radial nerve at the upper arm or elbow level and follow the branches outward along the forearm. The terminal branches of the three nerves in the hand and finger region – the digital nerves – may only be depicted sufficiently with a high resolution transducer (17–5 MHz).

The common finding of a more or less prominent thickening of a nerve segment – especially proximal of the site of nerve injury – is also an apparent feature of the traumatized nerves of the upper extremities. Such nerves appear more or less hypoechoic with a loss of the regular fascicular pattern on axial images. In addition sonography can provide information on the involvement of the surrounding tissues, e.g. nerve entrapment in between fracture fragments or riding of a nerve on the edge of a fracture fragment, encasing hematoma, etc. In several of our patients with traumatic nerve lesions, sonography played an important role in the decision making, whether to surgically inspect the nerve or not, sonography enabled differentiation of whether callus formation was encasing or simply displacing the nerve (Fig. 5.13). In the first case surgical removal was needed, while in the second conservative treatment was indicated (Bodner et al. 2001).

Complete or incomplete acute nerve dissections are visualized best on longitudinal scans, as the gap between the torn stumps can be depicted and even measured. In this regard sonography also enables exact location of the stumps in complete dissections, which is very important information for the surgeon. On sonography the proximal stump often appears thicker than the distal stump (Fig. 5.14). Chronic nerve dissections usually result in the formation of (stump) neuroma, which represents insufficient attempts of physiologic repair. Such lesions are often very painful (Tinel-Hoffmann sign) and the frequent pain episodes may – in addition to the loss of nerve function – reduce a patients quality of life.

In all cases a differentiation of complete from partial dissection should be attempted by careful evaluation of the texture of the nerve, its configuration and the integrity of the outer nerve sheath, as it might change the surgical approach. Nevertheless it is more important to differentiate dissections or avulsions (major nerve lesions) from lesions with preserved continuity (minor nerve lesions). In several studies we were able to show (Gruber et al. 2005, 2007b) that this basic information can change the further prognosis of an injured patient profoundly as necessary surgical intervention is performed earlier resulting in better outcome.

5.3.4 Therapy

Conservative treatment (physiotherapy, systemic anti-inflammatory drugs) is the method of choice in nerve palsy associated with traumatic fractures with resolving neurological symptoms and without previous sonographic evidence of a pathology advocating early surgery.

Primary surgical nerve inspection is required in nerve palsy associated with open bone fracture, in vascular injury or when bone debridement is needed. When the nerve is dissected or segments are damaged severely, primary nerve grafting is the method of choice. In most cases – when the clinical situation is more ambiguous – sonographic assessment may serve as a first line method for attempting a decision between conservative treatment or surgical intervention (Gruber 2003, 2005, 2007b).

Chronic dissections with neuroma formation are a therapeutic problem as the pain produced by the neuroma does not respond sufficiently to systemic therapy. In this context a sonographically guided instillation therapy – which is discussed in more detail in Chapter 7 of this book – can yield favorable results (Gruber et al. 2007a).

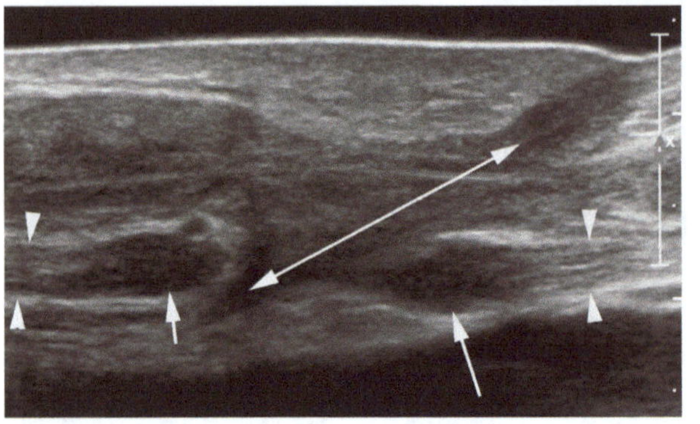

Fig. 5.14. Longitudinal sonogram through ulnar nerve (*arrowheads*) in the forearm of a patient who cut himself with a knife. The proximal (*long arrow*) and distal (*short arrow*) nerve stump is separated with interposition of scar tissue (*double headed arrow*) and slightly thickened (more so in the proximal stump) due to development of stump neuroma

5.4 Traumatic Nerve Lesions in the Lower Extremity

(H. Gruber)

5.4.1 Etiology

As in the upper extremity the nerves of the lower extremity are relatively exposed to traumatic injuries and injury mechanisms are quite similar: external forces with sharp or blunt injury or compromise by foreign bodies and internal forces such as fracture fragments, interposition between fragments or traction due to dislocation of bones. In the same way we have to distinguish acute primary lesions – acquired immediately at the time of injury – from secondary lesions that develop at a various interval after the inciting event. Thus nerves may also be impinged, partially or completely dissected, or simply present as swollen and edematous (Gruber et al. 2003). In secondary nerve palsy nerves may get progressively surrounded or displaced by scars or by fibrous or bony callus and externally obstructed.

The lower extremity is supplied by two main nerves: the femoral nerve for the ventral and the sciatic nerve for the dorsal side.

5.4.1.1
Femoral Nerve

The femoral nerve, which is formed out of the cranial roots of the lumbosacral plexus and, after piercing through the psoas muscle into the deep abdominal region, runs in a groove formed by the iliac and psoas muscle. This special relationship with the two muscles is why the femoral nerve often has rather a triangular than a round shape if scanned axially in the groin region (Gruber et al. 2003). While the nerve is only rarely injured in direct trauma, it is very prone to inadvertent iatrogenic damage: orthopedic hip replacement, gynecological procedures, hernia repair etc. A common finding is internal bleeding and edema with consecutive loss of function (Gruber et al. 2003) (Fig. 5.15a,b).

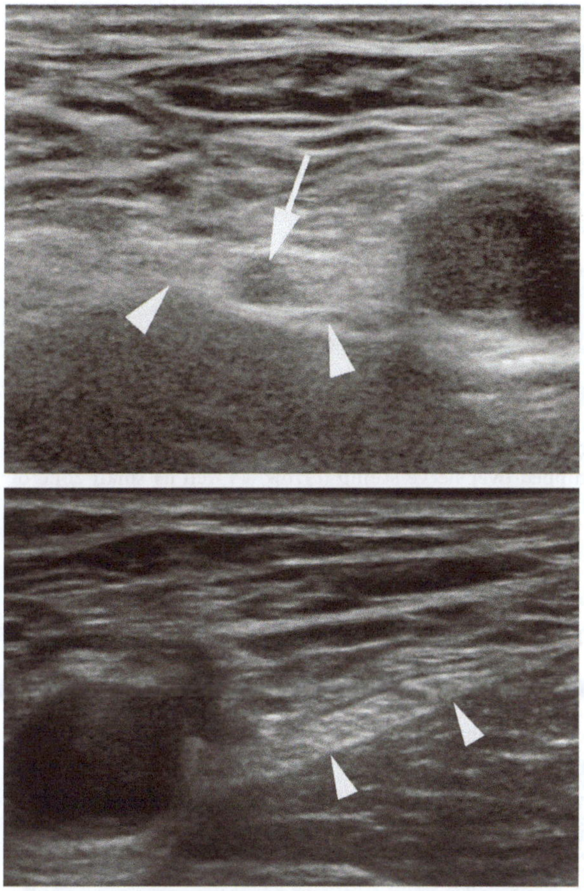

a

b

Fig. 5.15a,b. Transverse sonograms through femoral nerve (*arrowheads*) in a patient after hip surgery with demonstration of a small zone of internal bleeding and edema (*arrow* in **a**). **b** normal contralateral femoral nerve

5.4.1.2
Sciatic Nerve

The sciatic nerve undergoes very unspecific post-traumatic changes quite similar to those seen in other peripheral nerves. Along its course the nerve is protected by thick and strong groups of muscle, thus direct trauma is rare and occurs only with heavy impact of external forces (for example impalement injury) (Fig. 5.16). It may also suffer from displacement by intra- or intermuscular hematomas.

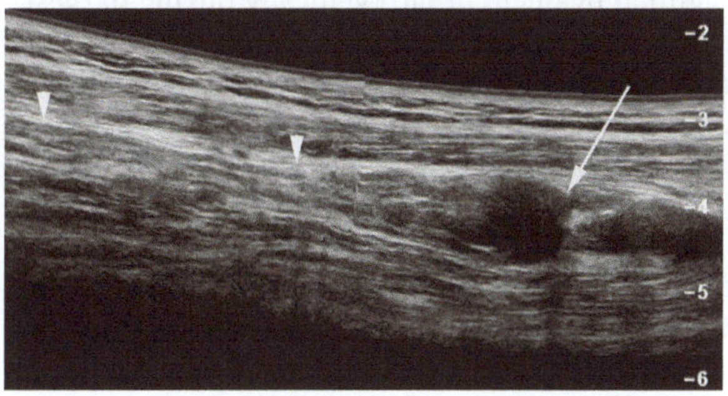

Fig. 5.16. Extended field of view sonogram through proximal sciatic nerve in a patient after a severe car accident with traction injury to the left thigh. Normal fascicular texture but somewhat wavy appearance is seen in the proximal section of the nerve (*arrowheads*). The stump after complete transection is markedly thickened due to terminal type neuroma (*arrow*)

5.4.1.3
Peroneal Nerve

The common peroneal nerve, after exiting from the sciatic nerve, takes an oblique course in the proximal popliteal fossa. It runs around the fibular head in a very superficial, exposed fibro-osseous tunnel and, running further distally in a very superficial layer, splits into a superficial and deep branch. Peroneal nerve injury is especially common in traumatic knee dislocation and occurs mainly in high speed accidents, in athletic sport injuries and in distinct fracture patterns (Kim and Kline 1996; Gruber et al. 2005). Various lesions of this nerve may be found at the "hot spot" at the fibular neck: overt stretching around the fibula induced by genicular varus trauma resulting in edemas, incomplete or complete dissection (Fig. 5.17) with or without preserved integrity of the outer nerve sheath (Fig. 5.18) – which may consecutively produce a so-called "neuroma in continuity lesion" (Gruber et al. 2007b) – and penetrating injuries or mere contusions due to a very exposed location.

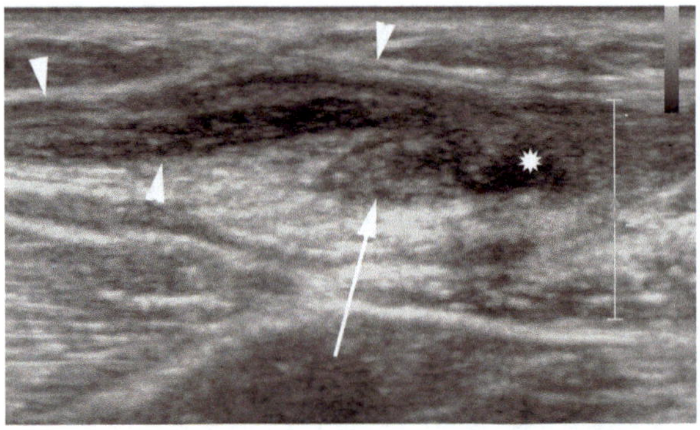

Fig. 5.17. Longitudinal sonogram in a patient after knee joint dislocation with complete peroneal palsy shows edematous proximal portion of peroneal nerve (*arrowheads*) and flipped over nerve stump (*arrow*) as well as small zone of internal bleeding and fascicular disruption (*asterisk*)

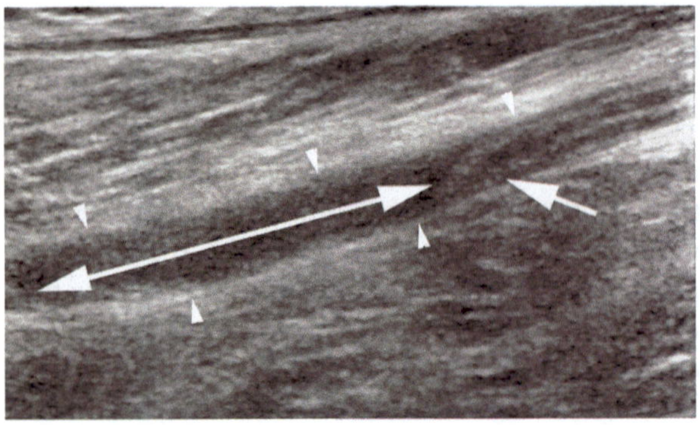

Fig. 5.18. Longitudinal sonogram in another patient after knee joint dislocation shows internal rupture of peroneal nerve with preserved outer nerve sheath (*arrowheads*). Notice small gap (*double-headed arrow*) and distal nerve stump (*arrow*)

5.4.1.4
Tibial Nerve

The tibial nerve – as the second terminal branch of the sciatic nerve – has a very protected course through the shank embedded between muscles, which is the reason why the nerve is almost always injured at the level of the ankle or bellow – in malleolar fractures with or without bone dislocations for example.

5.4.1.5
Lateral Femoral Cutaneous Nerve

The lateral femoral cutaneous nerve which enters the thigh region next to the ventral upper iliac spine, is often compromised by chronic compression by the inguinal ligament or iatrogenically during harvesting of a bone-graft at the iliac spine. Although the nerve is rarely dissected completely, severe neural edema may ensue, which leads to intense groin pain radiating into the thigh (Fig. 5.19).

5.4.2
Clinical Diagnosis

Clinically patients with traumatic nerve palsy in the lower extremity show motor deficits with impairment of motion and gait, especially in severe cases. More often, however, we find a combination of motor impairment with pain and sensory deficits in the typical region covered by the respective nerve. In up to 80% of cases nerve function recovers completely with conservative management, which is monitored with electrodiagnostic testing. When spontaneous regeneration of nerve function does not occur within 6 months, surgical inspection – as in other body regions – has for a long time been the only alternative to gain necessary information for further therapeutic decisions. Due to the already mentioned limitations, electrophysiological tests cannot provide us with an exact definition of the length nor the quality of nerve damage. This is especially problematic in peroneal nerve trauma associated with knee dislocation, where the damaged nerve segment may reach far more proximally than expected and may therefore be overlooked and underestimated during initial clinical assessment and surgery (Tomaino et al. 2000; Gruber et al. 2005). This was also the case in four of 12 patients in our own series of traumatic peroneal nerve palsies. Although not being avulsed completely such neural lesions may end up in severe neural fibrosis or in neuroma in continuity if complete axonal damage is the case (Gruber et al. 2007b).

5.4.3
Sonographic Findings

Patient position for sonographic nerve examinations in the lower extremity has to be chosen according to nerve of interest; while the femoral nerve is imaged in a normal supine position, a medial or lateral access is best for the tibial or peroneal nerve, with the sciatic nerve easily accessible in prone position. The choice of transducer depends on a patient's

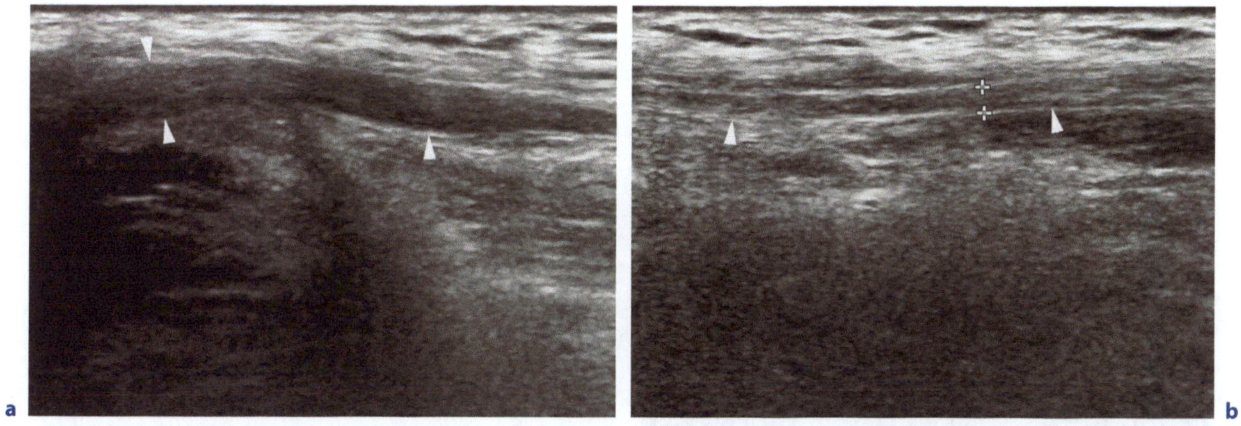

Fig. 5.19. (a) Longitudinal sonogram through lateral femoral cutaneous nerve (*arrowheads*) in a patient after hip surgery with marked edematous swelling of left sided nerve. **b** Normal contralateral nerve

build and the amount of soft tissues overlying the nerve. Usually 12–5 or 9–4 MHz broad band linear array transducers are used and a stand-off pad may improve image quality with imaging of the peroneal nerve at the fibular neck or the tibial nerve in the ankle region for example.

The femoral nerve is identified best in transverse scans in the groin region where it runs in the grove formed by the iliopsoas muscle lateral to the femoral vessels. Often its cross-sectional appearance is not oval but triangular; however, it always shows the typical echotexture known from most other peripheral nerves. It can be followed only some centimeters upward as it is shadowed by intra-abdominal gas-containing bowel. Further distally it splits into its terminal branches only some centimeters distal to the inguinal ligament.

The sciatic nerve is also identified best in a transverse plane and is found as a finger thick nerve structure embedded between the ischiocrural muscles of the thigh. At the level of the proximal popliteal fossa it splits into the peroneal and the tibial nerve. When from here the transducer is moved distally and laterally the common peroneal nerve is depicted running around the fibular head to pierce through the peroneal muscle group, by which it is often masked. The normal peroneal nerve is a rather small nerve presenting with just a few fascicles. However, when injured the nerve loses its typical sonographic fascicular pattern due to edema, vasocongestion or inner bleeding. In severe nerve damage the edema may even reach as proximal as the sciatic nerve. In these cases the sciatic nerve shows an abnormal hypoechoic texture of its lateral portion (Fig. 5.20), the part that later continues into the peroneal nerve.

Moving the probe centrally down from the sciatic nerve division, the tibial nerve is depicted neighboring the popliteal and then the posterior tibial vessels. It is embedded in the posterior shank muscles and points to the medial malleolar region. Here it is bent under the sustentaculum tali to reach the plantar region of the foot (its two terminal branches). The sural nerve, as one of the important sensory shank nerves, also forms at the division of the sciatic nerve to run distally next to the small saphenus vein. This thin cutaneous nerve often is transected during surgery (Fig. 5.21), such as in stripping of leg veins, for example, which can result in painful neuromas. The same may be true for the long sensory branch of the femoral nerve, the saphenus nerve. It runs next to the main stem of the large saphenus vein along the medial border of the leg and often undergoes the same lesions as the sural nerve (Fig. 5.22).

A "neuroma in continuity" is a frequent finding in peroneal nerve injury and represents a nodular hypoechoic structure of variable length along the course of the nerve resembling a pearl necklace (Fig. 5.23). Any neuroma formation indicates an at least incomplete chronic neural dissection. The sonographic diagnosis of an acute complete nerve dissection is straight forward with an apparent discontinuity of a nerve with pertinent nerve stumps (Figs. 5.14, 5.18). The stump can be embedded in hematoma or in chronic lesions in scar tissue.

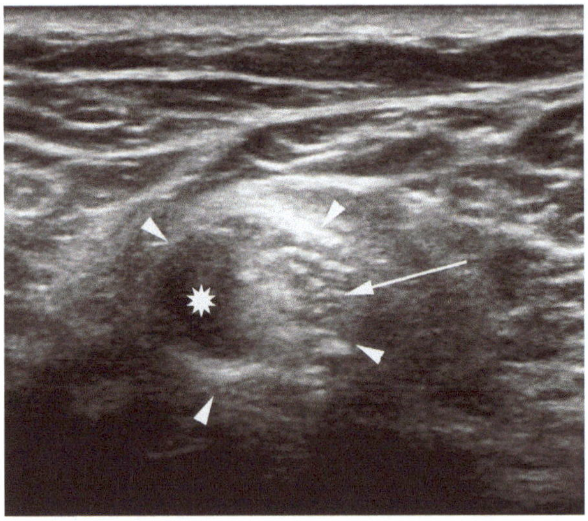

Fig. 5.20. Transverse sonogram through sciatic nerve (*arrowheads*) at the distal thigh level in a patient after knee joint dislocation and peroneal nerve palsy. Notice hypoechoic lateral portion due to internal rupture of the peroneal nerve elements (*asterisk*) but intact tibialis portion with regular echotexture (*arrow*)

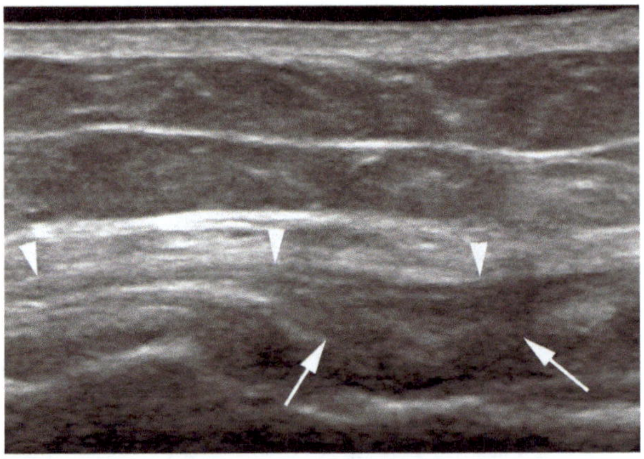

Fig. 5.22. Longitudinal sonogram through saphenus nerve (*arrowheads*) in another patient after venous stripping with compromise of the nerve by a close lying scar

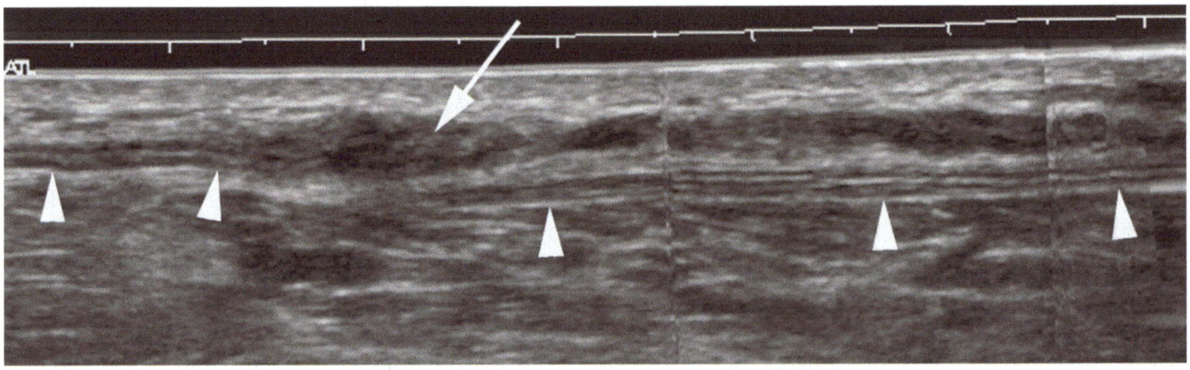

Fig. 5.21. Extended field of view sonogram through sural nerve in a patient after venous stripping with complete transection of the sural nerve (*arrowheads*) and a small terminal type neuroma in the proximal stump (*arrow*)

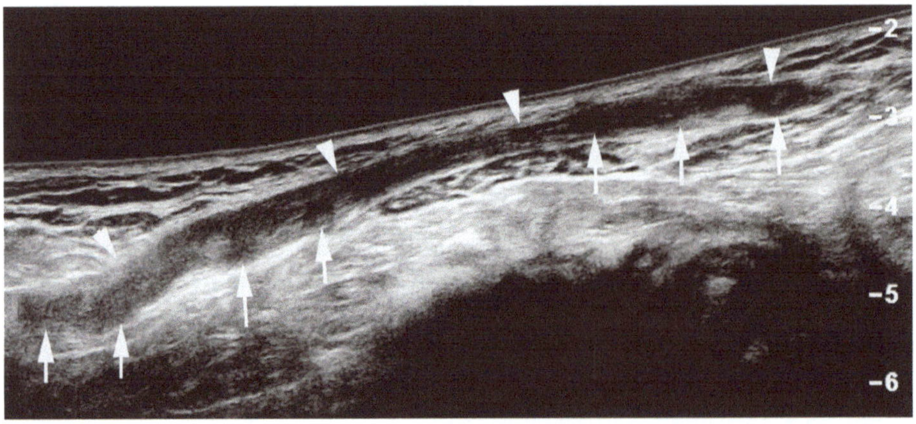

Fig. 5.23. Extended field of view sonogram through peroneal nerve (*arrowheads*) in a patient after knee joint dislocation shows a large neuroma in continuity with multiple small nodular neuromas along the nerve (*arrows*)

5.4.4 Therapy

Conservative management includes physiotherapy to strengthen the atrophic muscles, local steroid infiltration may bring relief in hypertrophic scar formation. However, any external compression of the nerve by scar tissue or callus formation requires surgical intervention. In general, surgical nerve inspection is indicated when electroneurographic testing shows no improvement of nerve function during conservative treatment, or when sonography shows signs of incomplete disruption such as extensive intraneural neuroma formation or complete nerve dissection. Chronic dissections with neuroma formation pose a therapeutic problem and may be an indication for sonographically guided instillation therapy (Gruber et al. 2007a) (see also Sect. 7.3).

5.5 Iatrogenic Nerve Lesions

(S. Peer)

Peripheral nerve lesions secondary to various surgical procedures are not uncommon. Some of these lesions may occur during surgical procedures, which are not primarily directed towards the nerve itself; inadvertent dissection of the nerve, traction, insertion of retractors and thermal injuries are the most common causative agents for this type of injury. Another large group of patients sustains peripheral nerve lesions in the course of nerve surgery: release of a nerve encased in a narrow osteofibrous tunnel, nerve suture after traumatic dissection, etc. In addition, secondary neural damage due to excessive scar formation or compression by hematomas also need to be considered. While the first kind of nerve injury has to be considered as truly iatrogenic, the second type may be regarded as an unfavorable postoperative result, due to occurring complications.

As already mentioned in the introduction to Chapter 5, true iatrogenic peripheral nerve lesions are a clinical as well as medico-legal problem, as the causal relationship between medical intervention and the nerve lesion is frequently not that easily established. Furthermore, detailed information about the type and extent of neural damage is crucial for the selection of adequate treatment.

In the next paragraphs we will present an overview of common postoperative/iatrogenic nerve lesions and typical sonomorphological findings.

5.5.1 Nerve Lesions in Association with Head and Neck Surgery

Various surgical procedures in the neck are associated with a potential risk for iatrogenic peripheral nerve damage. The nerve most commonly involved, which allows for sonographic assessment, is the accessory nerve. Surgical damage to other nerves in the neck region is either rare or the involved nerves are not easily examined with sonography, which is why we focus on sonography of the accessory nerve only.

5.5.1.1 Accessory Nerve Lesions

5.5.1.1.1 Clinical Considerations

The accessory nerve crosses the posterior cervical triangle in a superficial course, which makes it rather susceptible to injury. Historically, iatrogenic injury of this nerve has been one of the leading causes for trapezius paralysis. As early as in the 1940s accessory nerve injury in association with removal of tuberculous lymph nodes was reported (Wulff 1941). In general, any kind of surgery in the posterior cervical triangle can injure the nerve: Cervical lymph node biopsy, excision of benign masses or radical neck dissection for malignancy (Woodhall 1952; Harpf et al. 1999; Remmler et al. 1986). Besides iatrogenic injury still being the most common cause for trapezius paralysis, the nerve may rarely be injured in blunt or penetrating trauma to the neck during contact sports, or indirectly with traction injury to the upper extremity (Vastamaki and Solonen 1984).

The accessory nerve or cranial nerve IX is the only motor nerve innervating the trapezius muscle; however, it may be joined by proprioceptive branches from the second, third or fourth cervical nerve. In regard of this peculiar anatomical situation the leading clinical symptom for accessory nerve lesions is impaired trapezius muscle function; patients typically have an asymmetric neck line because of the atrophic trapezius and drooping of the shoulder girdle. Pain with prolonged use of the shoulder, or a constant feeling of a dull ache or heaviness about the shoulder are common complaints, patients have difficulties with overhead movements, heavy lifting, prolonged writing or driving a car (Wiater and Bigliani 1999). During active elevation of the arm winging of the scapula is observed as it is displaced laterally, rotating downward and outward. Characteristic findings include difficulty abducting the extremity above the horizontal plane and weakness during elevation against resistance.

Conventional imaging studies such as radiographs of the cervical spine and/or shoulder are hardly diagnostic but almost always obtained and serve the purpose of exclusion of coexisting bony pathology. Computed tomography and MRI are only indicated in cases where mass lesions with direct compromise of the nerve are suspected but even in this situation sonography may serve as a primary imaging study.

5.5.1.1.2 Sonography

The sonographic access to the accessory nerve is easy if some basic anatomic considerations are observed. The nerve is best identified at the lateral cervical triangle. After identification of the trapezius muscle and the sternocleidomastoid muscle, which aid as a guiding structure, the scanhead is moved upwards towards the location of the nerve, which lies superficially just underneath the skin. After identification of the nerve it is easily followed in its upward course to the spine and downwards along the trapezius muscle.

As the accessory nerve is a small nerve its sonographic appearance may not typically resemble the commonly known dotted pattern characteristic for bigger peripheral nerves, but be more like a single hypoechoic tubular structure (Bodner et al. 2002).

In the case of complete transection a gap in the continuity of the nerve may directly be shown with sonography (Fig. 5.24); however, this will sometimes be overshadowed by postoperative scar tissue which impairs direct visualization of the gaping within the nerve (Fig. 5.25). A loss of the normal nerve texture and outer diameter is nevertheless observed in these situations (Bodner et al. 2002).

While the existence of such a complete nerve transection is readily diagnosed with electrodiagnostic tests, the value of sonography in this situation is to establish the exact localization of nerve interruption, which is important information for planning surgical reconstruction. In particular, the distance between the nerve stumps and the shape of the stump, as well as the presence of additional scarring or neuroma formation in longer dating nerve lesions, is to be examined thoroughly during sonography (Fig. 5.26).

The latter is important information for the decision regarding primary nerve anastomosis or nerve grafting. While the therapy of complete transection is straightforward, incomplete nerve lesions may pose a clinical and therapeutic dilemma. In general, surgery is advocated by some authors if a nerve lesion does not show any clinical or electrodiagnostic signs of recovery within 3 months, whereas others advise exploration at 6–12 months after injury (Perlmutter and Apruzzese 1998). Another approach, especially with accessory nerve lesions, is to perform early microsurgical nerve repair (Wiater and Bigliani 1999), which may be especially feasible in patients where, according to sonographic studies, recovery with conservative management is not to be expected, such as injuries with interposition of scar tissue or organized hematoma (Grant et al. 1999; Peer et al. 2002). An early reconstruction spares the patient from long-lasting and, in this case, fruitless physical therapy and improves postoperative outcome in a situation where the muscle function of the trapezius is still good, with no muscular atrophy (Wiater and Bigliani 1999).

In chronic lesions of the accessory nerve sonography may not only be useful for evaluation of the nerve itself, but also for direct evaluation of trapezius muscle thickness (Fig. 5.27).

Again, this is critical information for surgical planning. With long-lasting trapezius muscle dysfunction, results of microsurgical nerve reconstruction will mostly depend on the state of the trapezius muscle (Bigliani et al. 1996). With severe muscular atrophy detected during sonographic exams a decision to perform an extensive muscle transfer, such as the Eden-Lange procedure will be more appropriate to receive good restoration of shoulder motion (Bigliani et al. 1996).

5.5.2 Nerve Lesions Associated with Orthopedic Surgery

Various orthopedic procedures (hip surgery, shoulder surgery, leg lengthening, etc.) may potentially harm a peripheral nerve in close proximity to the surgical access. Sometimes even nerves at a greater distance from the surgical access route may be damaged if retractors or hooks are inserted deeply into the soft tissues. Thus the sciatic nerve, for example, may be excessively stretched or even undergo direct injury during hip surgery. Rarely, the nerve may even be damaged directly by a surgical implant – we experienced radial nerves squeezed underneath a plate used for repair of humeral fractures and even a sciatic nerve encased by a circular wire used for fixation of a femoral shaft fracture.

In general, compared with nerve lesions in association with hip surgery, postoperative lesions after other orthopedic procedures are less frequent. Therefore, we will concentrate mainly on lesions in association with hip surgery and comment only briefly on the less frequent entities.

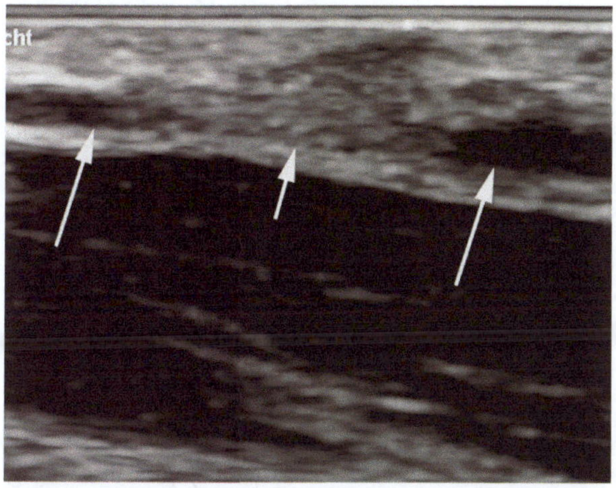

Fig. 5.24. Longitudinal sonogram through accessory nerve in a patient who underwent lateral cervical lymphadenectomy. Complete transection of accessory nerve with demonstration of a small gap (*short arrow*) and the separated and swollen nerve stumps (*long arrows*)

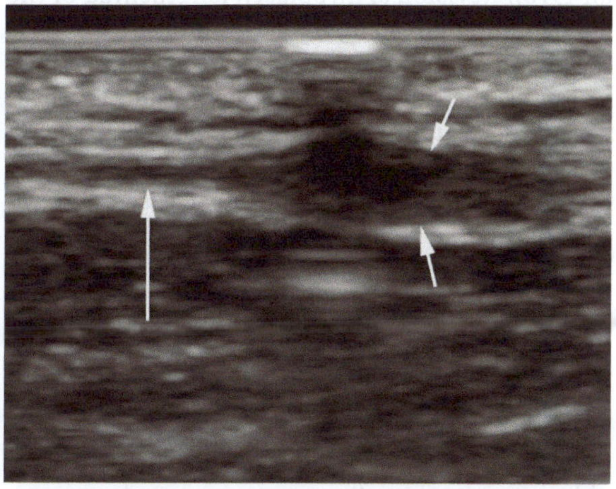

Fig. 5.25. Longitudinal sonogram through accessory nerve in a patient with iatrogenic accessory nerve palsy shows nerve (*long arrow*) impacted in scar tissue (*small arrows*). The continuity of the nerve was not reliably assessed in this patient

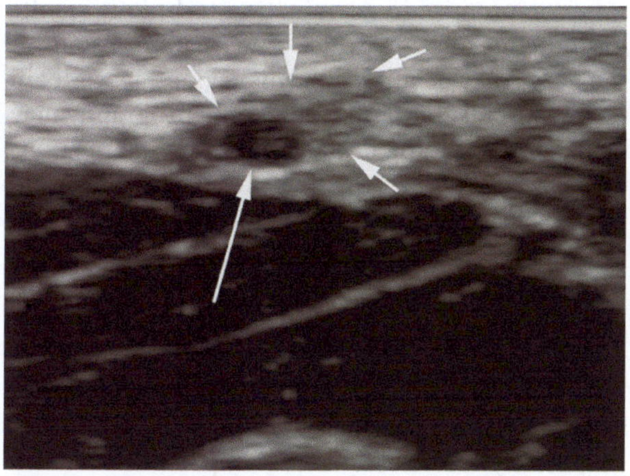

Fig. 5.26. Transverse sonogram through accessory nerve in a patient with accessory nerve palsy after lateral cervical lymphadenectomy. Swollen, edematous nerve stump (*long arrow*) is seen covered by scar tissue (*small arrows*)

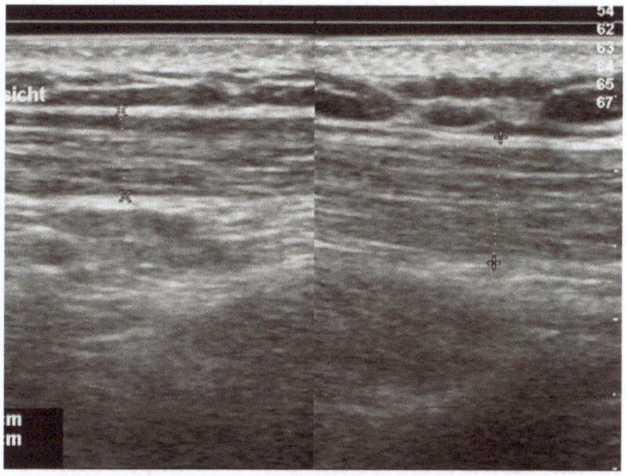

Fig. 5.27. Comparative measurement of trapezius muscle thickness in a patient with iatrogenic accessory nerve palsy showing reduction of muscle diameter in affected side (*left half* of image)

5.5.2.1
Total Hip Arthroplasty

5.5.2.1.1
Clinical Considerations

The clinical incidence of nerve palsy after primary total hip replacement (THR) is reported to range from 0.08% to 3.7% (Eggli et al. 1999). However, electrodiagnostic studies indicate that nerve damage may occur in up to 70% of cases (Weber et al. 1976). Revision arthroplasty, lengthening of the leg by more than 4 cm, dislocation of the hip during the operation, hemorrhage, direct injury by a retractor, the duration of the operation, the heat of polymerization as well as intrapelvic extrusion of cement have all been implicated, but the cause of the injury is uncertain in most cases. Several reports suggest that revision arthroplasty and leg lengthening are the most significant factors (Eggli et al. 1999; Oldenburg and Müller 1997). In the orthopedic literature there is also some dispute about an increased incidence of nerve lesions with various surgical approaches to the hip (i.e. direct lateral or posterior approach) and the direct lateral approach or Charnley transtrochanteric procedure is found to be more prone to the development of nerve injury (Weale et al. 1996). The reason for this lies in the use of sturdy self retaining retractors positioned anteriorly and posteriorly in this procedure, which may exert a considerable amount of traction on the soft tissues. Besides direct compromise of a nerve with the retractor an indirect type lesion may develop with excessive stretching of a nerve. Stretching of the nerve reduces the cross sectional area of the fascicles and increases intrafascicular pressure thus impairing blood flow in the perineural vascular plexus. Sunderland (1978) found that nerves are quite elastic structures and only stretching of 20%–35% is able to cause a functional nerve injury; however, this may occur in lengthening of the hip or with excessive stretching of soft tissues.

The nerves most commonly injured during hip surgery are the sciatic and femoral nerve (Gruber et al. 2005), but also the obturator nerve may be involved. Clinical findings range from causalgic pain in the distribution of the nerve to impairment of walking ability. In the postoperative situation the early clinical diagnosis of a nerve lesion is often difficult, as postoperative pain may be attributed to the procedure itself and the significance of the incidence of nerve injury reported in the literature is masked as only severe damage presents as a clinical complication. Nerve injury may vary from transient blocks in conduction to irreversible damage secondary to transection of the axons. While according to our experience complete lesions are very rare, most patients experience nerve damage to a certain bundle of fascicles within the sciatic or femoral nerve trunk. The latter type of lesions pose the biggest problems as far as differential diagnosis and treatment decisions are considered.

5.5.2.1.2
Sonography

In general, sonography may help in the diagnostic work-up of nerve lesions after THR in so far as direct evaluation of the nerve and its surroundings is feasible, thus enabling direct evaluation of hematomas or scars compressing a nerve, direct visualization of transected nerve bundles or localized nerve edema. However, visualization of the sciatic and femoral nerve with sonography is limited to certain anatomical regions, where the nerve is lying superficially with sufficient sonographic access. Access to the sciatic nerve is normally possible along the whole course of the nerve along the posterior thigh, where it lies on top of the adductor magnus muscle after having entered the thigh at the lower border of the gluteus maximus muscle. The more proximal course from the greater sciatic foramen underneath the gluteal muscles may only be examined with low frequency scan heads allowing to adjust the scan to the deep lying nerve. This necessary compromise in examination technique results in limited resolution, which is why subtle lesions of the nerve may be missed in this region especially in obese patients. In these cases MR-neurography may be used for imaging of the more proximal portions of the sciatic nerve, which has been shown to yield reliable results if specially optimized MR-sequences are applied (Maravilla et al. 1998).

The second commonly injured nerve during THR is the femoral nerve, which is much better accessible with sonography.

Lesions of the sciatic and femoral nerve attributed to THR may include the whole range of sonographically detectable nerve impairment known from other injuries, ranging from localized swelling of single fascicles, to partial interruption with neuroma formation (Fig. 5.28) and compression by scar tissue or hematoma (Fig. 5.29).

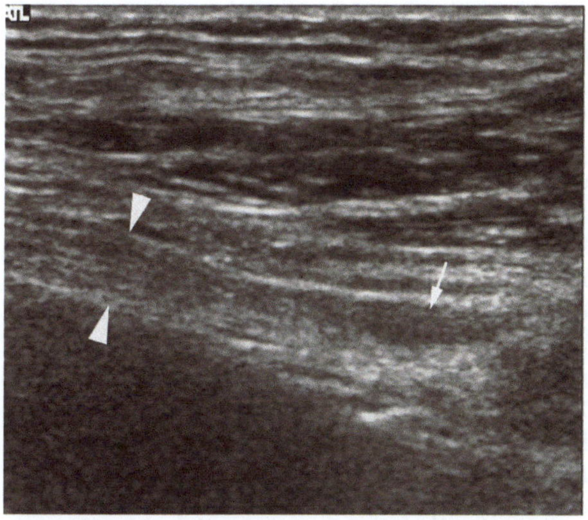

Fig. 5.28. Longitudinal sonogram through femoral nerve in a patient after hip surgery. A small hypoechoic nodule (*arrow*) consistent with a small traction neuroma is shown inside the otherwise normal femoral nerve (*arrowheads*)

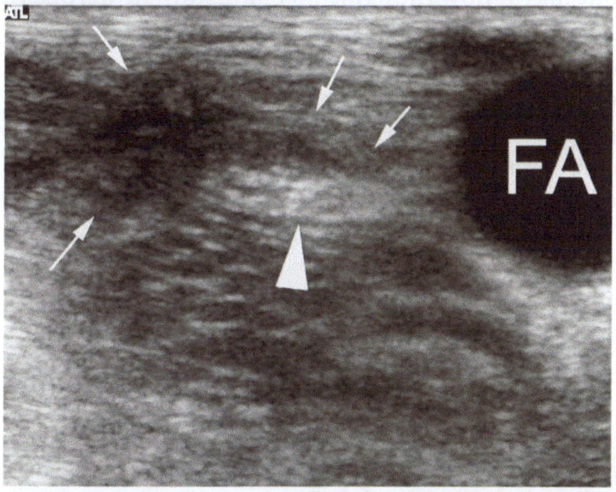

Fig. 5.29. Transverse sonogram through femoral nerve in a patient after total hip arthroplasty. Flattened femoral nerve (*arrowhead*) is seen lying on top of iliopsoas muscle. The nerve is compressed by a tight close lying scar (*small arrows*). *FA*, femoral artery

5.5.2.2 Shoulder Surgery

There are various reports on post-surgical damage of the axillary nerve or brachial plexus (Boardman and Cofield 1999), but despite shoulder surgery being a frequent procedure, these lesions are rare and there is only limited experience with sonographic assessment of the axillary nerve. While the axillary nerve may be identified with sonography at the back of the shoulder – where it appears at the dorsal aspect of the humerus entering from underneath the lower border of the teres minor muscle – it is not as easily assessed on its course through the axilla. A good guiding structure for identification of the axillary nerve is the posterior circumflex artery of the humerus. We aim for examination of this nerve following its course from the back of the shoulder to the axilla and upward to its origin from the posterior plexus fascicle, but in many cases it is not seen in its complete extent. This asks for a cautious interpretation of results, nevertheless pathology such as hematomas after shoulder dislocation with possible compromise to the nerve may be identified.

5.5.2.3 Peroneal Nerve Lesions

Direct surgical damage to the peroneal nerve is possible during leg lengthening procedures or correction osteotomies at the lower leg. Depending on the type of surgical procedure this may involve the common peroneal nerve or one of the peroneal nerve branches. While the common peroneal nerve is easily assessed with sonography (Peer et al. 2002), and the superficial branch may be followed almost down to the ankle, identification of the deep peroneal nerve is especially difficult in the post-surgical patient. Localized scaring or diffuse swelling of the leg with edema leads to sonographic artifacts with degradation of image quality, which especially affects visualization of the deep peroneal nerve on its course underneath the peroneus muscles. Typical peroneal nerve lesions include compression by scars (Fig. 5.30) or direct nerve damage due to inadvertent transection or traction injury (Fig. 5.31a,b).

5.5.2.4 Tibial Nerve Lesions

Lesions to the tibial nerve following orthopedic operations are rare; however, we encountered lesions associated with removal of osteosynthetic material, or external fixation of tibiotalar fractures.

The rationale for sonography in these cases is to differentiate direct nerve damage from a so-called post-traumatic tarsal tunnel syndrome. The latter is a condition similar to the idiopathic tarsal tunnel syndrome, and is due to reduction of space in the tarsal tunnel because of abutting periosteal callus, malpositioned fractures or organized hematoma.

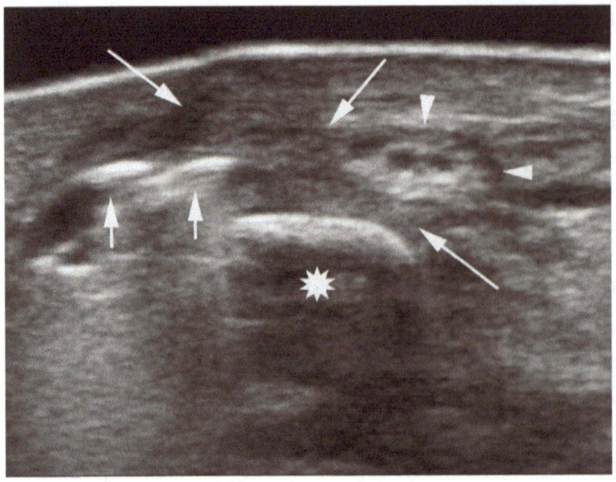

Fig. 5.30. Transverse sonogram through superficial peroneal nerve (*arrowheads*) at ankle level in a patient after fixation of a lateral ankle fracture. The nerve is swollen and encased by scar tissue (*long arrows*). *Asterisk*, distal fibular bone; *small arrows*, artifacts by plate and screws

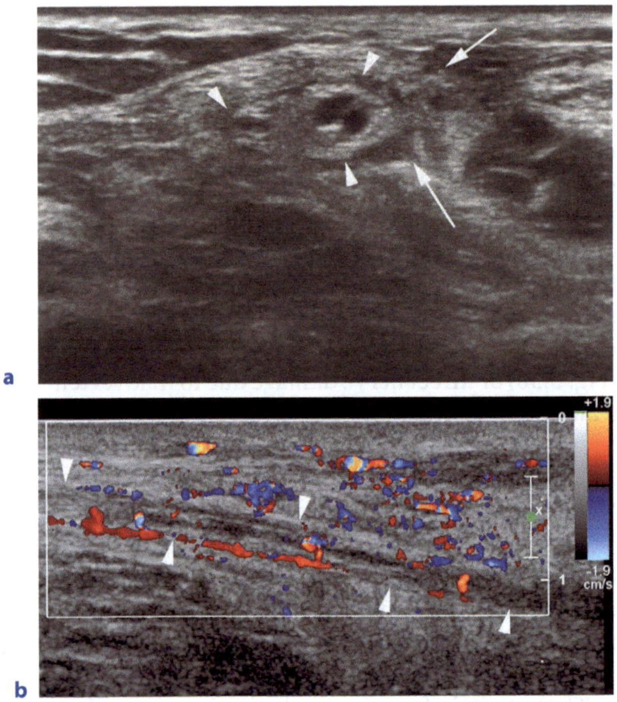

Fig. 5.31a,b. Transverse sonogram (**a**) and longitudinal color Doppler sonogram through common peroneal nerve in a patient after knee joint dislocation and operative revision. **a** Swelling of peroneal nerve (*arrowheads*) and compromise by small encasing scar. **b** Marked hypervascularization of nerve (*arrowheads*) and surrounding soft tissues due to unspecific neuritis

5.5.3 Nerve Lesions Following Fracture Repair

Fracture repair with the use of rods, wires and plates may result in postoperative nerve palsy either if a nerve is directly compromised by the fixation material or if there is hematoma and/or scar formation along the surgical access route. The main nerves affected are the radial nerve at its course along the surface of the humeral shaft, the ulnar nerve in the ulnar nerve groove and the peroneal nerve at its course around the fibular neck. Data in the literature about the frequency of such lesions is rare. As far as repair of humeral shaft fractures is concerned, lesions of the radial nerve caused by implanted material may be encountered in up to 20% of procedures (Cognet et al. 2002) and mainly occur after plate fixation. In these cases the nerve may be simply displaced or stretched by the plate (Fig. 5.32) or even be compressed underneath it (Fig. 5.33). Lesions to other nerves are very rare but may follow the same mechanism. The peroneal nerve may further be damaged during insertion of wires for placement of an external fixation device or leg extension. The resulting nerve damage ranges from simple edema to internal bleeding and complete transections.

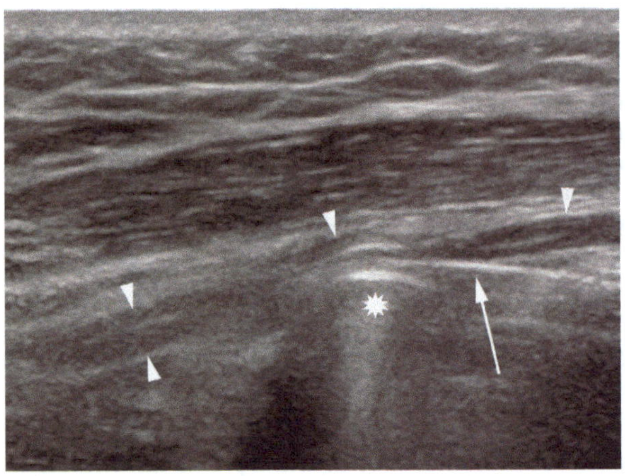

Fig. 5.32. Longitudinal sonogram through radial nerve (*arrowheads*) in a patient after humeral shaft fracture and plate fixation. Notice displacement of the nerve by the plate (*arrow*) and a screw (*asterisk*)

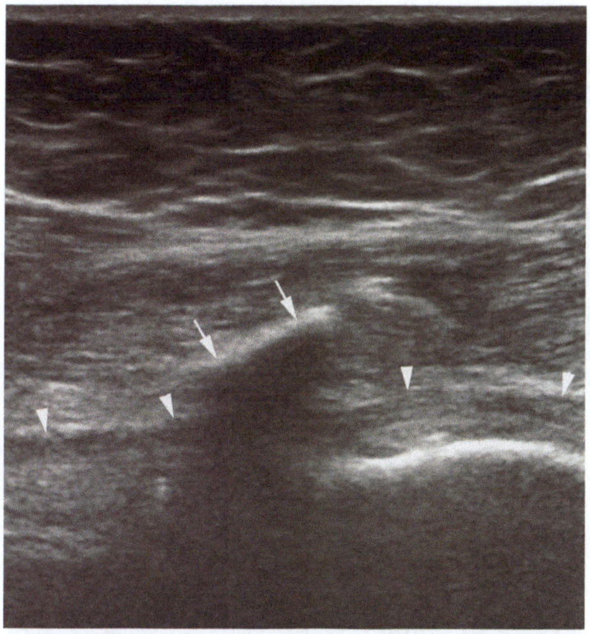

Fig. 5.33. Longitudinal sonogram through radial nerve in another patient after humeral shaft fracture and surgical repair shows displaced plate (*arrows*) with compression of the radial nerve (*arrowheads*) running underneath the plate

5.5.4 Miscellaneous Postoperative Lesions

Various other operative procedures may result in peripheral nerve lesions. General surgical procedures on the lower abdominal or inguinal region may result in damage to the ilioinguinal, iliohypogastric or genitofemoral nerve. During cardiac surgery median sternotomy is associated with a considerable risk of peri-operative damage to the brachial plexus, possibly due to excessive traction on the brachial plexus (Fig. 5.34) or compression of its medial cord by the first rib.

The harvesting of bone grafts from the iliac crest may be followed by meralgia paraesthetica due to injury of the lateral femoral cutaneous nerve. Simonetti and coworkers (1999) reported on sural nerve lesions in association with stripping of the small saphenus vein; furthermore, lesions to the sciatic and femoral nerve may follow various gynecologic operations (Fig. 5.35).

Nerve lesions due to local injections or punctures are rare, but may also be encountered even in minimal invasive procedures such as vaccinations in small children (Fig. 5.36).

In many of these aforementioned situations direct sonographic visualization of the involved nerve – even if it has a superficial course – is possible in certain circumstances only because of the small size of some nerves involved such as the iliohypogastric or ilioinguinal nerve. A sonographic evaluation of the site of post-surgical cutaneous scars is nevertheless useful in many situations, especially if neuroma formation is suspected in patients with operations dating back some weeks or months. The ability of sonography to depict neuromas has been shown in various studies (Graif 1995; Peer et al. 2001), and the sonographic features of these types of lesions are discussed in more detail in Chapter 5, Section 5.6.

5.5.5 Nerve Lesions Associated with Anesthesia

5.5.5.1 Peri-operative Nerve Lesions

Peri-operative nerve lesions can spoil an otherwise successful operation. The patient may be handicapped with some amount of functional disability and the medical team will possibly face litigation. The true incidence of peri-operative nerve damage still remains unclear and is probably under-reported. Such as in the case in direct surgical nerve injury the leading neurological symptom may appear minor to the attending physician compared with the clinical disorder that led to surgery, and therefore may be dismissed. The belief that such a minor lesion may be self-limited with full spontaneous recovery is widespread but often this is not the case.

Malpositioning of the patient on the operation table with subsequent stretching and/or compression of a nerve is today considered the most frequent cause for this type of injury, with direct needle trauma or chemical irritation being rare (Sawyer et al. 2000). With the first type of injury the ulnar nerve is most commonly involved as the ulnar nerve is rather susceptible to compression against the operating table especially when the forearm is extended and pronated (Fig. 5.37a,b). Another nerve which is frequently injured is the common peroneal nerve, which may be compressed between the head of the fibula and the operating table, or against a leg fixation device with the patient in the lithotomy position. Rarely also other peripheral nerves such as the median nerve may be compressed with the patient in a prone position (Fig. 5.38a,b).

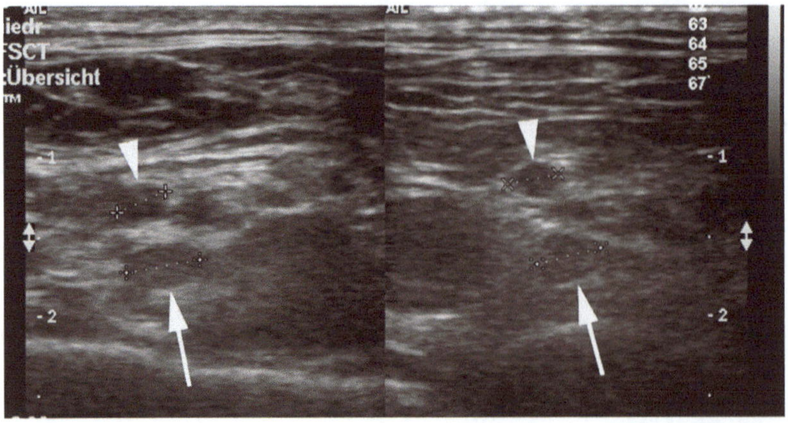

Fig. 5.34. Comparative transverse sonograms of brachial plexus (right side, left image; left side, right image) in a patient who underwent medial sternotomy for cardiac surgery and developed partial radial paralysis thereafter. In side by side comparison enlargement with edema of the right sided posterior plexus fascicle is seen (47 versus 41 mm; *short arrows*), while the medial fascicles show equal caliber (33 versus 32 mm; *arrowheads*)

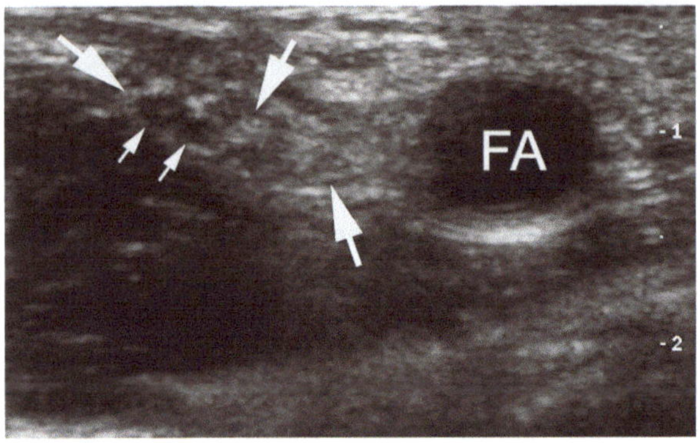

Fig. 5.35. Transverse sonogram through femoral nerve at level of inguinal canal in a patient after total hysterectomy and reconstructive operation of pelvic floor. Inside the otherwise normal femoral nerve (*large arrows*) two distinct hypoechoic nodules consistent with traction neuromas (*small arrows*) are demonstrated. *FA*, femoral artery

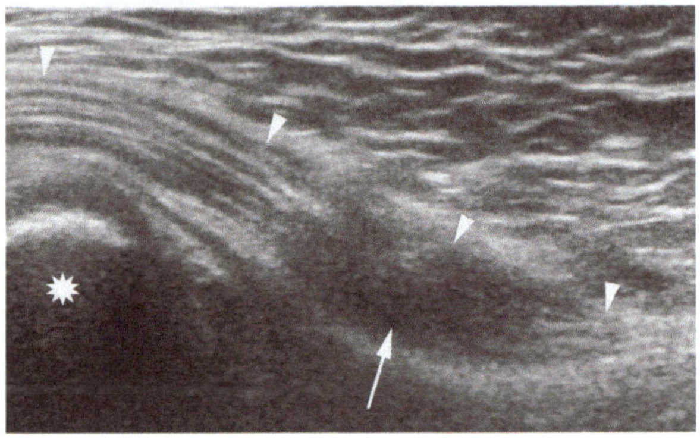

Fig. 5.36. Longitudinal sonogram through sciatic nerve (*arrowheads*) at its exit from underneath the gluteal muscles in a 1-year-old child who developed a sciatic nerve lesion after vaccination with intramuscular injection. Notice a small hypoechoic area with indistinct fascicular texture (*arrow*) inside the nerve. At surgical exploration internal hematoma was confirmed. *Asterisk*, ischial tuberosity

a

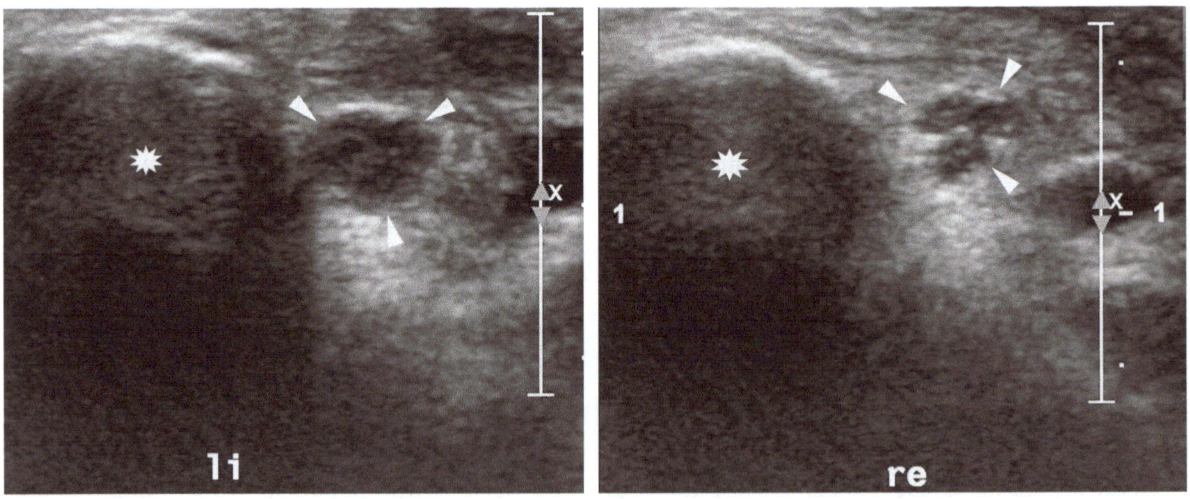

b

Fig. 5.37a,b. Transverse sonograms through ulnar nerve (*arrowheads*) at the level of the medial epicondyle (*asterisk*) in a patient, who developed ulnar nerve palsy after a set of operations with rather long duration. Marked swelling of ulnar nerve with loss of fascicular texture is noted **a** with side by side comparison. **b** Normal contralateral nerve

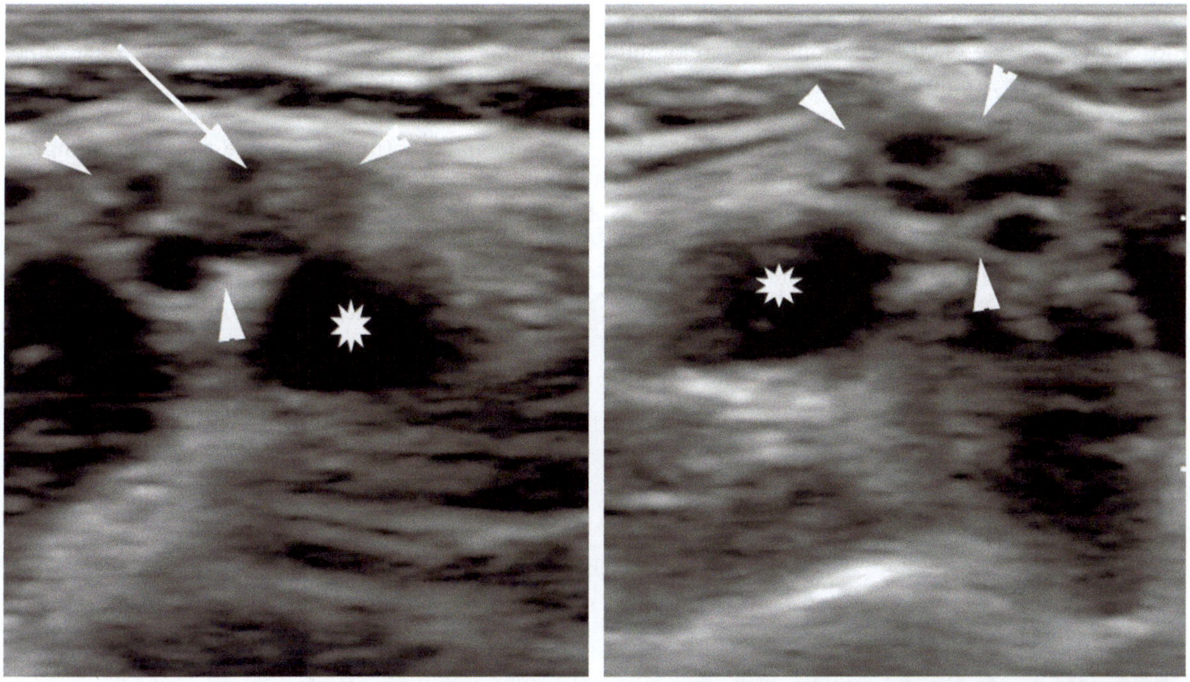

Fig. 5.38a,b. Transverse sonogram through median nerve (*arrowheads*) in a patient with median nerve palsy after an operation in prone position. **a** A small hypoechoic lesion is demonstrated consistent with traction edema (*arrow*). **b** Normal contralateral median nerve. *Asterisk*, brachial artery

Sonographic features in these types of nerve lesions are the same as compared to other types of traumatic nerve injury: Localized swelling of nerve fascicles with edema, hematoma, and in chronic nerve lesions scarring. The nerves commonly involved in association with anesthesia such as the ulnar or peroneal nerve are normally easy to assess with sonography due to their superficial course. As a general rule it is beneficial to compare the possibly damaged nerve with the unimpaired contralateral side, as findings with minor nerve lesions may only be subtle. A comparative study may also be advocated in regard to later legal issues, where exact documentation of site and extent of lesions is of outmost importance.

5.5.5.2 Nerve Lesions Associated with Regional Anesthesia

While regional anesthesia is associated with multiple benefits it also bares a certain risk of nerve damage which, generally speaking, may be avoided with meticulous technique and choice of material (Sawyer et al. 2000). In this regard we want to stress the value of sonography as a guidance for regional nerve blocks, which is discussed in more detail in Chapter 7, Section 7.2, of this book (Yang et al. 1998). The neurological sequels of nerve damage during anesthesia are quite unpleasant for the patient and spoil the experience of an otherwise successful operation. Data in the literature on the type and frequency of these lesions vary, which is mainly due to a change in the technique of the individual procedures and the risk factors of patients (obese patients, anticoagulants, etc.). Recent articles (Brull et al. 2007) report a neuropathy risk after peripheral nerve blocks of about 3%, with permanent neurological damage being extremely rare. However, we must keep in mind that due to under-reporting of adverse effects these figures may only partly reflect the true situation. Another reason for varying figures lies in the different thresholds of what investigators consider a significant neurological disturbance. A prospective study of transarterial axillary blocks for example found a 19% incidence of postanesthesia neurapraxia on the first postoperative day, falling to 5% at 2 weeks and clearing in all except one patient by 4 weeks (Urban and Urquhart 1994). At least some of this postanesthetic dysesthesia (which is quite frequent on day one after the operation) may just reflect residual blockade (Ben-David et al. 2006).

While there is some literature on the prevalence and clinical course of nerve lesions after regional anesthesia, there are no reports on the appearance of nerves after successful blocks or the type of nerve changes encountered in iatrogenic lesions. In the few cases we saw in our clinical routine, we experienced mainly edematous swelling of short nerve segments, close lying hematomas and even intraneural collections of liquid and/or intraneural bleeding with or without disruption of fascicular elements (Fig. 5.39a,b).

5.6 The Postoperative Nerve

(S. Peer)

The rationale for sonographic assessment of postoperative nerves is straight forward: Incomplete recovery of clinical symptoms after surgical exploration, decompression or microsurgical reconstruction of a peripheral nerve. As is true for other organ systems typical and transient postoperative findings have to be differentiated from unfavorable development with the need for further intervention. In respect to iatrogenic nerve lesions it is important to have an adequate knowledge of the postoperative evaluation of a nerve. Typical postoperative changes, such as short lasting edema and/or hypervascularization of a nerve, the formation of hematomas or scars have to be differentiated from incomplete surgical repair with persistent transection of nerve bundles or development of neuroma.

5.6.1 Normal Findings in Postoperative Nerves

The spectrum of imaging findings in postoperative nerves depends on the type and extent of surgery performed; in external neurolysis a nerve is isolated from surrounding tissues, which in many instances is simply performed to allow for direct inspection of the nerve and intraoperative electrodiagnostic testing. In the same way a nerve known to be surrounded by scar tissue may be released. As the outer sheath of the nerve and the nerve fascicles are not involved in this type of surgery postoperative changes in uncomplicated follow-ups are only subtle. With only minimal surgical disturbance of the nerve sonographic studies may be normal or show only mild nerve edema with loss of normal fascicular pattern.

The latter is thought to represent a common and non-specific reaction of a nerve to minor compromise, which may occur in the post-surgical setting and is most probably caused by transient stretching of the nerve during the operation. The same reaction is also known from nerve compression syndromes such as carpal tunnel disease, nerves subjected to direct blunt trauma and various other pathologies and represents a disturbance of localized microvascular blood flow in the epi- and perineurium. There is a gradual transition from mere loss of fascicular pattern to localized swelling of nerve fascicles with increase of outer nerve diameter, related to more pronounced edema and hypervascularization. In these more advanced states a differentiation between a self-limited postoperative finding and a persistent impairment of the nerve may be difficult and the value of sonography lies mainly in the exclusion of external reasons for nerve swelling such as encasing scars. As a general rule we may observe a gentle tapering of a nerve to normal size above and below a level of swelling in transient edema and an abrupt change in nerve caliber in nerves hampered by scars (Fig. 5.40a,b).

Persistent nerve edema and swelling of fascicles may commonly be seen as a complication after release and transposition of a nerve, when the extrinsic blood supply of the nerve is severed. As for the ulnar nerve the extrinsic vessels (superior and inferior ulnar collateral artery and posterior ulnar recurrent artery) may be transected during release of the nerve in patients with cubital tunnel syndrome (Balogh et al. 1997; Prevel et al. 1993). Due to a localized disturbance of blood supply in the postoperative nerve a persistent clinical impairment follows and sonographically this may appear as a persistent and pronounced edema of the nerve.

With internal neurolysis the nerve and its sheath is directly involved in surgery and this procedure is mainly used for reconstruction of partial nerve lesions requiring a split repair in which functioning nerve fascicles are separated from nonfunctioning transected elements or scarred intraneural tissue. In this procedure a risk for inadvertent damage of still functioning nerve elements exists and postoperative scar formation close to the nerve surface may exert deleterious effects on nerve recovery (Mackinnon and Dellon 1988).

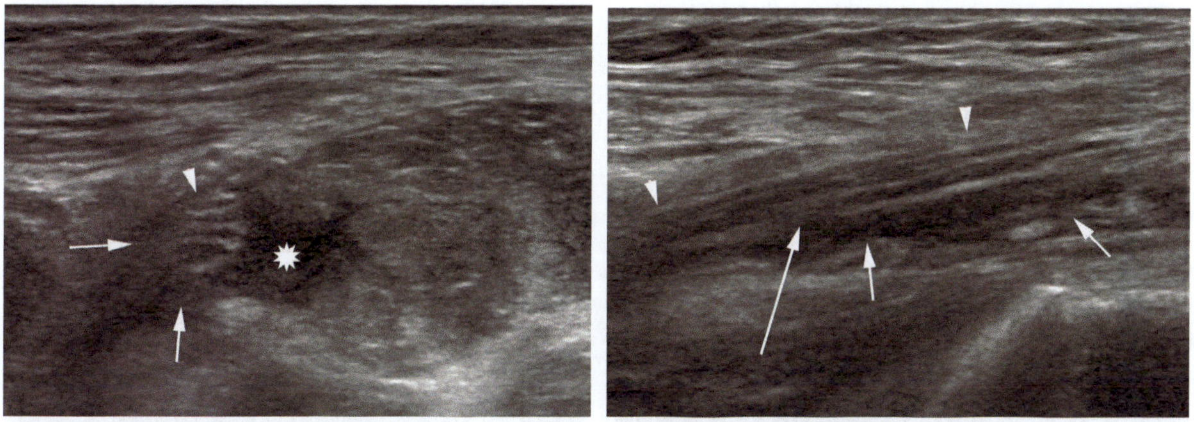

a b

Fig. 5.39a,b. Transverse (**a**) and longitudinal (**b**) sonogram through femoral nerve (*arrowhead*) in a patient who developed femoral nerve palsy after a three-in-one or "Winnie-block". **a** Notice edema with small hematoma inside the psoas muscle (*asterisk*) and compromise of the nerve by close lying hematoma (*arrows*). **b** Hematoma underneath the nerve consistent with (**a**) is demonstrated (*small arrows*) and there is a short zone of disrupted outer epineurium (*long arrow*)

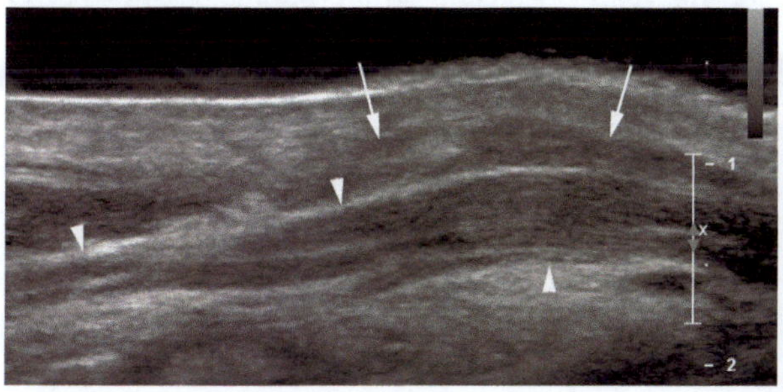

a

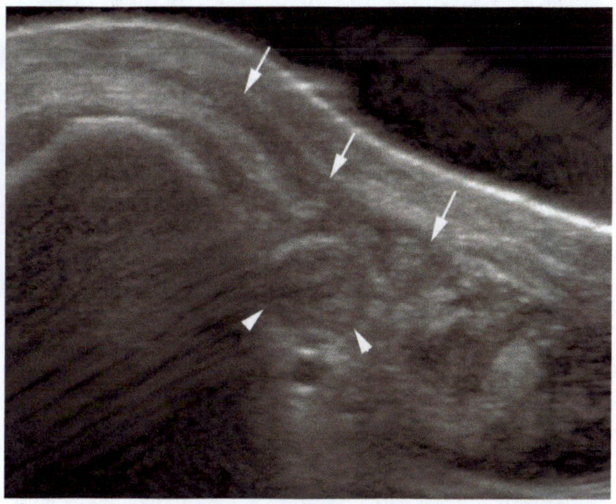

b

Fig. 5.40a,b. Longitudinal (**a**) and transverse (**b**) sonogram through ulnar nerve after decompression of the ulnar nerve groove in a patient with cubital tunnel syndrome. The ulnar nerve (*arrowheads*) is markedly swollen and compromised by a close lying scar (*arrows*)

With complete traumatic transection of a nerve or after resection of nerve tumors a more extensive surgical procedure with approximation of the nerve ends is required. The choice of reconstruction depends on the distance of the gap between the nerve stumps after resection of all irreversibly traumatized tissue. Given a small gap an end-to-end anastomosis is generally preferred; however, significant tension on the approximated ends has to be avoided by all means. If this is not achieved, then the gap is bridged with interposition of nerve grafts, usually harvested from superficial sensory nerves, such as the sural nerve or the medial brachial and antebrachial cutaneous nerve. In both types of surgical repair the nerve (or nerve and graft) ends are anastomosed with fine monofilament sutures placed within the external or internal epineurium. Despite being only very thin these sutures are constantly seen on sonographic exams of reconstructed peripheral nerves (Fig. 5.41) and should not be mistaken for pathology, such as fibrotic changes or tiny calcifications in granulation tissue for example.

The sonographic examination of internal neurolysis or complete nerve reconstruction should always attempt to define the continuity of reconstructed elements. According to our experience with sonography in a large series of patients who received nerve reconstruction after partial or complete traumatic transection this is only partly achieved. While the integrity of the outer epineurium or the continuity of the nerve in total may be achieved in most cases (Fig. 5.42), an evaluation of the continuity of single fascicles is often not possible (Fig. 5.43). True discontinuity of a reconstructed nerve due to loosening of sutures is readily established in many cases and may either be partial or complete (Fig. 5.44).

This is most probably due to a somewhat oblique course of proximal and distal fascicles, which hampers the achievement of a sonographic scan alignment, that directly shows both fascicles in continuity. A certain increase in nerve diameter is generally seen at the level of nerve suture, which is a normal finding as long as it appears mild and fusiform (Fig. 5.43).

An irregular bulging of the nerve surface or single nerve elements on one surface, however, should raise a suspicion of partial incomplete fusion of nerve fascicles and neuroma formation (Fig. 5.45a,b). The latter is especially true if an additional fibrous mass lesion exists.

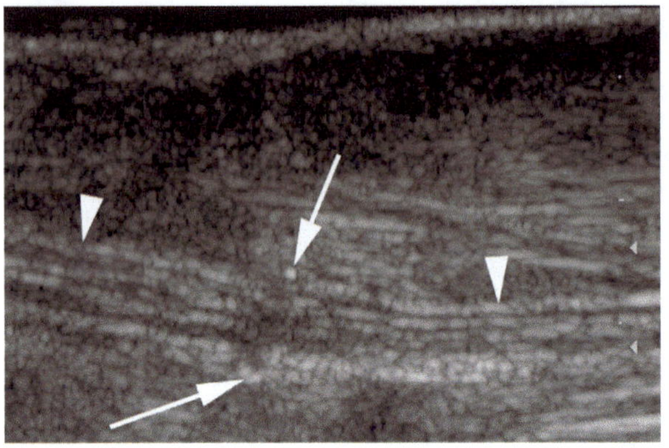

Fig. 5.41. Longitudinal sonogram through median nerve (*arrowheads*) in a patient with forearm amputation and replantation. Tiny echogenic foci, which are caused by suture material are seen on both sides of the site of nerve suture (*arrows*). Note that there is no increase in nerve diameter at suture site and good continuation of single nerve fascicles in this reconstruction (clinically the patient showed excellent restitution of nerve function)

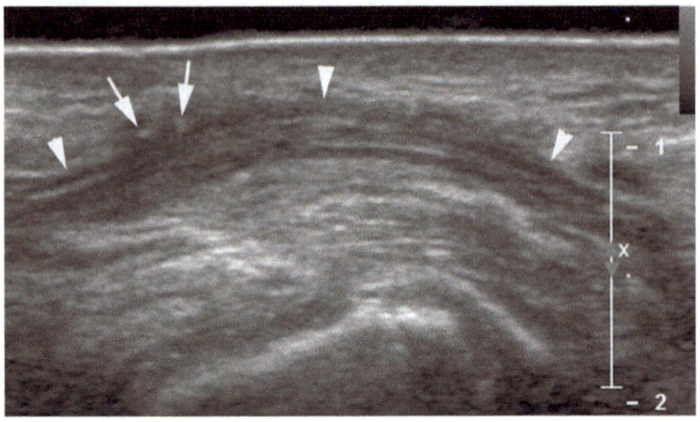

Fig. 5.42. Longitudinal sonogram through median nerve (*arrowheads*) in a patient after sharp transection of the nerve shows established continuity at the site of the anastomosis (*arrows*, suture artifacts), with very good continuity of single fascicles

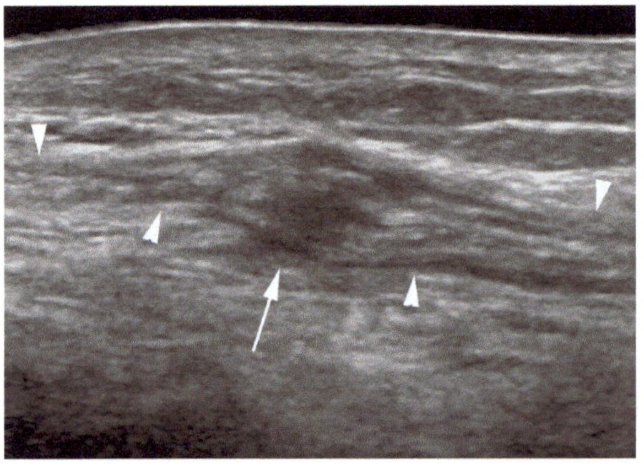

Fig. 5.43. Longitudinal sonogram through median nerve in a patient after hand transplantation and clinically good median nerve function shows apparent continuity of the outer nerve sheath (*arrowheads*) but continuity of single fascicular elements cannot be readily established (*arrow*)

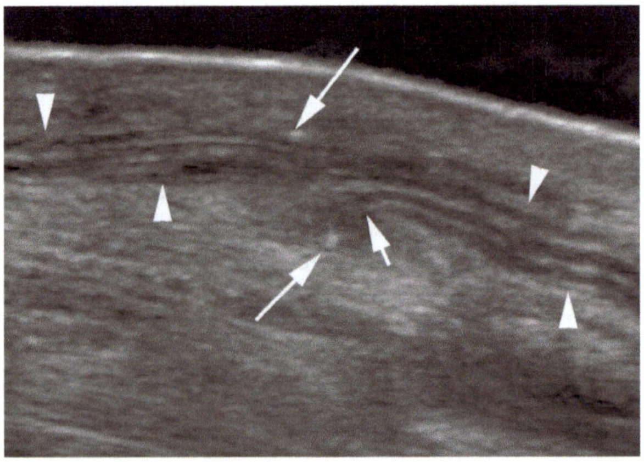

Fig. 5.44. Longitudinal sonogram through ulnar nerve (*arrowheads*) in a patient with sharp transection of the nerve and intrafascicular repair. Only partial continuity has been established with demonstration of a discontinuous nerve portion (*small arrow*) because of loosened sutures. *Long arrows*, suture artifacts

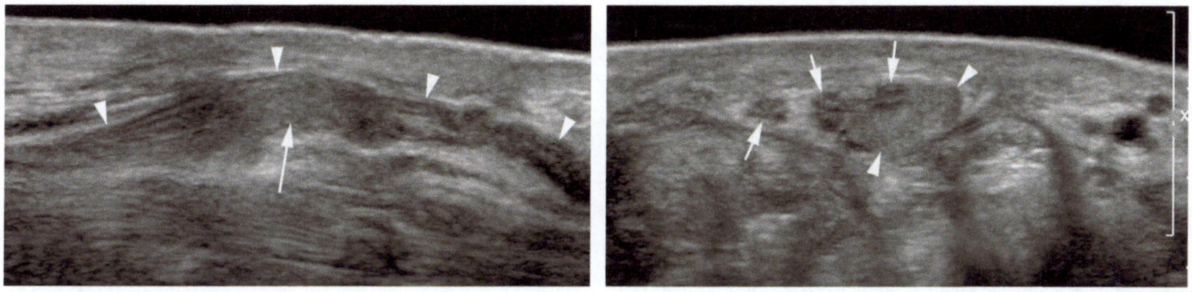

Fig. 5.45a,b. Longitudinal (**a**) and transverse (**b**) sonogram through median nerve in a patient with sharp transection of the nerve and intrafascicular repair. **a** Eccentric, slightly hypoechoic nodular mass consistent with neuroma (*arrow*) is demonstrated inside the otherwise continuous nerve (*arrowheads*). **b** Eccentric neuroma (*arrowheads*), normal median nerve bundles (*arrows*)

5.6.2 Postoperative Scaring

Postoperative scaring is a common problem after reconstructive nerve surgery and sonography has proven helpful in early detection of scars in patients with bad recovery after nerve repair (Peer et al. 2001). Scaring may also follow external neurolysis or surgery not primarily directed to a nerve itself (fracture repair, vascular surgery, etc.). While the mechanism of nerve compression by an overlying scar is easily understood, other pathophysiologic influences have to be considered, which may lead to a more refined sonographic examination technique. A nerve encased by a scar not only experiences compression with an apparent decrease of nerve diameter on sonography, but may also have tight adhesions between outer epineurium and the scar tissue. In the case of a close lying scar the nerve with an adhesion may even have a fairly normal or even bigger diameter (due to edema) compared to more proximal or distal nerve portions (Fig. 5.46a,b).

In this situation scar tissue can cause persistent pain as well as delayed recovery of sensory and motor deficits because of constant traction on the nerve due to limited possibility for longitudinal translation during movement of an extremity. A functional sonographic examination with close inspection of longitudinal nerve motion at the site of suture during passive or active movement should therefore be attempted in postoperative patients to rule out compromise due to adhesions.

A nerve with too large a gap between nerve stumps, which is reconstructed by direct anastomosis, will react developing an intraneural scar due to constant traction on the rejoined fascicles. These fibrotic changes must not be confused with neuroma formation, which has a completely different pathophysiologic reason. However, intraneural scars and neuromas may hardly be differentiated with sonography based on the echotexture of the pathological tissue elements. Only the shape and course of these lesions may aid in the differential diagnosis. We do not consider a low specificity in this differential a big draw back of sonography, as a second surgical exploration will normally be adequate for treatment of both types of lesions. The mechanism of neuroma formation and its sonographic work-up will be discussed in the next paragraph.

5.6.3 Neuroma Formation

Neuroma formation is common in traumatic peripheral nerve lesions and may develop in two distinct settings. Firstly, it may constitute a direct result of the trauma. If an incomplete nerve lesion undergoes a trial of conservative treatment, there may be partially damaged axons, which try to reestablish continuity by sprouting of axons and Schwann cells at the proximal stump. The success of this restitution mechanism depends on the integrity of the axonal or fascicular outer sheath. If this is also impaired, axonal overgrowth results, as sprouting axons and Schwann cells lack a pathway to reach their distal target. A typical example for this type of injury is traction neuroma, which – as the name already suggests – is a consequence of excessive stretching of a nerve. Traction neuroma is easily visualized with sonography, and constitutes an ovoid or spindle-shaped mass inside a peripheral nerve. This mass is of variable size depending on the amount of nerve elements involved. With only single fascicles involved, the outer diameter of the nerve

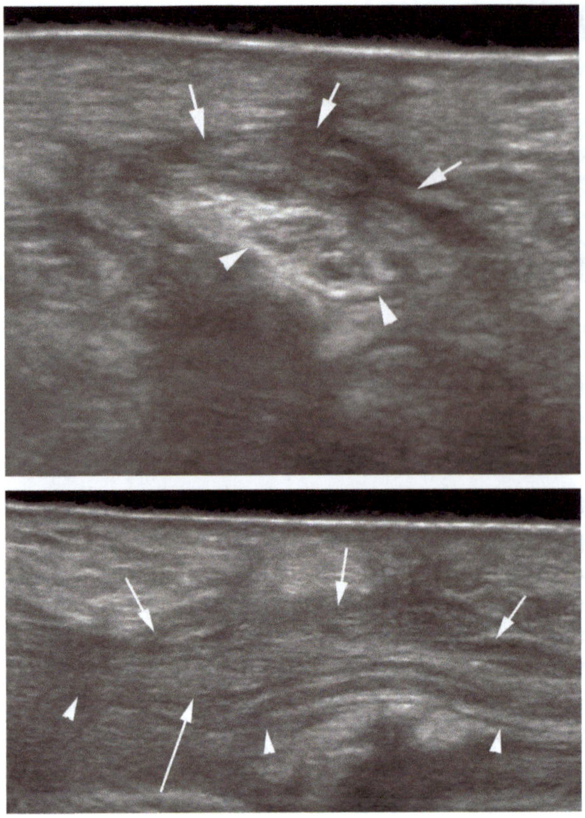

a

b

Fig. 5.46a,b. Transverse (**a**) and longitudinal (**b**) sonogram through tibial nerve (*arrowheads*) in a patient after repair of an ankle fracture shows marked scar formation (*arrows*) with encasement of the slightly swollen nerve

may appear fairly normal or only slightly enlarged, due to coexisting edema. Inside the nerve a hypoechoic bulbous mass can be detected. If the whole nerve is involved, normal fascicular echotexture is replaced by a mass enlarging the nerve diameter, but the outer nerve sheath if not impaired may appear normal. The latter type of injury is commonly seen in traction injuries of the brachial plexus (motor vehicle accidents). Examples for these types of lesions are shown in the chapters on nerve lesions of the plexus, upper and lower extremity.

The second mechanism for the development of neuroma is post-surgical. Focal external or intraneural scaring may impair the reestablishment of nerve continuity and result in neuroma formation (Fig. 5.45a,b). In this regard neuroma is a major complication of surgical interventions and research on surgical techniques which help to reduce the incidence of post-surgical neuroma is ongoing. Thus resection of nerve stumps to functioning neural tissue, microsurgical adaptation of fascicles and epineural sheaths (with or without grafting) and the avoidance of traction are main concerns. The sonographic appearance of this type of neuroma is fairly similar to post-traumatic neuroma. According to our own hitherto unpublished experience the sensitivity of sonography in the detection of post-traumatic and post-surgical neuroma is very high. The necessity to define the extent of nerve involvement, as well as the exact localization and size of neuroma in respect to further surgical intervention is clear.

References

Alan CH (2000) Functional aspects of primary nerve repair. Hand Clin 16:67–72

Balogh B, Vass A, Piza-Katzer H (1997) Ist eine Vorverlagerung des N. ulnaris beim Sulcus nervi ulnaris-Syndrom wirklich indiziert. Handchir Mikrochir Plast Chir 29:133–139

Ben-David B, Barak M, Katz Y, Stahl S (2006) A retrospective study of the incidence of neurological injury after axillary brachial plexus block. Pain Practice 6:119–123

Bigliani LU, Compito CA, Dualde XA, Wolfe IN (1996) Transfer of the levator scapulae, rhomboid major, and rhomboid minor for paralysis of the trapezius. J Bone Joint Surg 78A:534–540

Birch R, Raji AR (1991) Repair of median and ulnar nerves. Primary suture is best. J Bone Joint Surg Br 73:154–157

Birch R, Bonney G, Dowell J, Hollingdale J (1991) Iatrogenic injuries of peripheral nerves. J Bone Joint Surg [Br] 73:280–285

Boardman ND, Cofield RH (1999) Neurologic complications of shoulder surgery. Clin Orthop 368:44–52

Bodner G, Buchberger W, Schocke M et al. (2001) Radial nerve palsy associated with humeral shaft fracture: evaluation with US-initial experience. Radiology 219: 811–816

Bodner G, Harpf C, Gardetto A et al. (2002) Ultrasonography of the accessory nerve. J Ultrasound Med 21:1159–1163

Brull R, McCartney C, Chan V, El-Beheiry H (2007) Neurological complications after regional anesthesia: contemporary estimates of risk. Anesth Analg 104:965–967

Carvalho GA, Nikkhah G, Matthies C, Penkert G, Samii M (1997) Diagnosis of root avulsions in traumatic brachial plexus injuries: value of computerized tomography myelography and magnetic resonance imaging. J Neurosurg 86:69–76

Cognet JM, Fabre T, Durandeau A (2002) Persistent radial palsy after humeral diaphyseal fracture: cause, treatment, and results. 30 operated cases. Rev Chir Orthop Reparatrice Appar Mot 88:655–662

De Laat EA, Visser CP, Coene LN, Pahlplatz PV, Tavy DL (1994) Nerve lesions in primary shoulder dislocations and humeral neck fractures. A prospective clinical and EMG study. J Bone Joint Surg Br 76:381–383

Doi K, Otsuka K, Okamoto Y et al. (2002) Cervical nerve root avulsion in brachial plexus injuries: magnetic resonance imaging classification and comparison with myelography and computerized tomography myelography. J Neurosurg 96:277–284

Eggli S, Hankemayer S, Müller ME (1999) Nerve palsy after leg lengthening in total replacement arthroplasty for developmental dysplasia of the hip. J Bone Joint Surg [Br] 81:843–845

Graif M (1995) Peripheral nerves. In: Fornage BD (ed) Musculoskeletal ultrasound. Churchill Livingston, New York, pp 73–98

Grant GA, Goodkin R, Kliot M (1999) Evaluation and surgical management of peripheral nerve problems. Neurosurgery 44:825–840

Gruber H, Peer S, Kovacs P, Marth R, Bodner G (2003) The ultrasonographic appearance of the femoral nerve and cases of iatrogenic impairment. J Ultrasound Med 22:163–172

Gruber H, Peer S, Meirer R, Bodner G (2005) Peroneal nerve palsy associated with knee luxation: evaluation by sonography-initial experiences. AJR Am J Roentgenol 185:1119–1125

Gruber H, Glodny B, Bendix N, Tzankov A, Peer S (2007a) High-resolution ultrasound of peripheral neurogenic tumors. Eur Radiol (in print)

Gruber H, Glodny B, Galiano K, Kamelger F, Bodner G, Hussl H, Peer S (2007b) High-resolution ultrasound of the supraclavicular brachial plexus-can it improve therapeutic decisions in patients with plexus trauma? Eur Radiol 17:1611–1620

Haber HP, Sinis N, Haerle M, Schaller HE (2006) Sonography of brachial plexus traction injuries. AJR Am J Roentgenol 186:1787–1791

Harpf C, Rhomberg M, Rumer A, Hussl H (1999) Iatrogenic lesion of the accessory nerve in cervical lymph node biopsy. Chirurg 70:690–693

Hayamizu K, Naito K, Ito K (1995) Ultrasonography for traction injuries of the brachial plexus. Nippon Igaku Hoshasen Gakkai Zasshi 55:873–877

Jaquet JB, Luijsterburg AJ, Kalmijn S, Kuypers PD, Hofman A, Hovius SE (2001) Median, ulnar, and combined median-ulnar nerve injuries: functional outcome and return to productivity. J Trauma 51:687–692

Kim DH, Kline DG (1996) Management and results of peroneal nerve lesions. Neurosurgery 39:312–319

Mackinnon SE, Dellon AL (1988) Nerve repair and nerve grafts. In: Surgery of the peripheral nerve. Thieme, New York, pp 89–129

Maravilla KR, Aagaard BDL, Kliot M (1998) MR neurography – imaging of peripheral nerves. MR Imaging Clin 6:179–194

Martinoli C, Bianchi S, Santacroce E, Pugliese F, Graif M, Derchi LE (2002) Brachial plexus sonography: a technique for assessing the root level. AJR Am J Roentgenol 179:699–702

Noble J, Munro CA, Vannemredy SSV et al. (1998) Analysis of upper and lower extremity peripheral nerve injuries in a population of patients with multiple injuries. J Trauma 45:116–122

Oldenburg M, Müller RT (1997) The frequency, prognosis and significance of nerve injuries in total hip arthroplasty. Int Orthop 21:1–3

Perlmutter GS, Apruzzese W (1998) Axillary nerve injuries in contact sports: recommendations for treatment and rehabilitation. Sports Med 26:351–361, review

Peer S, Bodner G, Meirer R, Willeit J, Piza-Kratzer H (2001) Evaluation of postoperative peripheral nerve lesions with high resolution ultrasound. AJR Am J Roentgenol 177:415–419

Peer S, Kovacs P, Harpf C et al. (2002) High resolution sonography of lower extremity peripheral nerves: anatomic correlation and spectrum of pathology. J Ultrasound Med 21:315–322

Penkert G, Carvalho GA, Nikkhah G et al. (1999) Diagnosis and surgery of brachial plexus injuries. J Reconstr Microsurg 15:3–8

Prevel CD, Matloub HS, Zhong Y et al. (1993) The extrinsic blood supply of the ulnar nerve at the elbow: an anatomic study. J Hand Surg 18A:433–438

Remmler D, Byers R, Scheetz J et al. (1986) A prospective study of shoulder disability resulting from radical and modified neck dissections. Head Neck Surg 8:280–286

Robinson LR (2000) Traumatic injury to peripheral nerves. Muscle Nerve 23:863–873

Sawyer RJ, Richmond MN, Hickey JD, Jarrat JA (2000) Peripheral nerve injuries associated with anaesthesia. Anaesthesia 55:980–991

Seddon HJ (1975) Surgical disorders of the peripheral nerves, 2nd edn. Churchill Livingstone, New York

Sheppard DG, Iyer RB, Fenstermacher MJ (1998) Brachial plexus: demonstration at US. Radiology 208:402–406

Simonetti S, Bianchi S, Martinoli C (1999) Neurophysiological and ultrasound findings in sural nerve lesions following stripping of the small saphenus vein. Muscle Nerve 22:1724–1726

Steinmann SP, Moran EA (2001) Axillary nerve injury: diagnosis and treatment. J Am Acad Orthop Surg 9:328–335

Sunderland S (1978) Nerves and nerve injuries, 2nd edn. Churchill Livingstone. New York

Tomaino M, Day C, Papageorgiou C, Harner C, Fu FH (2000) Peroneal nerve palsy following knee dislocation: pathoanatomy and implications for treatment. Knee Surg Sports Traumatol Arthrosc 8:163–165

Urban MK, Urquhart B (1994) Evaluation of brachial plexus anesthesia for upper extremity surgery. Reg Anesth 19:175–182

Vastamaki M, Solonen KA (1984) Accessory nerve injury. Acta Orthop Scand 55:296–299

Weale AE, Newman P, Ferguson IT, Bannister GC (1996) Nerve injury after posterior and direct lateral approaches for hip replacement. J Bone Joint Surg [Br] 78:899–902

Weber ER, Daube JR, Coventry MB (1976) Neural and vascular injury in total hip arthroplasty. J Bone Joint Surg [Am] 58:66–69

Wiater JM, Bigliani LU (1999) Spinal accessory nerve injury. Clin Orthop 368:5–16

Wilbourn AJ (1998) Iatrogenic nerve injuries. Neurol Clin 16:55–82

Woodhall B (1952) Trapezius paralysis following minor surgical procedures in the posterior cervical triangle. Ann Surg 136:375–380

Wulff HB (1941) Treatment of tuberculous cervical lymphoma: late results in 230 cases treated partly surgically. Acta Chir Scand 84:343–366

Yang WT, Chui PT, Metreweli C (1998) Anatomy of the normal brachial plexus revealed by sonography and the role of sonographic guidance in anesthesia of the brachial plexus. AJR Am J Roentgenol 171:1631–1636

Yoshikawa T, Hayashi N, YamamotoS et al. (2006) Brachial plexus injury: clinical manifestations, conventional imaging findings, and the latest imaging techniques. Radiographics 26[Suppl 1]:133–143

Tumors and Tumor-Like Lesions

Gerd Bodner and Siegfried Peer

CONTENTS

G. Bodner, MD
Professor, Department of Radiology, St. Bernards Hospital, Europort 1–4, Gibraltar
S. Peer, MD
Professor, Department of Radiology, Section for Diagnostic and Interventional Sonography, Innsbruck Medical University, Anichstrasse 35, 6020 Innsbruck, Austria

6.1 Introduction

Peripheral nerve tumors are uncommon, nerve sheath tumors, schwannoma and neurofibromas being the most frequent. Their clinical signs and symptoms are often unspecific, which is why they may pose a diagnostic problem; this is particularly true for the neck, where a palpable mass is often mistaken for an enlarged lymph node by the referring clinician. Several neurogenic tumors can affect the musculoskeletal system, including traumatic neuroma, Morton's neuroma, neural fibrolipoma, nerve sheath ganglia, neurilemmoma, neurofibroma and malignant peripheral nerve sheath tumors (Murphey et al. 1999). In general the diagnosis of such a lesion is based on the detection of a mass in association with neurologic signs. It is important, however, to delimitate musculoskeletal lesions with secondary nerve involvement from lesions directly derived from neurogenic tissue. In this regard imaging may be helpful, but only if the applied method has the potential to establish the diagnosis by demonstration of a lesion in direct continuity with a peripheral nerve.

Furthermore, an exact description of the intrinsic imaging appearance and location of a lesion is necessary, as these may present clues for the final differential diagnosis (Fig. 6.1).

According to our experience sonography is a valuable diagnostic tool for these purposes, as it is a generally available and cheap method, which allows for direct evaluation of these mostly superficially lying tumors (Gruber et al. 2007). In most cases the association with a peripheral nerve is easily established and with the application of color Doppler, power Doppler and spectral wave analysis a lesion's malignant potential may even be realized (Bodner et al. 2002).

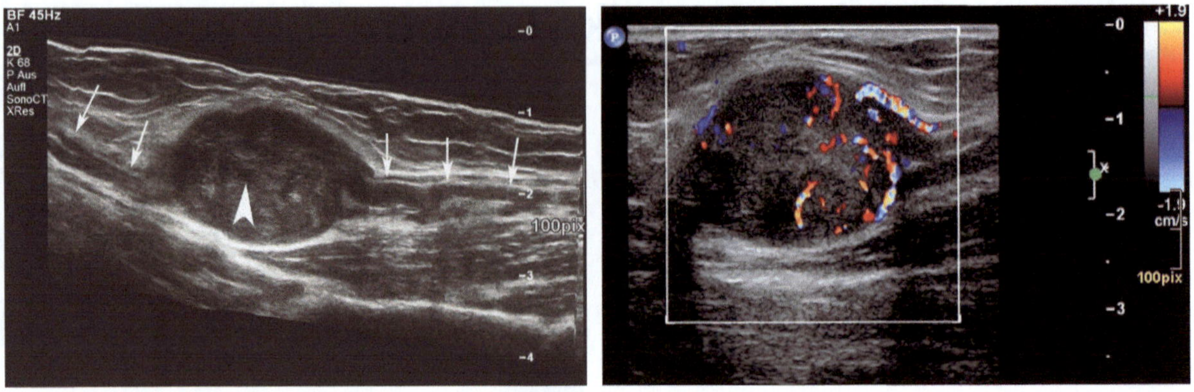

a b

Fig. 6.1a,b. Longitudinal sonogram (**a**) and color Doppler sonogram (**b**) in a patient with a firm palpable mass at the left forearm. A well defined lesion with hypoechoic echotexture is seen, which shows direct continuity with the median nerve (*arrows* in **a** and **b**), the lesion arising from the surface of the nerve. Within the tumor small cystic areas are noted (*white arrow*). **b** Color Doppler sonography reveals multiple tumor vessels. The combination of findings is characteristic for a Schwannoma

6.2 Benign Peripheral Nerve Tumors

Classically, benign peripheral nerve tumors have been divided into schwannoma (neurilemmoma) and neurofibroma, which constitute the most frequent benign nerve tumors (Weiss and Goldblum 2001). While these tumors are similar in appearance and contain cellular elements related to normal Schwann cells, some distinguishing clinical and pathologic features exist. Other rare benign neural tumors include granular cell tumor, nerve sheath myxoma and extracranial meningioma. Clinically all benign tumors present as a slow growing mass, with or without pain. Sometimes a Tinel sign can be shown by tapping on the tumor or neurological deficit can appear as a sign of nerve compression.

6.2.1 Schwannoma (Neurilemmoma)

6.2.1.1 Clinical Introduction

Schwannoma most commonly affects patients aged 20–40 years (but may also appear in the older age group) and constitutes approximately 5% of all benign soft tissue neoplasms (Murphey et al. 1999). It occurs equally in both genders. Predilection areas are the flexor surface of the upper and lower limb and the neck area. It mainly appears as a solitary lesion, rarely the tumor presents in a plexiform or multinodular form. The lesion shows non-aggressive features including slow growth and small size, pain and neurologic symptoms are unusual, except in larger tumors. At clinical examination the lesion is freely mobile to palpation except at the site of nerve attachment.

At pathologic analysis the schwannoma has a size of 2–5 cm and shows a true capsule – which allows for easy surgical enucleation – and a fusiform shape, because of the nerve entering and exiting the mass.

In larger nerves the mass has an eccentric location in relationship to the involved nerve, which is an important sonographic criterion for its differentiation from neurofibroma. Histologically the lesion derives from the nerve sheath and may appear in a solid and myxoid form. It is distinguished at immunohistochemical analysis from neurofibroma by intense staining for S-100 protein.

Degenerated schwannoma (also called ancient schwannoma) may show a high amount of cystic degeneration, central hemorrhage and calcification, which is attributed to its slow growth.
Malignant transformation in a schwannoma is extremely rare (Weiss and Goldblum 2001).

The treatment of schwannoma is usually surgical enucleation of the lesion after incision of the epineurium, which because of the eccentric location of the tumor in contrast to neurofibroma, normally allows sparing of the native nerve.

6.2.1.2
Sonography

Sonographic visualization of benign peripheral nerve tumors depends on the location of the tumor. Deep lying tumors at a depth of more than 3 cm below the skin surface are better visualized with a 4- to 7-MHz broad band linear probe, whereas superficially lying tumors are best investigated with 5- to 17-MHz broad band linear probes.

Many reports in the literature describe the sonographic appearance of peripheral nerve tumors in various locations (Johnston and Beggs 1994; Beggs 1999; Martinoli 1996; Lin 1999; Giovagnorio and Martinoli 2001; Peer et al. 2002; Reynolds et al. 2004; Bendix et al. 2006), and in fact the earliest reports on the application of sonography for imaging of peripheral nerves focused on the evaluation of nerve tumors (Hughes and Wilson 1986; Fornage 1988).

The typical sonographic appearance of a benign peripheral nerve tumor in general is a well defined mass with an oval or fusiform shape (Fig. 6.1a). This shape is considered to be the number one imaging feature, which should raise the suspicion for a peripheral nerve tumor – as it is caused by the tubular entering and exiting of a nerve in a typical nerve distribution (Murphey et al. 1999). In a small tumor arising from a superficial nerve, however, the sonographic demonstration of a connection to a nerve is unlikely due to the small size of the affected nerve.

Because of the uniform cellular pattern of schwannoma a homogeneous echotexture is found in most tumors. In general they show a medium to low echogeneity (Reynolds 2004); however, schwannomas with hyperechoic echotexture have also been reported in the literature (Simonovsky 1997). In our experience all larger schwannomas showed small cystic areas within the tumor (Fig. 6.1a). Whereas Reynolds et al. (2004) stated that schwannomas cannot be distinguished from neurofibromas, in our experience, and also according to Beggs (1999), larger tumors with a more myxoid matrix frequently show cystic internal changes.

A large schwannoma with pronounced degenerative changes is also called an “ancient schwannoma”. It shows a high amount of cystic degeneration, central haemorrhage and calcification, as a sign for slow and long growth (Lin et al. 1999; Isobe 2004; Bendix 2006) (Fig. 6.2).

The advantage of sonography for the differential diagnosis of schwannoma and neurofibroma is the demonstration of the tumor originating at an excentric location relative to the nerve, which is typical for schwannoma (Fig. 6.1a). This is especially true for tumors larger than 2 cm.

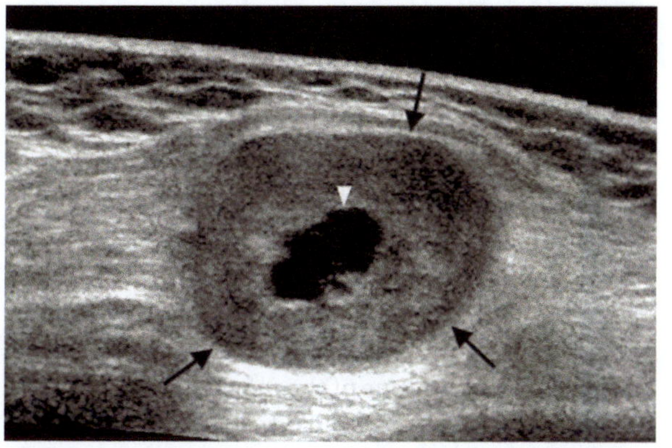

Fig. 6.2. Longitudinal sonogram of the right chest wall. Long standing palpable mass (*arrows*) showing well defined tumor margins with a central cystic area. Core needle biopsy confirmed the diagnosis of ancient schwannoma

Just like other neurogenic tumors affecting the peripheral nerve schwannomas may demonstrate high vascularity on color Doppler studies (Fig. 6.1b).

6.2.2
Neurofibroma

6.2.2.1
Clinical Introduction

Neurofibromas share the same features as schwannomas, as far as predilection for age and gender are concerned. They are classically divided into three groups depending on their appearance: localized, diffuse or plexiform. The plexiform and sometimes also the diffuse form are closely associated with Morbus Recklinghausen (Neurofibromatosis type 1).

The localized neurofibroma is the most common, accounting for approximately 90% of lesions, and mainly affects young patients of any gender. Macroscopically it has a fusiform appearance with entering and exiting of a nerve. Often it affects rather superficially lying small nerves of the extremities. Histologically neurofibroma shows wavy, elongated cells within bands of collagen. Tumor vascularity is usually rich. Rarely myxoid cells appear within the tumor, but they are never as prominent as in schwannoma. Treatment of neurofibroma is normally surgical and, in contrast to schwannoma,

implies reconstruction with nerve grafting if a deep nerve is involved.
The diffuse form of neurofibroma primarily affects children and young adults and is most frequently found in the adipose subcutaneous tissue of the neck region. In most cases (up to 90%) this is a solitary lesion not associated with neurofibromatosis.

Neurofibromatosis, first described by von Recklinghausen, is an inherited autosomal dominant genetic disease and affects one in 3000 births, which is why it constitutes one of the most common genetic disorders. The classic clinical triad consists of cutaneous lesions, skeletal deformities and mental deficiency. First characteristic signs appear in early childhood: café au lait spots, pigmented hamartomatous lesions of the iris (Lisch nodule) and osseus lesions. Neurofibromas can be found in virtually any nerve and any body including visceral organs (Roos and Muckway 1995) and constitute the hallmark of neurofibromatosis.

All three types of neurofibromas may appear in neurofibromatosis; however, only the plexiform neurofibroma is pathognomonic and it usually appears in an early stage, even before other cutaneous signs of neurofibromatosis may occur. This tumor has a tortuous internal appearance, with separation of single nerve fascicles by endoneural tumor material. The lesion may induce a massively hypertrophic and disfigured limb, called Elephantiasis neuromatosa, which is probably caused by the hypervascular condition of the tumor. Neurofibromas in association with neurofibromatosis type 1 (Morbus Recklinghausen) may undergo malignant transformation in 2% 29% of cases. Treatment of patients with neurofibromatosis is often nonsurgical because of the multiplicity of lesions or reserved for symptomatic lesions.

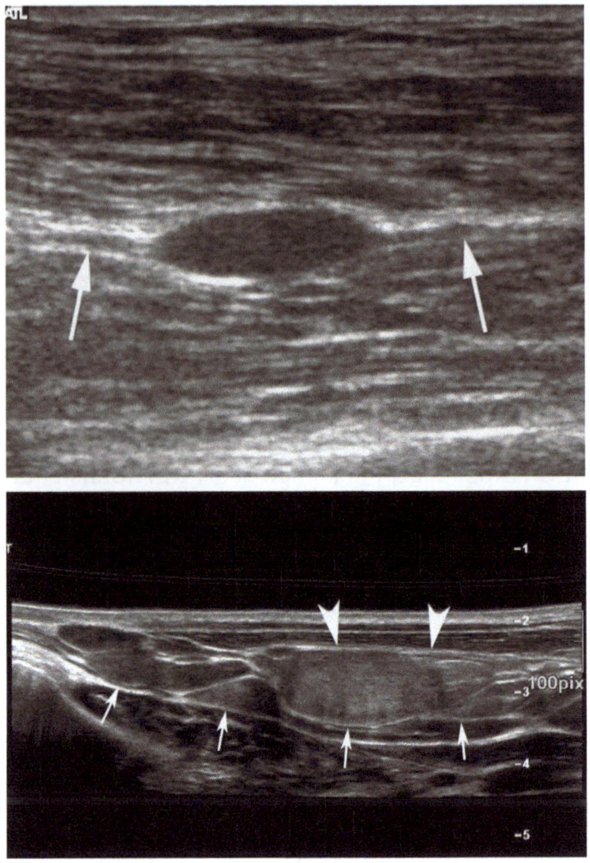

a

b

Fig. 6.3. a Longitudinal sonogram acquired at the proximal thigh in a female patient with neurofibromatosis type I. A small hypoechoic spindle shaped mass is demonstrated in continuity with a tiny femoral nerve branch (*arrows*), consistent with a small neurofibroma. **b** Sonographic extended view along the left upper arm showing multiple well defined nodules along the median nerve in a patient with fibromatosis type 1. Note that the largest nodule has a hyperechoic echogenicity (*arrowheads*) compared to the other, more hypoechoic nodules (*arrows*)

6.2.2.2 Sonography

The sonographic appearance of localized solitary neurofibromas is more or less the same as in neurofibromatosis. In patients with neurofibromatosis type I, small tumors without any clinical relevance are frequently detected along peripheral nerves. The individual tumors have an oval shape with mostly hypoechoic texture and may either be well defined or also somewhat ill defined (Simonovsky 1997; Gruber et al. 2007). Rarely hyperechoic echogenic nodules are also seen. In severe forms, chain-like nodules along the affected nerves are found (Fig. 6.3b).

The plexiform neurofibroma invariably shows a pathognomonic appearance with multiple large fascicles, separated by isoechoic tissue (Fig. 6.4). Fast growing and especially malignant neurofibromas may show central necrosis, calcifications, or cystic formation and ill defined margins (Fig. 6.5).

A target sign known as a distinct MRI feature of neurofibroma on T2 weighted sequences was also reported for sonography (Lin et al. 1999). This finding, however, has not been confirmed to date in larger series. Despite rather typical sonographic criteria of neurofibroma, which were also apparent in our own series of 11 patients with neurofibromatosis type 1, there is considerable overlap of sonographic

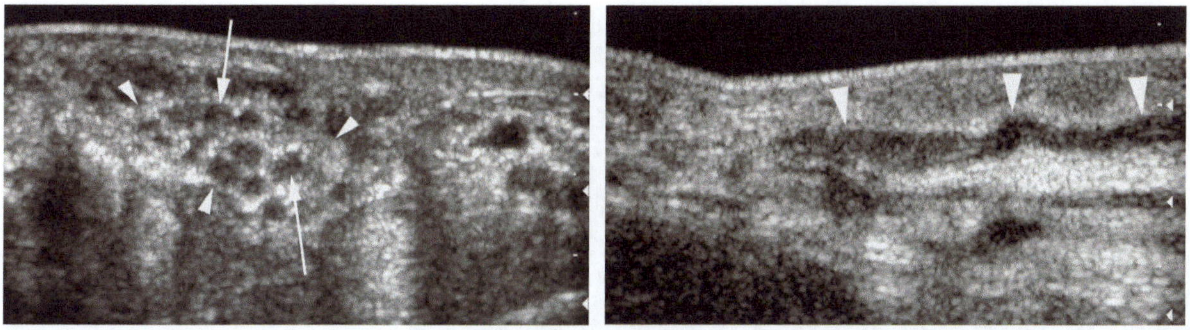
a b

Fig. 6.4a,b. Transverse (**a**) and longitudinal (**b**) sonogram acquired at the right hand in a patient with plexiform neurofibroma. The median nerve (*arrowheads* in **a**) is enlarged with multiple, enlarged, hypoechoic fascicles (*arrows* in **a**). Single fascicles are elongated and distorted (*arrowheads* in **b**)

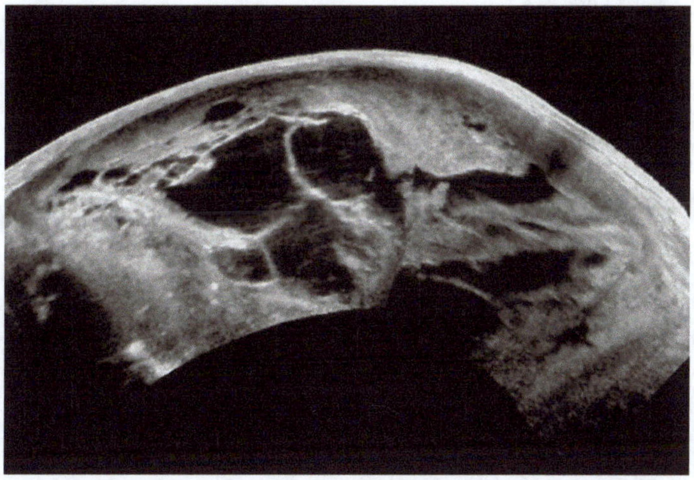

Fig. 6.5. Malignant neurofibroma in neurofibromatosis I. Panoramic view of a huge tumor at the right shoulder with a maximum outer diameter of 35 cm. The echotexture appears very inhomogeneous with multiple cystic, necrotic areas

features. Gray scale sonography alone is therefore not considered reliable enough to correctly differentiate benign from malignant nerve tumors, and sonography guided needle biopsy should be performed.

Most peripheral nerve tumors show a high vascularity, which can be assessed with color Doppler sonography and spectral wave analysis. In a study regarding differentiation of malignant and benign soft tissue tumors we were able to differentiate malignant from benign tumors by analyzing the vascular architecture and spectral wave analysis (Bodner et al. 2002). In a series of 79 soft tissue tumors we investigated seven nerve tumors. Gray scale information such as echogenicity or echo pattern did not have any significant value for differential diagnosis; however, color Doppler sonography was able to demonstrate an anarchic vascular architecture in malignant neurogenic tumors (Fig. 6.6), containing stenosed and occluded vessels, self loops and trifurcations. Especially stenosed vessels showed a high systolic velocity of more then 100 cm/s; a flow velocity below 20 cm/s indicated a distally occluded tumor vessel. The combination of anarchic vessel architecture with these spectral characteristics resulted in a sensitivity of 94% and specificity of 93% in the differentiation of malignant from benign tumors.

6.2.3 Granular Cell Tumor

Granular cell tumor is a rare, benign nerve tumor that is more common in women than men, and appears in the 4th and 5th decade, found more frequently in the African population.

It is mostly found in the subcutis, lesser in the submucosa or muscle, but it can appear virtually in any site of the body and organ. In up to 10% of patients the tumor appears on multiple sides. Malig-

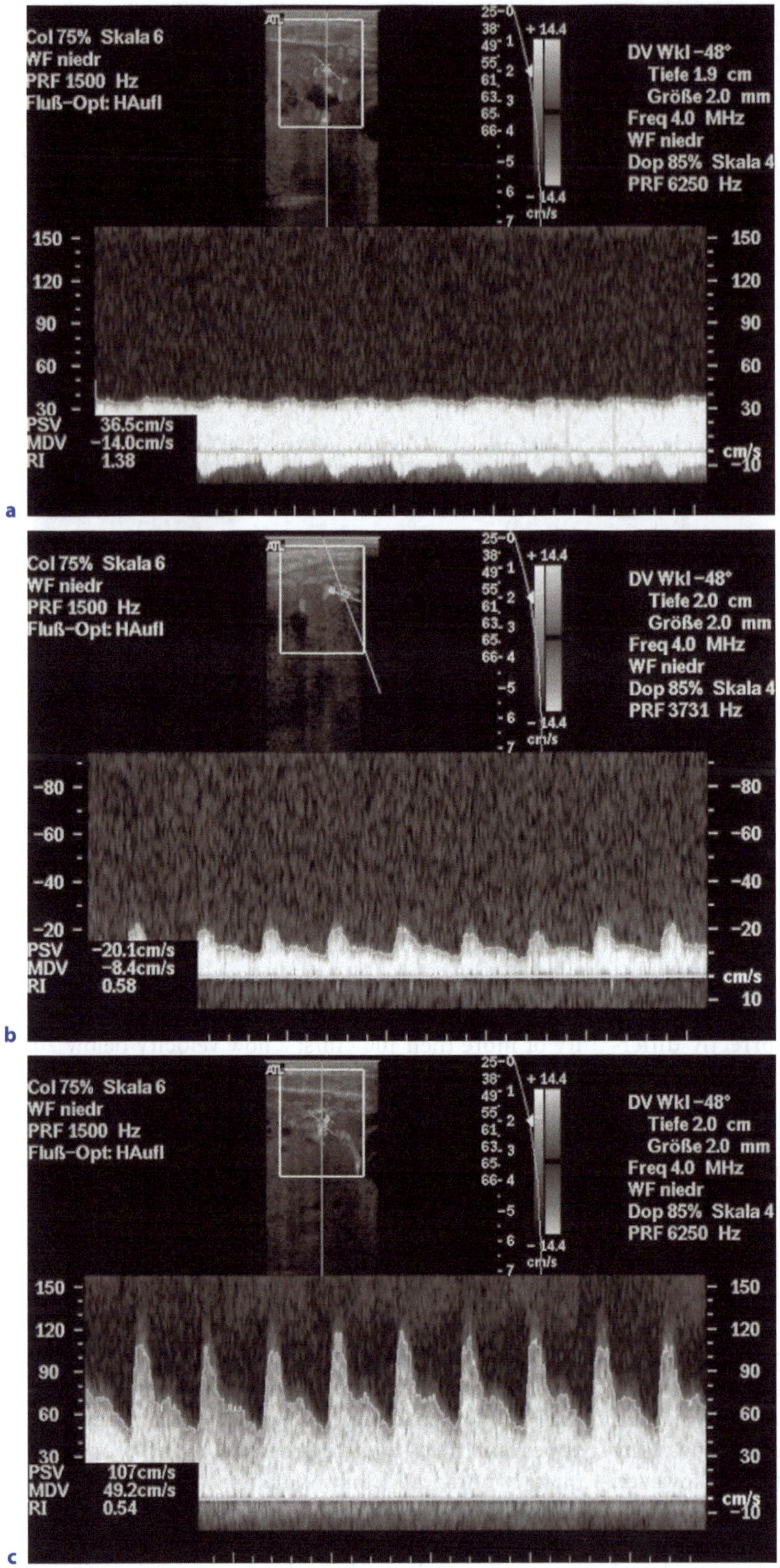

Fig. 6.6a–c. Color Doppler sonograms and spectral wave analysis in a patient with malignant neurofibroma. **a** An arteriovenous shunt with high velocity undulating waveform is demonstrated. **b** Inside the same lesion an arterial vessel with low velocity is demonstrated. **c** Several vessels with high velocity "stenotic" wave forms are demonstrated

nant granular cell tumor is extremely rare. The tumor is only rarely found in continuity with a peripheral nerve, therefore the diagnosis will less likely be made by sonographic findings. We encountered one case where the continuity of the tumor with a peripheral nerve was readily established (Fig. 6.7) (GRUBER et al. 2007).

6.3 Malignant Peripheral Nerve Tumors

Malignant peripheral nerve tumors account for 5%–10% of all soft tissue sarcomas, they may arise from the nerve sheath, perineural cells and fibroblasts. Lesions mainly affect major nerve trunks such as the sciatic nerve or brachial plexus. Patients more frequently present with local pain or neurologic symptoms compared to benign tumors. Some of these lesions are secondary tumors, which appear after local radiotherapy. Typically those tumors grow fast and reach a large size. Local recurrence after surgical removal is about 40%. Metastatic spread, especially to the lung occurs in up to 68% and the overall 5-year survival rate is 43.7% (WANEBO et al. 1993), depending on the size and location of the tumor.

Sonographic experience with imaging of malignant peripheral nerve tumors is limited; a distinction based on gray scale imaging alone is practically impossible except with the demonstration of malignant features such as invasive growth. The concept of color Doppler and spectral wave analysis for the differentiation of benign and malignant lesions has been discussed in the previous paragraph.

6.3.1 Clear Cell Sarcoma

Clear cell sarcoma is an extremely rare tumor that has the ability to produce melanin but it is distinguished from the skin melanoma by its deep location, almost always in conjunction with aponeurotic or tendon like structures (ENZINGER 1968). Young women are more affected then men. GANDOLFO et al. (2000) described a clear cell sarcoma at the foot; the tumor appeared as a well defined, hypoechoic mass attached to the lateral plantar complex, color Doppler sonography showed rich tumor vascularity.

6.4 Non-neural Tumors Within Nerve Sheath

6.4.1 Nerve Sheath Ganglion

Intraneural ganglia are rare lesions, most frequently affecting the large nerves about the knee (mainly the common peroneal nerve) (LEIJTEN et al. 1992; MASCIOCCHI et al. 1992; YAMAZAKI et al. 1999; KATZ and LENOBEL 1970), involvement of sciatic nerve, the tibial nerve at the ankle or the ulnar nerve at the elbow has also been reported (PEER et al. 2002; PUIG et al. 1999).

It has been shown by SPINNER et al. (2003, 2007) that those ganglions arise from the joint rather then from the nerve sheath itself. Joint fluid leaks into the sheath of a joint nerve branch by a small capsular gap and is then pumped into the nerve sheath of the main nerve, partially dissecting the epineurium

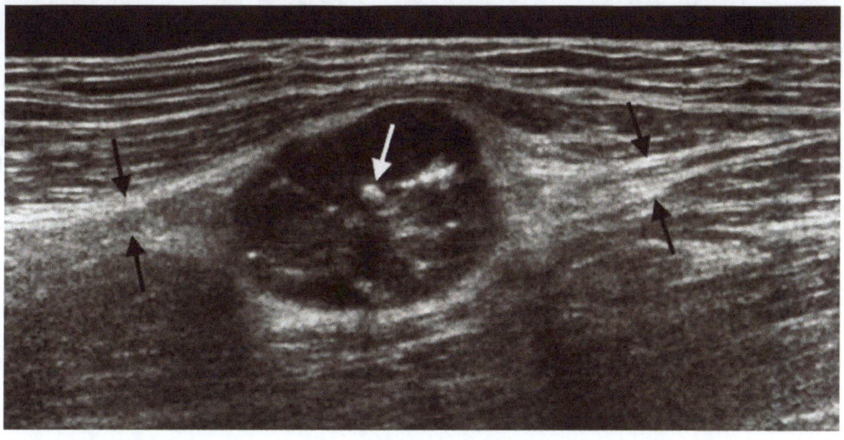

Fig. 6.7. Longitudinal sonogram showing a well defined hypoechoic mass between the subcutaneous soft tissues and the quadriceps muscle in the left thigh. The tumor had a slow growth and was well palpable. The tumor shows multiple small calcifications and continuity to a small peripheral nerve (*arrows*). Core needle biopsy revealed granular cell tumor

(Spinner 2003, 2007), The fluid then extends along the course of the nerve, by compressing and displacing the nerve fascicles and forming an intra-nerval ganglion (Fig. 6.8).

Depending on the size of the ganglion patients either present with a palpable mass or with neurological symptoms only. From a histological viewpoint these lesions show myxoid changes together with a peripheral fibrotic lining. Sonography typically reveals a cystic, well-defined globular lesion, sometimes septated with anechoic echotexture and posterior acoustic shadowing (Figs. 6.8, 6.9). Surgical enucleation is the most appropriate treatment. Intraneural ganglia should be differentiated from a simple Baker cyst arising from the medial joint space, extending to the lateral border and displacing the sciatic or tibial nerve.

We realized similar findings of compressing the tibial nerve inside the tarsal tunnel by a tibiotalar joint ganglion (Peer et al. 2002) (Fig. 6.9).

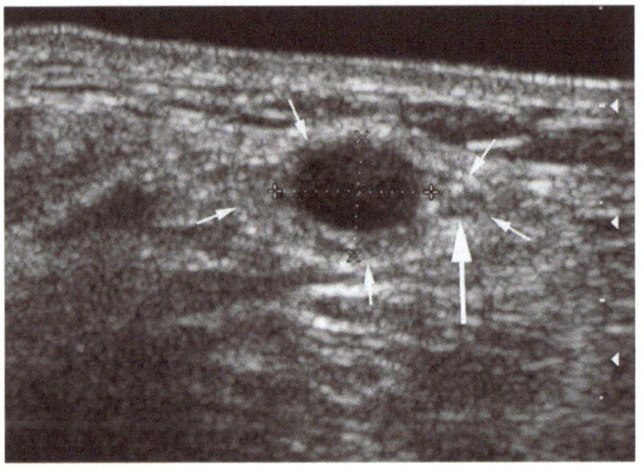

Fig. 6.8. Transverse sonogram of common peroneal nerve in a patient with a palpable popliteal mass, pain and numbness in the dorsal aspect of the foot and muscle weakness in the peroneus as well as tibialis anterior muscles. A round hypoechoic mass with well defined margins and posterior acoustic enhancement and close relationship to the nerve (*long arrow*) is revealed by sonography. A thin hyperechoic line (the outer nerve sheath) shows direct continuity with the outer layer of the ganglion (*small arrows*) confirming a nerve sheath ganglion

a
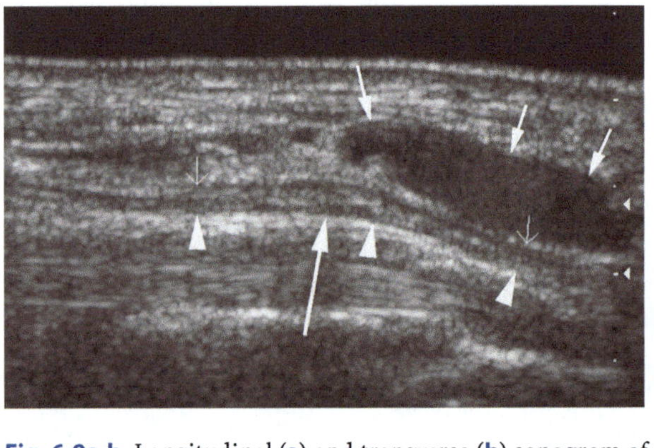
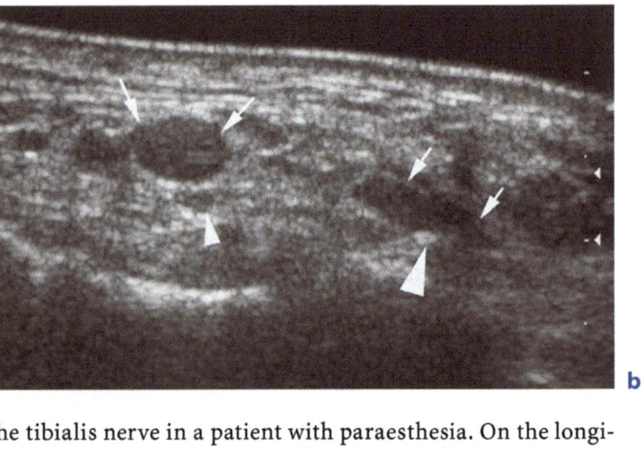
b

Fig. 6.9a,b. Longitudinal (**a**) and transverse (**b**) sonogram of the tibialis nerve in a patient with paraesthesia. On the longitudinal scan the tibialis nerve (*arrowheads* in **a** and **b**) shows a bowing course just proximal to the medial tibiotalar joint. At the right margin of the image a spindle shaped hypoechoic lesion with well defined margins (*small arrows* in **a** and **b**) lies close to the nerve surface. The nerve diameter is slightly enlarged due to congestive edema (compression by the ganglion) just proximal to the upper pole of the ganglion (*long arrow* in **a**). Part of the ganglion (*small arrows* in **b**) is visualized in close connection to the distal margin of the tibial metaphysis (*large arrowhead* in **b**) confirming its articular extension

6.4.2 Neural Fibrolipoma

Neural fibrolipoma was initially described by Mason in 1952, and various synonyms, such as fibrolipomatous hamartoma of nerve, perineural and intraneural lipoma, have been used for this rare lesion (Silverman and Enzinger 1985; Toms et al. 2006). Hypertrophy of fatty tissue and fibroblasts in the epineurium of a nerve is considered the most probable cause for the development of fibrolipoma; however, the exact pathogenesis is still unclear.

The typical presentation is in a patient less than 30 years of age, often at birth or in early childhood with a slowly growing mass with or without pain or neurological deficit. The upper extremity is most commonly involved (78% – 96% of cases) with a predilection for the median nerve. Involvement of the lower extremity, ulnar or radial nerve, or the brachial plexus is rare. A localized soft, slowly enlarging mass in the wrist or forearm, with or without accompanying pain, is usually present. Neurologic symptoms consistent with carpal tunnel disease may be the leading finding in lesions involving the median nerve. About one third up to two thirds of patients have coexisting macrodactyly and bone overgrowth.

On sonographic examinations the involved nerve is grossly enlarged, with a cable-like appearance on transverse scans, which is caused by the hypoechoic bands resembling the fascicles embedded in hyperechoic surrounding fatty tissue (Fig. 6.10) (Murphey et al. 1999). In a series of 15 cases Toms et al. (2006) described evenly interspersed fat and neural bundles within the tumor. The presence of fat may help to differentiate neural fibrolipoma from plexiform neurilemmas. The fascicles within the neural lipoma do not appear to be tortuous as seen in plexiform schwannomas, but rather cable-like.

Surgical resection is hampered by the fact that the tumor sometimes diffusely infiltrates the fascicles; this distinguishes the tumor from circumscribed lipoma within the nerve sheath.

Other tumors which occasionally can be found along the peripheral nerves include true lipomas, lymphomas and hemangiomas.

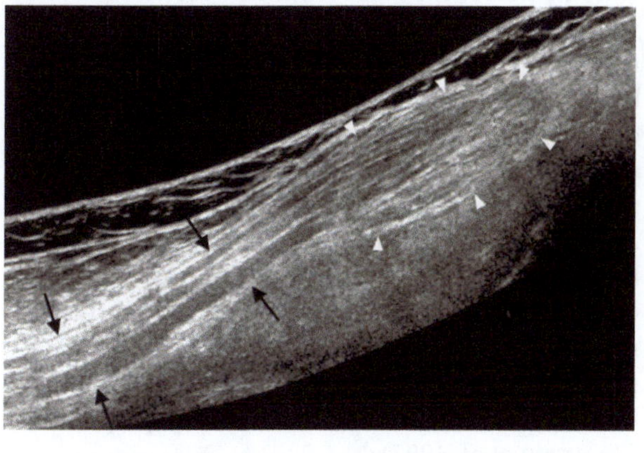

Fig. 6.10. Longitudinal sonogram at the right thigh showing a cable-like appearance of the sciatic nerve over an extent of approximately 12 cm (*black arrows*). At the distal part of the nerve an oval shaped and well defined mass is noted (*white arrows*), Tumor resection revealed fibrolipoma

6.4.3 Peripheral Nerve Hemangioma

Hemangiomas of peripheral nerves are extremely rare; most hemangiomas that are found along the peripheral nerves probably infiltrate the affected nerve rather then originate from the nerve (Purcell 1945). Depending on the involvement of the affected nerve, weakness and pain are the predominant clinical signs. Sonography shows tortuous vessels between the nerve fascicles, with fascicles appearing edematous. Typically for hemangiomas, phleboliths may be found along the tumor vessels.

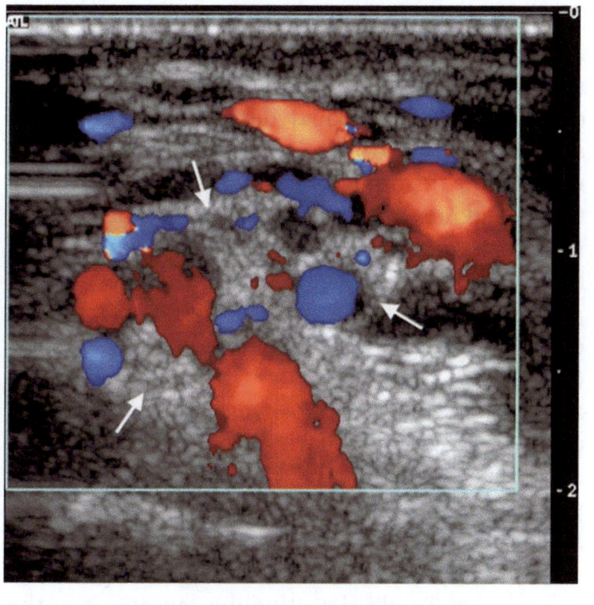

Fig. 6.11. Transverse sonogram at the forearm in a patient with slow growing hemangioma. Color Doppler sonogram showing multiple tumor vessels between the nerve fascicles of the median nerve, the fascicles appear thickened (*arrows*)

6.5 Neuroma

6.5.1 Morton's Neuroma

6.5.1.1 Clinical Introduction

Morton's neuroma is not a neoplasm in its true sense. The entity was first described by Thomas Morton in 1876, who reported on 12 patients with "a peculiar and painful affection of the fourth metatarsophalangeal articulation" (Morton 1876). The exact pathophysiological mechanism for this entity is still undetermined; however, suggested reasons include repetitive microtrauma and nerve entrapment. While Morton himself favored a mechanical pathomechanism with squeezing of the nerve between the metatarsal heads, Mulder (1951) and others suggested an influence of abnormal metatarsal mobility with subsequent enlargement of the intermetatarsal bursa (Mulder 1951; Bossley and Cainey 1980). The latter replaces the plantar nerve and accompanying vessels, which results in a state more prone to pinching of these structures (Bossley and Cainey 1980).

Morton's neuroma, which clinically represents a fusiform enlargement of a digital branch of the medial or lateral plantar nerve, consists of perineural fibrosis, local vascular proliferation, edema of the endoneurium and axonal degeneration (Shereff and Grande 1991). Most commonly the digital nerve in the third intermetatarsal space is involved, the second intermetatarsal space being affected less frequently and involvement of other digital nerves being rare. There is enlargement of the digital nerve just proximal of its terminal bifurcation and just distal to the level of the intermetatarsal ligament (Fig. 6.12).

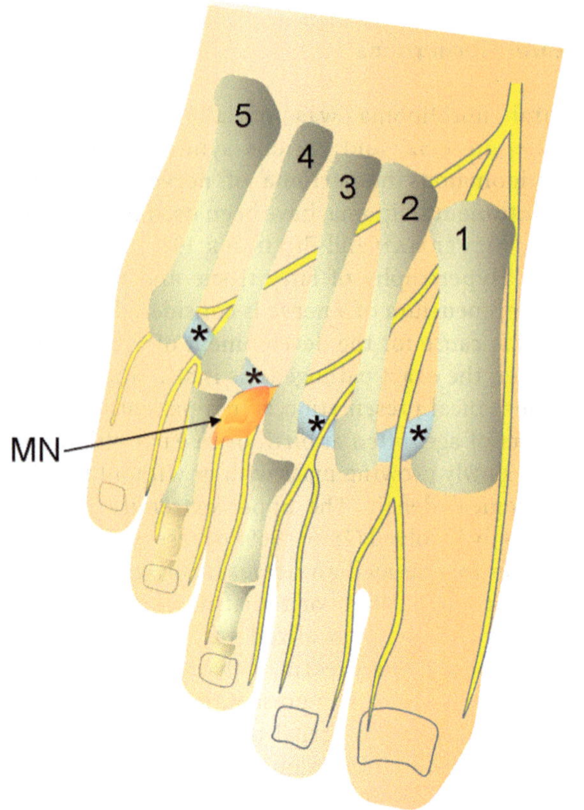

Fig. 6.12. Schematic drawing of the forefoot showing the course of the digital nerves between the metatarsal bones (*1–5*) and the intermetatarsal ligaments (*asterix*). Typical location for Morton's neuroma (*MN*) formation is between the 3rd and 4th and the 2nd and 3rd intermetatarsal space

Patients typically suffer from a sharp, burning pain originating at the level of the metatarsal heads and radiating to the toes. Tingling sensations and paresthesias in the same distribution are common. Symptoms are worsened by walking and relieved by rest. During physical examination typical signs, such as a positive Tinel's sign (tingling sensations in the distal distribution of a nerve with light taping on the affected part of the nerve trunk) and Mulder's sign (a palpable click when the metatarsals are squeezed together with simultaneous application of pressure to the sole of the foot) may be seen (Mulder 1951). Dorsiflexion of the toes results in worsening of pain, while plantar flexion causes some relief. Morton's neuroma is palpable in one third of patients only, but associated synovial cysts may be clinically evident. Women are more commonly affected, which is attributed to the more flexible state of the female foot and the habit of wearing high heels (Morton 1876). Asymptomatic lesions are common with a prevalence of 33% reported in an MRI study of 57 patients (Bencardino et al. 2000). The only observable difference between symptomatic and asymptomatic patients is the size of the lesion, with neuromas less than 5 mm in diameter considered asymptomatic (Zanetti et al. 1997).

The treatment of Morton's neuroma ranges from the use of orthotic devices and local steroid or alcohol injections to surgical resection in cases resistant to conservative management (Llanos et al. 1999).

6.5.1.2
Sonography

REDD and coworkers (1989) first reported on the potential of sonography for the detection of Morton's neuroma. Meanwhile various clinical studies have confirmed their initial experience with reported sensitivities for the sonographic detection of neuromas between 93% and 98% (QUINN et al. 2000; REDD et al. 1989; SHAPIRO and SHAPIRO 1995).

Recommendations on the best sonographic examination technique vary among authors: While the initial results of REDD and coworkers (1989) have been achieved with the patient in a sitting position scanning from the dorsal aspect of the foot, recent studies more commonly favor a plantar approach with the patient lying prone on the examination couch. The reasoning for the dorsal approach may derive from the commonly favored dorsal approach in surgery for Morton's neuroma, and was thought to yield better image quality, as the thick fibrotic plantar pad resulting in some amount of sonographic artifacts can be avoided. However, the dorsal approach is only effective with vigorous plantar flexion of the toes, which enables delivery of the neuroma into the intermetatarsal space. Like other researchers we use the dorsal approach only in cases where the plantar approach results in equivocal findings. With the plantar approach we use a good amount of transmission gel together with a standoff pad, which substantially improves image quality. With the non-imaging finger pressure is exerted on the dorsal aspect of the scanned intermetatarsal space splaying the metatarsals, which allows for a better sonographic access to the intermetatarsal tissues. A 12-MHz or higher linear array transducer is recommended.

The typical sonographic appearance of Morton's neuroma is a well defined, hypoechoic, fusiform mass in relation with the plantar neurovascular bundle classically of the third digital interspace. As the plantar digital nerve courses plantar to the intermetatarsal ligament, the typical location for neuroma is in the lower aspect of the intermetatarsal space and in between the metatarsal heads (Figs. 6.13, 6.14) (PEER et al. 2002; QUINN et al. 2000).

However, according to QUINN and coworkers (2000) there is some amount of variation in the localization of intermetatarsal mass lesions found with sonography. In their sonographic study of 27 patients with surgically confirmed neuromas, they detected a mass either located plantar with dorsal extension or in a completely dorsal location in 18 patients. Only nine surgically confirmed neuromas where entirely plantar. This seems anatomically counterintuitive at first sight, given the location of the neurovascular bundle. Two possible explanations for this finding have to be considered: Firstly, according to the early work of MULDER (1951) a neuroma may be located more dorsally because of coexisting abnormal metatarsal mobility with subsequent splaying of metatarsals and widened digital interspaces. Secondly, the dorsally extending mass may be an enlarged intermetatar-

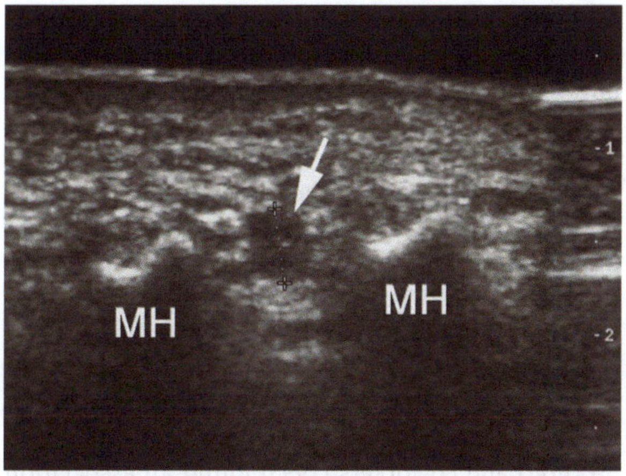

Fig. 6.13. Transverse sonogram in a patient with typical symptoms for Morton's neuroma. At the level of the metatarsal heads (*MH*) a small 0.6-cm globular mass with hypoechoic echotexture is seen, consistent with a small Morton's neuroma (*arrow*)

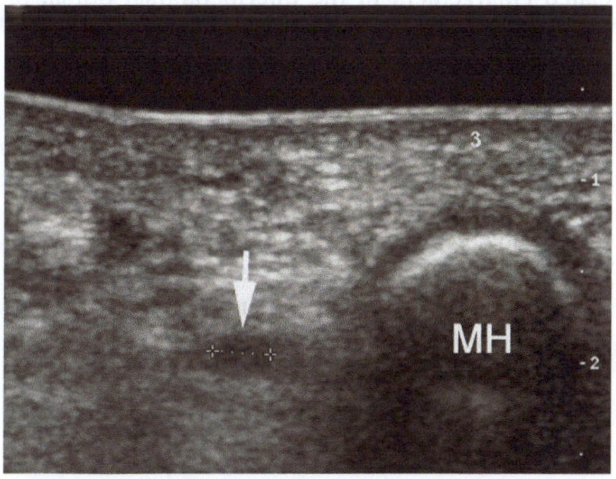

Fig. 6.14. Transverse sonogram in another patient with symptoms suggestive for Morton's neuroma reveals a small nodular lesion with only 4 mm diameter (*arrow*) adjacent to the third metatarsal head (*MH*). Despite its small size this lesion was symptomatic

sal bursa, which because of its equal echotexture is sometimes difficult to discern from a neuroma. This bursa is present in each interspace dorsal to the deep transverse intermetatarsal ligament and is found to be intimately related with Morton's neuroma during surgery. Inflammation of the bursa has also been proposed to be a causative factor in the pathogenesis of Morton's neuroma and associated clinical symptoms (Mulder 1951; Bossley and Cainey 1980). According to Shapiro et al. (1995) the enlarged fluid filled bursa may be discerned if a lesion with anechoic center and posterior acoustic enhancement is revealed in the dorsal compartment of an intermetatarsal space. Shapiro and coworkers (1995) found an association between an enlarged bursa and a small 2- to 4-mm diameter neuroma in 10% of patients. So we have to keep in mind that a hypoechoic mass in the intermetatarsal space visualized with sonography in a patient suspected for having Morton's neuroma may in fact be: (a) a true neuroma, (b) a neuroma with an associated enlargement of the intermetatarsal bursa, or (c) an enlarged bursa in association with a small size neuroma (less than 5 mm), which is not distinguished separately from the bursa. This has some implications for the sonographer on examination technique:

- Always try to establish a continuity between the neuroma and a digital nerve, as this will raise the specificity of the sonographic examination. However, this is not always accomplished due to the small size of the plantar nerves (in 55% of true neuromas in the study of Quinn et al. 2000). But with state of the art equipment (i.e. high frequency transducers) this will probably be achieved in a higher percentage of patients.
- Give a close inspection to the echotexture of an intermetatarsal mass and search for liquid components, or posterior acoustic enhancement suggesting a fluid filled bursa. In contrast, the neuroma itself is of hypoechoic or mixed echotexture, sometimes it may even show hyperechoic areas consistent with interspersed fat.
- A larger mass should always raise the suspicion of an enlarged bursa (normally a neuroma only rarely exceeds 20 mm in length) (Quinn et al. 2000).
- Because of the intimate relationship of Morton´s neuroma and an enlarged intermetatarsal bursa the actual size of the neuroma may be overestimated.

In conclusion, sonography is valuable for the diagnosis of Morton´s neuroma, with a sensitivity close to MR imaging, if a tailored examination is performed. Besides its diagnostic capabilities sonography may also serve as a tool for the guidance of local corticoid or alcohol instillation.

6.5.2
Friction Neuroma

Lesions (friction neuroma) similar to Morton's neuroma are sometime found along the nerves in the hand (Weiss and Goldblum 2001). They are very much related to occupational injuries to the nerve in patients who repeatedly perform the same finger movement. Typically they are found along the digital nerve of the thumb.

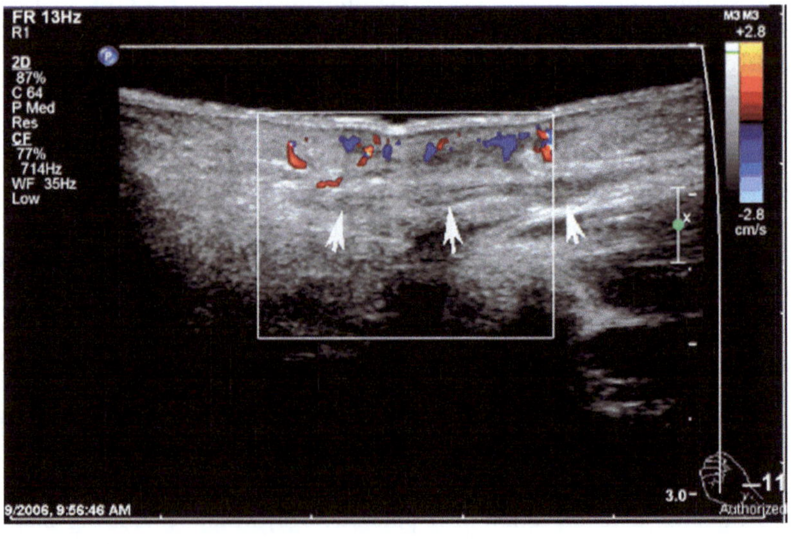

Fig. 6.15. Longitudinal scan in a patient with long standing numbness in the inner side of the thumb. The digital nerve shows irregular thickening (*arrows*) over an extent of 1 cm. Color Doppler sonography shows increased vascularity within the skin and subcutaneous soft tissues

The appearance of a friction neuroma in the hand is similar to a Morton's neuroma. The friction neuroma shows a fusiform swelling when scanned along the course of the digital nerve (Fig. 6.15) and round shaped in a transverse scan.

6.5.3
Traumatic Neuroma

6.5.3.1
Clinical Introduction

Depending on their pathogenesis neuromas may be divided into posttraumatic and postsurgical lesions (see also Chap. 4). Traumatic neuromas develop after complete or partial transection of a peripheral nerve, and regarding their location this group may further be divided into intraneural or terminal neuromas. While intraneural traumatic neuromas develop in an otherwise intact nerve trunk because of minor trauma (mainly traction injuries), or as a result of chronic irritation and friction, terminal neuromas are always a result of severe trauma with partial avulsion, disruption or total transection of a nerve. Postsurgical neuromas most commonly appear in the lower extremities after leg amputation and in the head and neck region related to tooth extraction, or after surgical nerve reconstruction. Neuromas develop within 1–12 months after the initial event and vary in size, depending on the size of the involved nerve and the amount of impaired nerve tissue.

The typical clinical findings in patients with neuroma are a localized soft tissue mass and pain, which is in most cases reproduced with tapping on the mass (positive Tinel's sign). At histologic analysis neuromas show a mixture of various cellular elements including Schwann cells, axons, endo- and perineural elements, wrapped in dense collagenous, fibrotic tissue (Kransdorf and Murphey 1997). The disorganization of the neural tissue allows for histologic differentiation of neuroma from neurofibroma.

6.5.3.2
Sonography

Given a patient's history the sonographic diagnosis of neuroma is straightforward and the differential diagnosis hardly problematic. In the typical clinical setting a bulbous mass in association with a nerve stump (Fig. 6.16) or arising from the lateral aspect of a nerve with partially discontinuous fascicles (Fig. 6.17), or a spindle shaped mass inside a nerve (Fig. 6.18) is consistent with neuroma. The diagnostic clue is the demonstration of a nerve in direct continuity with the mass.

The echotexture of neuromas is hypoechoic and more or less homogeneous, lesion margins are generally well defined, however some irregularity, which is probably due to multidirectional cell proliferation, has been reported (Martinoli et al. 1996). Also scarring around the nerve stump may cause irregular margins.

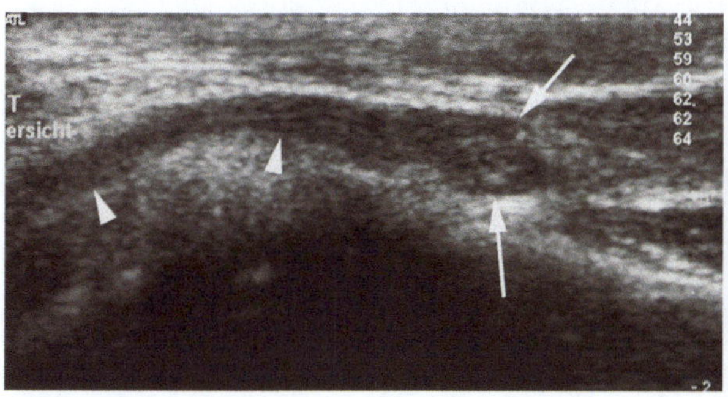

a

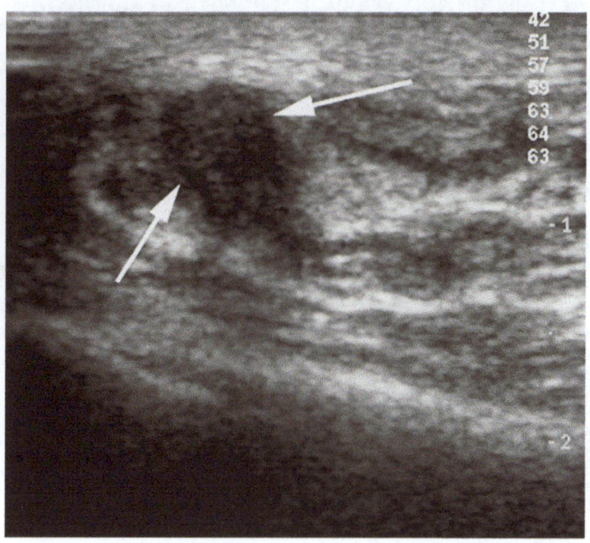

b

Fig. 6.16a,b. Longitudinal (**a**) and transverse (**b**) sonogram in a patient with traumatic amputation of the arm in a motor vehicle accident. The ulnar nerve (*arrowheads* in **a**) tapers in a bulbous hypoechoic mass consistent with stump neuroma. In the transverse plane the diagnosis is not readily established, however a localized enlargement of the nerve is seen (*arrows* in **b**)

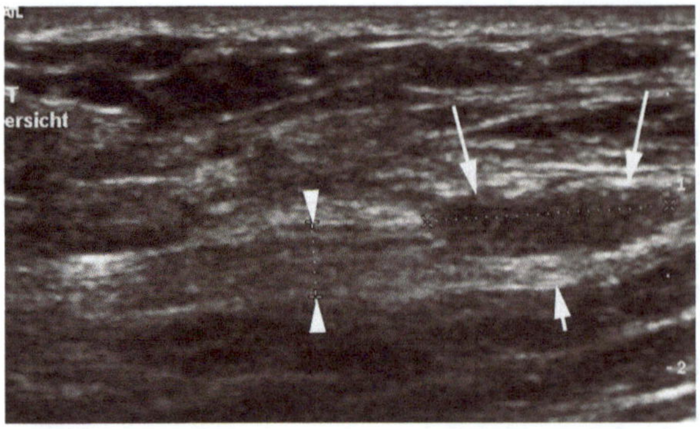

Fig. 6.17. Longitudinal sonogram through the distal portion of the sciatic nerve in a patient with a femoral shaft fracture and traumatic lesion of the sciatic nerve. A spindle shaped neuroma (*long arrows*) is seen located in the lateral bundle of the sciatic nerve (*arrowheads*) with otherwise continuous nerve fascicles in the lower aspect of the nerve (*short arrow*)

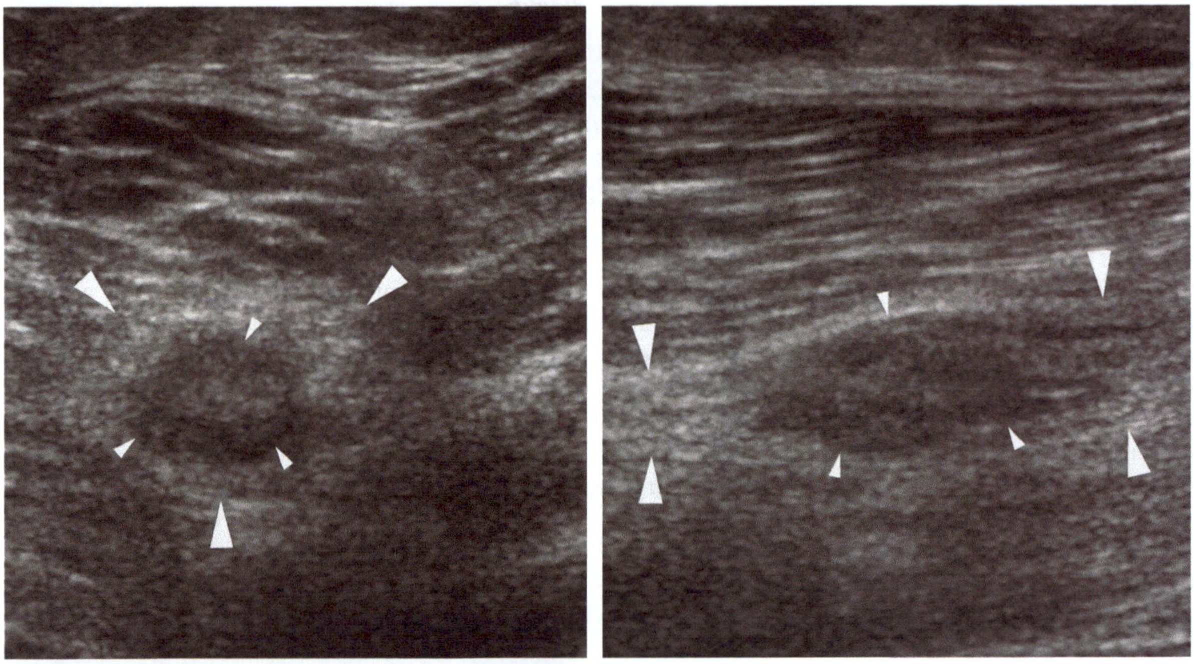

a b

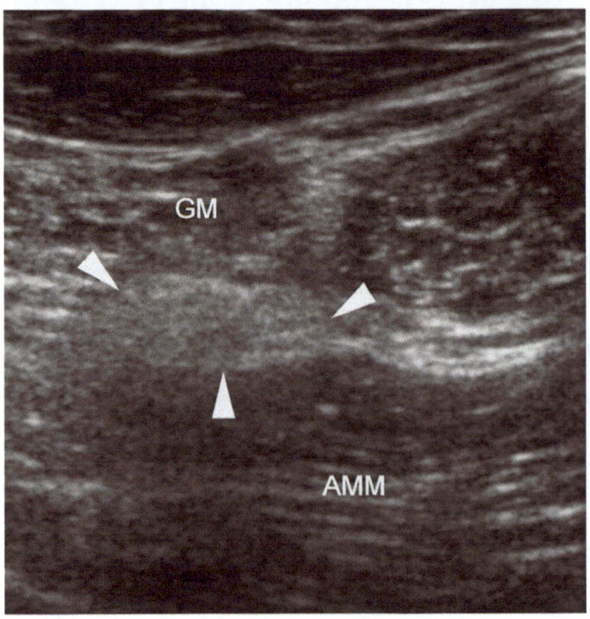

c

Fig. 6.18a–c. Transverse (**a**) and longitudinal (**b**) sonogram through the lower thigh in a female patient, who received resection of a sciatic nerve neurofibroma with end-to-end anastomosis of nerve stumps. The patient suffered from burning pain in the lateral aspect of the foot and the fifth toe with hypaesthesia, and electrophysiologic testing revealed a lesion of the suralis portion of the sciatic nerve. There is marked enlargement of the sciatic nerve (*large arrowheads* in **a** and **b**) due to a fusiform, hypoechoic intraneural mass (*small arrowheads* in **a** and **b**) consistent with postoperative neuroma. Compare normal appearing sciatic nerve proximal to the lesion (**c**). *GM*, gluteus muscle; *AMM*, adductor magnus muscle

Based on the nonspecific intrinsic echotexture of neuromas alone a differentiation against other lesions is hardly possible, which is why the demonstration of continuity with a nerve and knowledge of patient history is of the utmost importance. The latter, however, may sometimes be difficult if very small nerves at the fingers or toes are involved.

Sonography is especially helpful in patients with phantom pain after amputation, because of its ability to identify an underlying neuroma and thus rule out other reasons for the development of phantom pain, such as recurring tumor and localized inflammation or abscess formation among others. In addition, sonography may guide local therapy with instillation of corticoids, analgesics or phenol (see also Chap. 7).

References

Beggs I (1999) Sonographic appearances of nerve tumors. J Clin Ultrasound 27:363–368

Bencardino J, Rosenberg ZS, Beltran J et al. (2000) Morton's neuroma: is it always symptomatic. AJR Am J Roentgenol 175:649–653

Bendix N, Wolf C, Gruber H, Bodner G (2005) Ultrasound of tumours and tumour-like lesions of peripheral nerves. Ultraschall Med 26:318–324 (German)

Bodner G, Schocke M, Rachbauer F et al. (2002) Differentiation of malignant and benign musculoskeletal tumors: combined color Doppler ultrasonography, power Doppler ultrasonography and spectral wave analysis. Radiology 223:410–416

Bossley CJ, Cainey PC (1980) The intermetatarsophalangeal bursa: its significance in Morton's metatarsalgia. J Bone Joint Surg [Br] 62-B:184–187

Fornage BD (1988) Peripheral nerves of the extremities: imaging with ultrasound. Radiology 167:179–182

Gandolfo N, Martinoli C, Cafiero F et al. (2000) Malignant melanoma of soft tissues (clear cell sarcoma) of the foot. Is MRI able to perform a specific diagnosis? Report of one case and review of the radiological literature. Anticancer Res 20:3993–3998

Giovagnorio F, Martinoli C (2001) Sonography of the cervical vagus nerve: normal appearance and abnormal findings. AJR Am J Roentgenol 176:745–749

Gruber H, Glodny B, Bendix N, Tzankov A, Peer S (2007) High-resolution ultrasound of peripheral neurogenic tumors. Eur Radiol 17:2880–2888

Hughes DG, Wilson DJ (1986) Ultrasound appearances of peripheral nerve tumors. Br J Radiol 59:1041–1043

Isobe K, Shimizu T, Akahane T, Kato H (2004) Imaging of ancient schwannoma. AIR Am J Roentgenol 183(2):331–336

Johnstone AJ, Beggs I (1994) Ultrasound imaging of soft-tissue masses in the extremities. J Bone Joint Surg Br 76:688–689

Katz MR, Lenobel MI (1970) Intraneural ganglion cyst of the peroneal nerve. J Neurosurg 32:692–694

Kransdorf M, Murphey MD (1997) Neurogenic tumors. In: Imaging of soft tissue tumors. Saunders, Philadelphia, pp 235–273

Llanos LF, Vila J, Nunez-Samper M (1999) Clinical symptoms and treatment of the foot and ankle nerve entrapment syndromes. Foot and Ankle Surgery 5:211–218

Leijten FS, Arts WF, Puylaert JB (1992) Ultrasound diagnosis of an intraneural ganglion cyst of the peroneal nerve. J Neurosurg 76:538–540

Lin J, Jacobson JA, Hayes CW (1999) Sonographic target sign in neurofibroma. J Ultrasound Med 18:513–517

Martinoli C, Serafini G, Bianchi S et al (1996) Ultrasonography of peripheral nerves. J Peripheral Nervous System 1:169–174

Masciocchi C, Innacoli M, Cisternino S et al. (1992) Myxoid intraneural cysts of external popliteal ischiadic nerve. Eur Radiol 14:52–55

Mason ML (1953) Presentation of cases. In: Proceedings of the American Society for Surgery of the Hand. J Bone Join Surg [Am] 35:273–275

Morton TG (1876) A peculiar and painful affection of the fourth metatarsophalangeal articulation. Am J Med Sci 71:37–45

Murphey MD, Smith WS, Smith SE et al. (1999) From the archives of the AFIP: imaging of musculoskeletal neurogenic tumors: radiologic-pathologic correlation. RadioGraphics 19:1253–1280

Mulder JD (1951) The causative mechanisms in Morton's metatarsalgia. J Bone Joint Surg [Br] 33-B:74–95

Peer S, Kovacs P, Harpf C et al. (2002) High resolution sonography of lower extremity peripheral nerves: anatomic correlation and spectrum of pathology. J Ultrasound Med 21:315–322

Puig S, Turkof E, Sedivy R et al. (1999) Sonographic diagnosis of recurrent ulnar nerve compression by ganglion cysts. J Ultrasound Med 18:433–436

Quinn TJ, Jacobson JA, Craig JG, van Holsbeeck (2000) Sonography of Morton's neuromas. AJR Am J Roentgenol 174:1723–1728

Redd RA, Peters VJ, Emery SF et al. (1989) Morton Neuroma: sonographic evaluation. Radiology 171:415–417

Reynolds DL Jr, Jacobson JA, Inampudi P, Jamadar DA, Ebrahim FS, Hayes CW (2004) Sonographic characteristics of peripheral nerve sheath tumors. AJR Am J Roentgenol 182:741-744

Roos KL, Muckway M (1995) Neurofibromatosis. Dermatol Clin 13:105–111

Shapiro PP, Shapiro SL (1995) Sonographic evaluation of interdigital neuromas. Foot Ankle 16:604–606

Shereff MJ, Grande DA (1991) Electron microscopic analysis of the interdigital neuroma. Clin Orthop 271:296–299

Silverman TA, Enzinger FM (1985) Fibrolipomatous hamartoma of nerve: a clinicopathologic analysis of 26 cases. Am J Surg Pathol 9:7–14

Simonovsky V (1997) Peripheral nerve schwannoma preoperatively diagnosed by sonography: report of three cases and discussion. Eur J Radiol 25:47–51

Spinner RJ, Atkinson JL, Tiel RL (2003) Peroneal intraneural ganglia: the importance of the articular branch. A unifying theory. J Neurosurg 99:330–343

Spinner RJ, Amrami KK, Wolanskyj AP et al. (2007) Dynamic phases of peroneal and tibial intraneural ganglia forma-

tion: a new dimension added to the unifying articular theory. J Neurosurg 107:296–307
Wanebo JE, Malik JM, Vandenberg SR et al. (1993) Malignant peripheral nerve sheath tumors: a clinicopathological study of 28 cases. Cancer 71:247–252
Weiss S, Goldblum J (2001) Enzinger and Weiss's soft tissue tumors, 4th edn. Mosby, St Louis
Yamazaki H, Saitoh S, Seki H (1999) Peroneal nerve palsy caused by intraneural ganglion. Skeletal Radiol 28:52–56
Zanetti M, Strehle JK, Zollinger H et al. (1997) Morton neuroma and fluid in the intermetatarsal bursae on MR images of 70 asymptomatic volunteers. Radiology 203:516–520

Interventional Techniques

7

Peter Kovacs and Hannes Gruber

CONTENTS

P. Kovacs, MD
Department of Radiology, Innsbruck Medical University, Anichstrasse 35, 6020 Innsbruck, Austria
H. Gruber, MD
Associate Professor, Department of Radiology, Innsbruck Medical University, Anichstrasse 35, 6020 Innsbruck, Austria

Sonography is able to detect peripheral nerve lesions smaller than 1 cm, which is the critical size to be detected with MR or CT. Thomas et al. (1999) proved not only the unrivaled resolution power of sonography but also the precision by which interventions can be performed at the peripheral nerves. Due to this and to the fact that sonographic interventions are always real-time procedures, where the sonographer watches and controls the situation at any time, sonography is presented here as the state-of-the-art modality to perform accurate interventional procedures in peripheral nerve system.

7.1 Sonographically Guided Biopsy of Neural Lesions

Patients often present with palpable soft-tissue masses of very different characters. In this context tumors of the peripheral nervous system are not that rare as assumed (Kransdorf 1995a). Kransdorf showed that, of the malignant soft tissue masses, up to 6% are malignant peripheral nerve tumors and about 10% of the benign soft tissue masses are neurofibromas or schwannomas. In the 16- to 25-year-old patient group about 25% of the soft tissue masses are originating from peripheral nervous tissue (Kransdorf 1995b).

Even small peripheral tumorous lesions may be highly symptomatic as they tend to alter the function of the according peripheral nerve. If such tumors are located in the retroperitoneum they tend to produce more unspecific and diffuse symptoms which lead – before all in malignant cases – to rather bad early detection-rates.

As good therapy must always be based on an accurate diagnosis, fine-needle aspiration biopsies are procedures which are very simple to perform but with clear restrictions (Singh et al. 2004). It is reported that in experienced hands an accuracy of up to 95% can be expected. Referring to our institutional pathologists these results are very questionable as a high diagnostic uncertainty remains in many cases of fine-needle aspiration biopsies. Thus we prefer percutaneous core needle biopsies (PCNB) by which much more tissue is gained which is at least partially preserved in its tissue structure. Also for this procedure a sufficient palette of biopsy-material – i.e. coaxial needles, cutting needles – at different lengths and sizes is available. As this procedure is also less invasive than open biopsy, at least a very low complication rate is to be expected (Ogilvie et al. 2006). If performed image-guided, it proves to be a very accurate diagnostic tool (Dupuy et al. 1998) and if guided sonographically it becomes – as well as very accurate in even tiny structures – a very simple and time-sparing procedure (Torriani et al. 2002).

Like sonographically guided PCNB in other disorders, for the biopsy of neural lesions aseptic measures are also mandatory: after a relaxed positioning of the patient with a preserved accessibility to the lesion of interest, we begin with skin cleansing with a suitable disinfectant. Thereafter the coverage with sterile drapery follows. Under sonographic real-time control, extensive local anesthesia is performed subcutaneously along the planned approach for the aiming biopsy device and at the neural lesion. Subsequently a coaxial core needle – of a suitable size for the size of the nerve tumor – is advanced towards the lesion of interest and the central mandrin is removed. The relative positioning of this needle should be cleared with the responsible surgeon so that no additional area is contaminated unnecessarily. This additional pre-interventionally positioned "channel" for the biopsy-gun produces a most atraumatic biopsy-procedure, which is more comfortable for the patient, and if biopsy is performed in a malignant lesion (which is often unknown in advance), a needle tract seeding with often untoward consequences for the patient can be prevented (Hansen et al. 1995). By subsequent use of a suitable biopsy gun we then obtain tissue samples of the tumor under sonographic real-time control (Fig. 7.1). The tissue fragments are immediately preserved in a container for subsequent assessment by the pathologist. However, it must be kept in mind that PCNB carried out even by experienced investigators, may involve sampling error due to biopsy of non-diagnostic tumor parts in up to 80% of the cases (Shives 1993). Thus

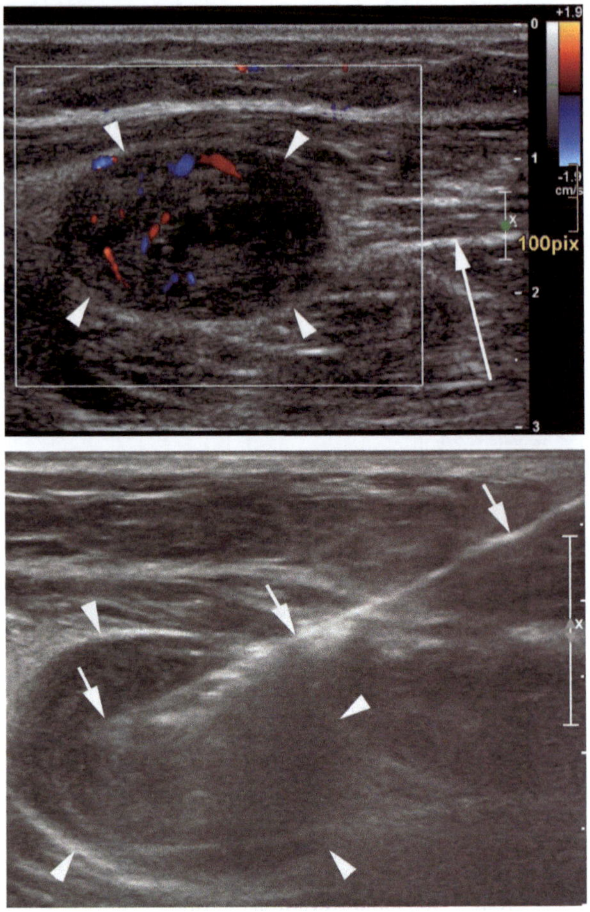

a

b

Fig. 7.1a,b. Sonographic guided biopsy of nerve tumor. **a** Vascularized schwannoma (*arrowheads*) of a muscle nerve (*long arrow*) within soleus muscle. **b** Core needle biopsy (*short arrows*) of the schwannoma (*arrowheads*) using 14 G coaxial biopsy system

an adequate number of tissue samples must be obtained and samples should be extracted from vital – usually visibly vascularized – tumor sites.

Finally, after removal of the coaxial-needle, a band-aid for the cutaneous puncture and a mild local compressive dressing is usually sufficient.

7.2 Sonographically Guided Regional Anesthesia

Anesthesiologists primarily use anatomical landmarks and nerve stimulators to perform regional anesthesia. According to the motto "No paresthesia, no anesthesia" (MOORE 1954) the needle is advanced blindly as close as possible to the nerve. Nerve stimulators have been an important – and for a long time the only – tool to control the advancement of the needle to the nerve. However, they are only applicable for anesthesia of nerves with sensory elements, whereas mere motor nerves without sensory function, such as the femoral nerve, will not produce sufficient paresthesia induced by nerve stimulation. However, such guidance procedures deal with the risk of intraneural injections. The potential harmful effect on the nerve fibers is the reason why Moore's motto is still under debate (GRAF and MARTIN 2001; BUCKENMAIER and BLECKNER 2005).

Sonographic guided regional anesthesia can be performed on any nerve, which can be depicted clearly by sonography (MARHOFER et al. 2005). The clinical use of sonographic guidance for regional anesthesia became very popular among anesthesiologists in the last few years and is no longer limited to regions with a complex topography. Sonography is applied to delineate the nerve structures themselves and to administer anesthetic under direct, visual control, and should avoid unintended complications such as intraneural injection or punctures of vessels and organs. It increases the success rate of the block and leads to a faster block onset compared to conventional techniques (CHAN et al. 2003). The minimum effective dose of anesthetic used can be significantly reduced, which leads to reduced systemic toxicity (MARHOFER et al. 1998; SANDHU et al. 2006a).

The type of transducer used depends on the region of concern and the depth of the nerve to be anesthetized (MARHOFER and CHAN 2007). The needle can be inserted in two ways, but actually only one mode can be recommended: at the short side of the transducer and advanced parallel to the sonographic section plane (in-plane needle approach), which always results in a complete depiction of the needle at its path towards the nerve. The insertion perpendicular to the transducer (out-of-plane needle approach), is a very unreliable and potentially harmful procedure as the needle tip becomes visualized just before reaching the target unless the transducer is not continuously tilted in relation to the tip of the needle (Fig. 7.2). Thus to avoid unintended puncture of vessels, muscles or organs, a test-bolus of local anesthetics or saline often has to be injected repeatedly during needle insertion. Such deposits allow less harmful advancement of the needle to reach the intended neural parts by this insertion technique.

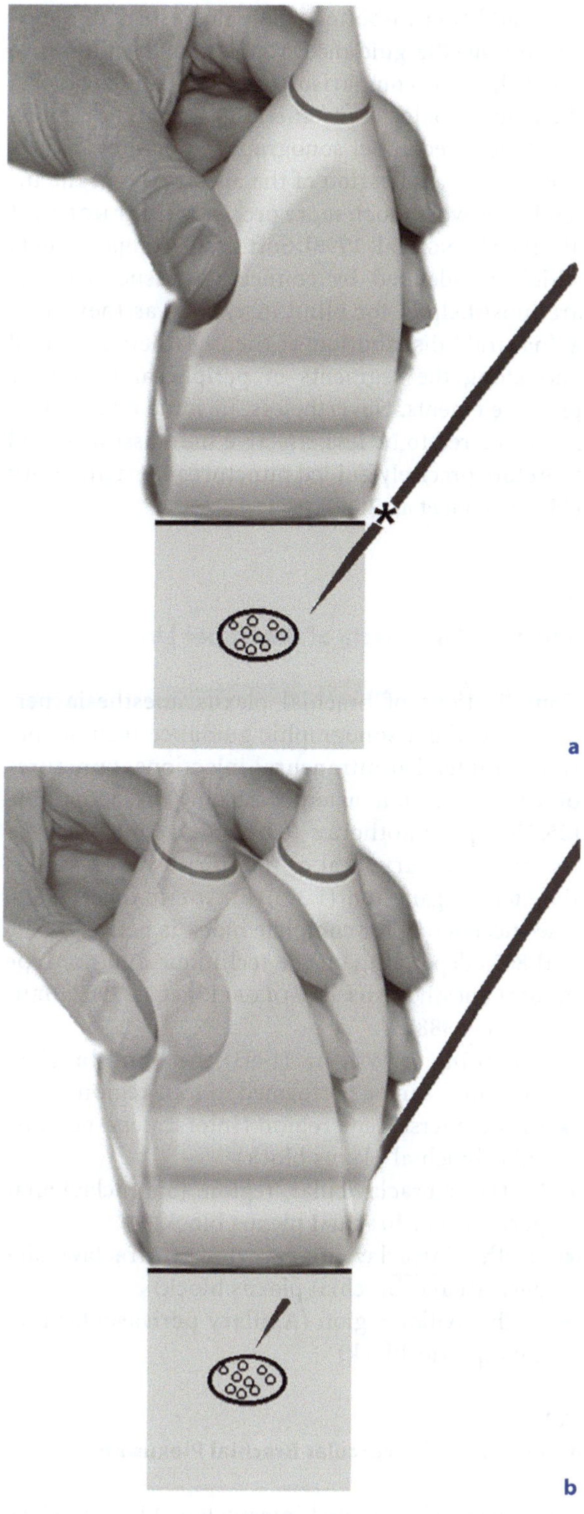

Fig. 7.2a,b. Injection techniques. **a** In-plane needle approach: The needle is inserted at the small side of the transducer (*asterisk*) and advanced diagonally within the sonographic section pla ne. **b** Out-of-plane needle approach: If the needle is inserted perpendicular to the transducer, it needs to be tilted continuously following the tip of the needle

In addition to better technical results of sonographic needle guidance, reports in the literature showed, that in comparison with non-guided blocks, the amount of local anesthetics used can be significantly reduced under sonographic guidance. This is because the application of the anesthetics at the intended nerve is much more precisely (Marhofer et al. 1998; Yang et al. 1998). Soft tissue compartments which are defined by connective tissues sheaths are most helpful for blind insertions as they favor a "natural" distribution of the anesthetics around and along the segments of peripheral nerves or plexus elements. Nevertheless, in some regions this is considered to be less effective than assumed and therefore precisely guided punctures are mandatory (Marhofer et al. 2000).

7.2.1 Regional Anesthesia of the Upper Limb

Complications of brachial plexus anesthesia performed without sonographic guidance include, besides unintended intraneural injections, punctures of the subclavian artery resulting in hematoma (25.7%), pneumothorax (0.6%–5%), and block of the recurrent laryngeal or phrenic nerve as well as the stellate ganglion (1.3%) (Bridenbaugh 1988). The success rate for complete block is between 70% and 80% depending on the technique and the type of local anesthetic used (Goldberg et al. 1987; Bedder et al. 1988).

According to Winnie (1993) the blind brachial plexus block can be performed in four regions:

- In the interscalene region (Interscalene perivascular brachial plexus block)
- In the supraclavicular region (Supraclavicular perivascular brachial plexus block)
- In the infraclavicular region (Infraclavicular perivascular brachial plexus block)
- In the axillar region (Axillary perivascular brachial plexus block)

7.2.1.1 Interscalene Perivascular Brachial Plexus Block

For sonographic guided interscalene block the brachial plexus is imaged between the anterior and middle scalene muscles, where in transverse sections it appears as a chain of hypoechoic nodules (Kapral et al. 1994) representing the spinal roots in the superior and the trunks of the plexus in the inferior interscalene region (Yang et al. 1998).The position of the transducer for sonographic access to this region is depicted in Figure 7.3. The known success rate blocks under real-time sonographic guidance ranges from 95% (Kapral et al. 1994) to 100% (Ting and Sivagnanaratnam 1989) without any severe complications reported. Compared to sonographically, only controlled procedures success is more accurate and frequent (98% vs 77%) including a prolonged duration of anesthesia (Jandrasits et al. 1998).

Yang et al. (1998) report unintended incomplete blocks in 6 of 15 patients, but with analgesia achieved in all patients postoperatively. However non-guided techniques are known to allow for a success rate of 75% for postoperative anesthesia at most (Tuominen et al. 1989).

7.2.1.2 Supraclavicular Perivascular Brachial Plexus Block

In the supraclavicular region the hypoechoic nodules representing the fascicles of the plexus accompany the subclavian artery (Fig. 7.4). For the approach to the plexus the patient lies supine with the arm in a neutral position and the head turned slightly to the opposite side (Kapral et al. 1994). In contrast to non-guided techniques with a success rate of 72% at most (Moorthy et al. 1991), sonographic guidance succeeds in 95% of patients (Kapral et al. 1994).

7.2.1.3 Infraclavicular Perivascular Brachial Plexus Block

For infraclavicular block the brachial plexus is scanned with a perpendicular transducer-position directly below the clavicle depicting the fascicles surrounding the axillary artery (Fig. 7.5). Ootaki et al. (2000) reported here a success rate for a complete block in 95% of patients. Complete sensory and motor blocks were achieved in 100% in the musculocutaneous and medial antebrachial cutaneous nerves, in 96.7% in the median nerve and in 90%–95% in the ulnar and radial nerve, respectively. Sandhu et al. (2006b) retrospectively analyzed 1146 cases of infraclavicular blocks and reported successful blocks in 99.3% (n=1138). Six patients had incomplete blocks, two patients needed additional local anesthetic supplementation. Subtotal blocks may be due to variations in the anatomy of the brachial plexus, concerning the individual organization and branching of the subsequent peripheral nerves.

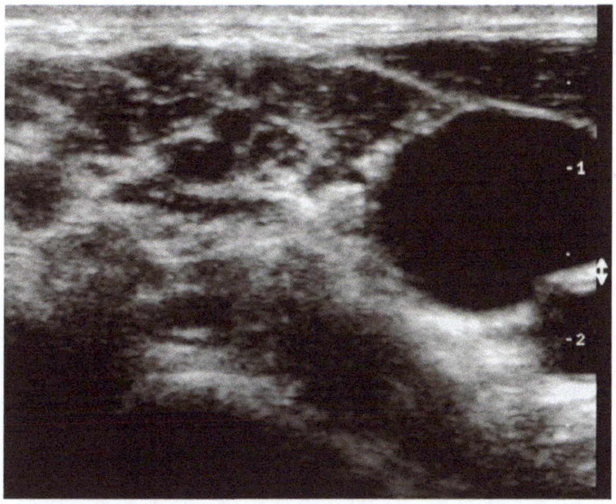

a

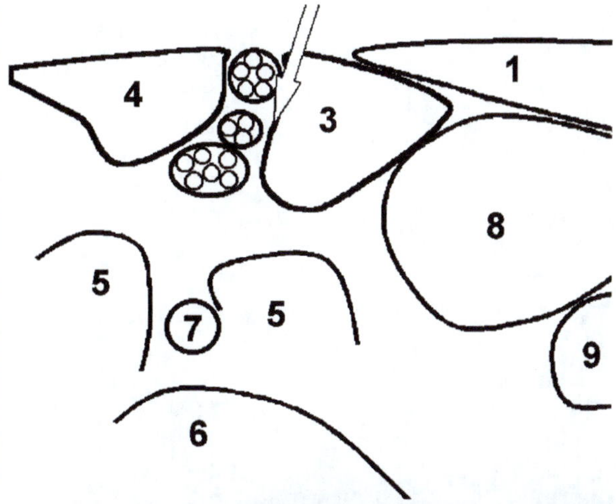

b

Fig. 7.3a–c. Sonographic guided interscalene brachial plexus block. **a** Sonogram. **b** Corresponding line drawing and recommended position of needle (*arrow*). **c** Position of the transducer in transverse plane with site of needle insertion medial to the transducer (*asterisk*). Posterior to the sternocleidomastoideus muscle (*1*) and proximal to the clavicle (*2*) the brachial plexus is depicted between the anterior (*3*) and the middle scalene muscle (*4*). The roots forming the plexus appear between the tubercles of the transverse process (*5*) of the cervical vertebra (*6*). Vertebral artery (*7*), internal jugular vein (*8*), common carotid artery (*9*)

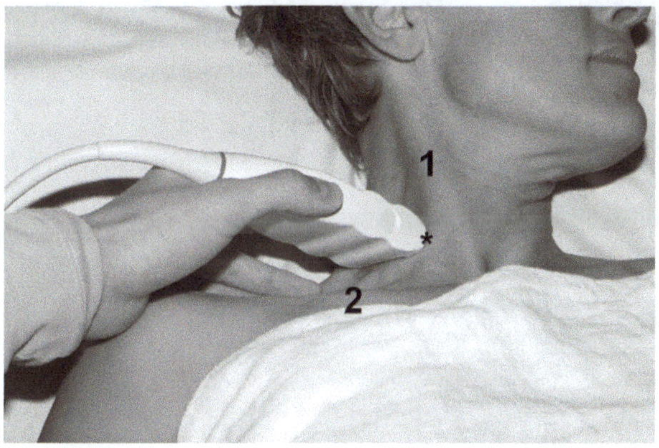

c

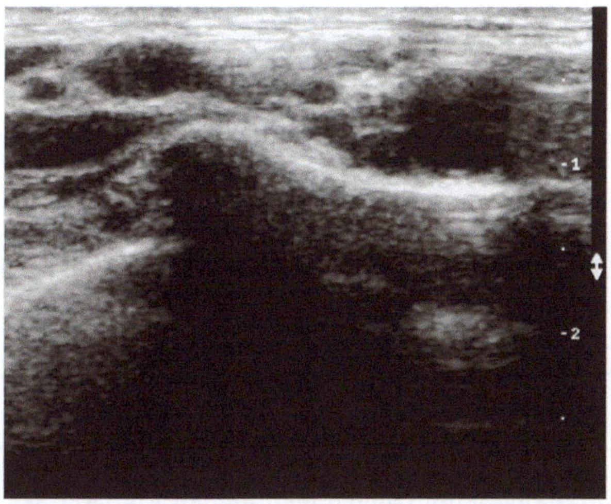

a

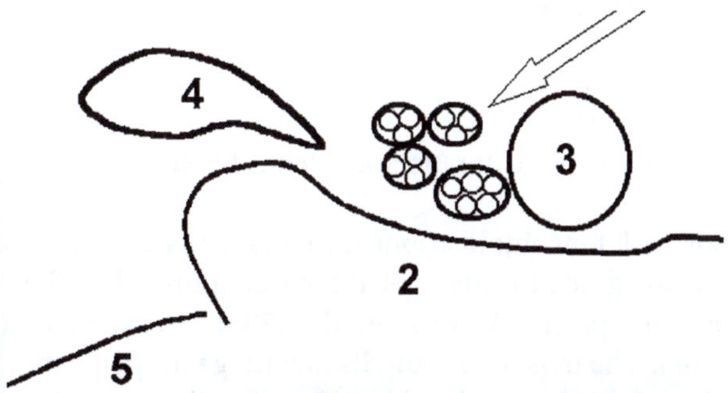

b

Fig. 7.4a–c. Sonographic guided supraclavicular brachial plexus block. **a** Sonogram. **b** Corresponding line drawing and recommended position of needle (*arrow*). **c** Position of the transducer in transverse plane with site of needle insertion medial to the transducer (*asterisk*). Sternocleidomastoideus muscle (*1*). Just above the clavicle (*2*) the forming fascicles of the brachial plexus are accompanied by the subclavian artery (*3*). Ventral border of the trapezius muscle (*4*), parietal pleura (*5*)

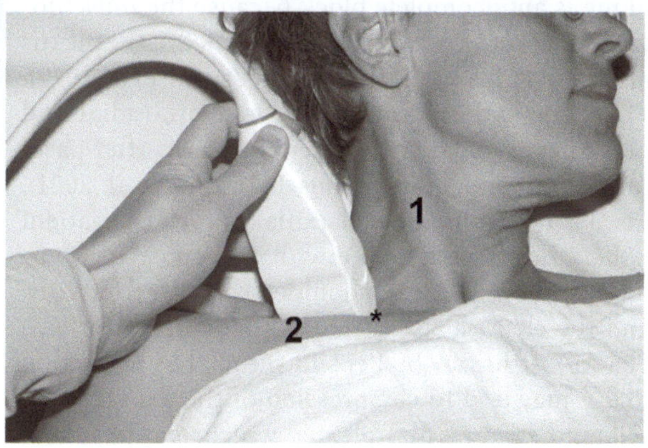

c

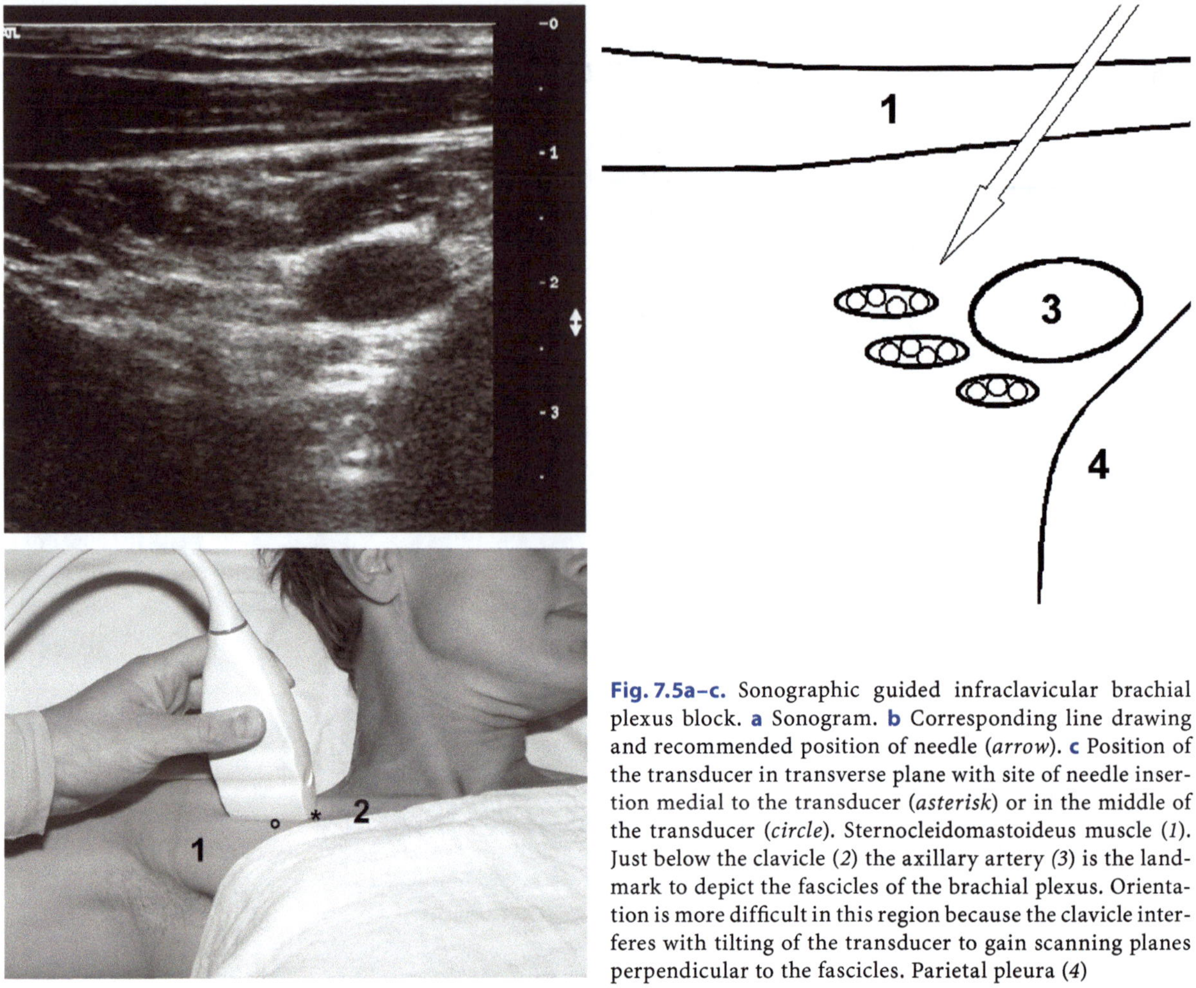

a

b

c

Fig. 7.5a–c. Sonographic guided infraclavicular brachial plexus block. **a** Sonogram. **b** Corresponding line drawing and recommended position of needle (*arrow*). **c** Position of the transducer in transverse plane with site of needle insertion medial to the transducer (*asterisk*) or in the middle of the transducer (*circle*). Sternocleidomastoideus muscle (*1*). Just below the clavicle (*2*) the axillary artery (*3*) is the landmark to depict the fascicles of the brachial plexus. Orientation is more difficult in this region because the clavicle interferes with tilting of the transducer to gain scanning planes perpendicular to the fascicles. Parietal pleura (*4*)

7.2.1.4 Axillary Perivascular Brachial Plexus Block

Low risk for complications is reported in general for the non guided axillary perivascular approach to the brachial plexus (Winnie et al. 1979; Bridenbaugh 1988). The most common disadvantage in this technique is an incomplete block because the musculocutaneous and axillary nerves often leave the plexus proximal to the site of the block (Winnie et al. 1979). The same may be true for the median, radial and ulnar nerve which usually begin to form after passing the minor pectoralis muscle (Retzl et al. 2001). For a sonographic guided axillary block the patient is best positioned supine with the upper arm abducted about 90°, the shoulder rotated externally, and the elbow flexed at 110° ("Cleopatra position", Fig. 7.6). It has to be kept in mind that abduction to 90° may lead to compression of the axillary vessels and the brachial plexus, which may result in an insufficient spread of the applied anesthetics. If this is suspected a slight adduction of the upper arm is recommended to improve a better spreading after injection. Kapral et al. (1994) in their series reported no severe complications and a complete block in 95% of the patients.

7.2.2 Regional Anesthesia of the Lower Limb

At the lower limb sonographic guidance is described for following regions:

- Psoas compartment block (Kirchmair et al. 2001, 2002)
- 3-in-1 block in the inguinal region (Marhofer et al. 1997, 1998)
- Sciatic nerve block
- Pudendal nerve block in the gluteal region (Gruber et al. 2001; Kovacs et al. 2001)

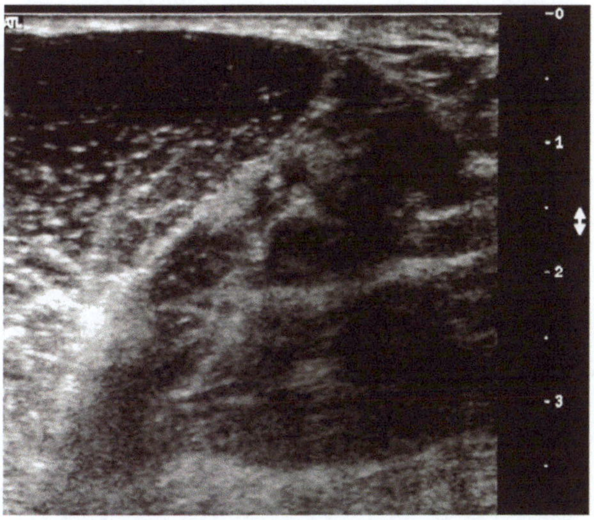

a

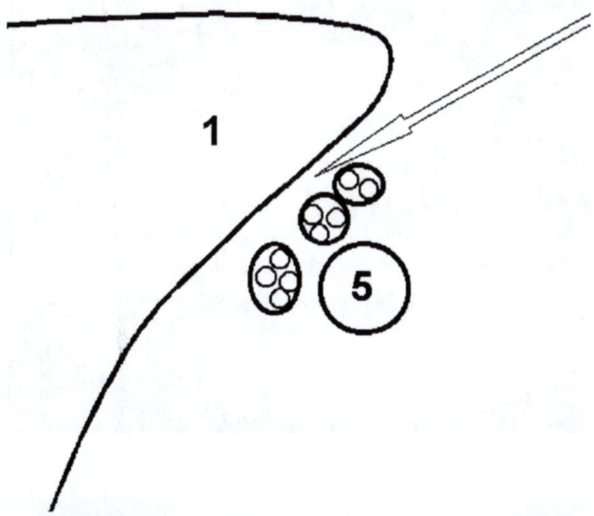

b

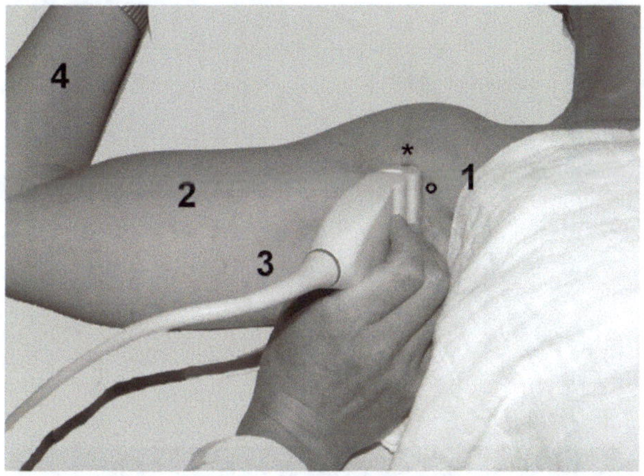

c

Fig. 7.6a–c. Sonographic guided axillar brachial plexus block. **a** Sonogram. **b** Corresponding line drawing and recommended position of needle (*arrow*). **c** Position of the transducer in transverse plane with site of needle insertion medial to the transducer (*asterisk*) or in the middle of the transducer (*circle*). Distal to the pectoralis minor muscle and deep to the pectoralis major muscle (*1*) the brachial plexus and the axillary artery (*5*) enter the groove between the biceps brachii (*2*) and the triceps brachii muscle (*3*). Note abduction in shoulder joint and position of forearm (*4*)

7.2.2.1
Psoas Compartment Block

The psoas compartment block is used to reach the spinal nerve roots forming the lumbar plexus within the psoas major muscle and is usually performed at the level of L4–5, because non-guided anesthetic instillations at the levels L2–3 and L3–4 often result in unintended renal punctures with consecutive subcapsular and intrarenal bleeding (Aida et al. 1996). Kirchmair et al. (2002) showed that a sonographic guided advancement of the needle into the psoas major muscle can be done at negligible risk in the L2–3 and L4–5 level. The instillation is performed at the sitting patient and the needle is inserted into the skin 4–5 cm lateral to the spinous processes, guided through the erector spinae muscle into the posterior part of the psoas major muscle under real-time control (Figs. 7.7 and 7.8). In cadaver specimens only 1 out of 48 attempts failed.

7.2.2.2
3-in-1 Block

The so-called 3-in-1 block is used to block off the femoral, the lateral femoral cutaneous and the obturator nerve by the administration of a single injection of local anesthetics in the inguinal region (Winnie et al. 1973). The sonographic guidance for this block is performed with the patient positioned supine and the leg rotated externally about 15°. The needle is inserted 2 cm distal to the inguinal ligament and advanced through the intermuscular fascial space (Marhofer et al. 1997, 1998), which separates the femoral nerve and the iliopsoas muscle from the femoral vessels (Fig. 7.9), to meet all intended nerves. In contrast to the stimulator guided technique – with a success rate lower than 80% – sonographic guidance succeeds in 95% of cases and allows one to administer less volume of local anesthetics (Marhofer et al. 1998). The needle tip positioned eas-

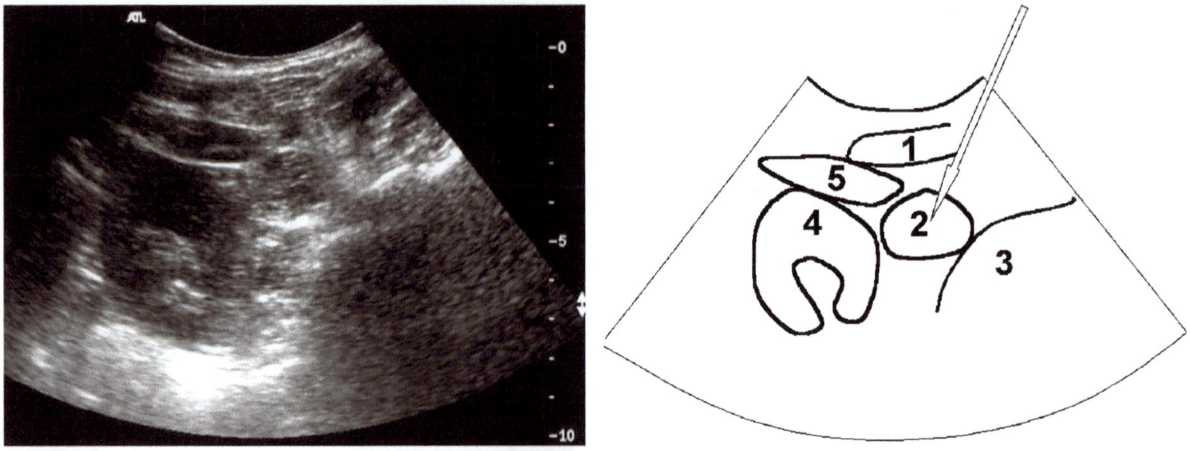

a b

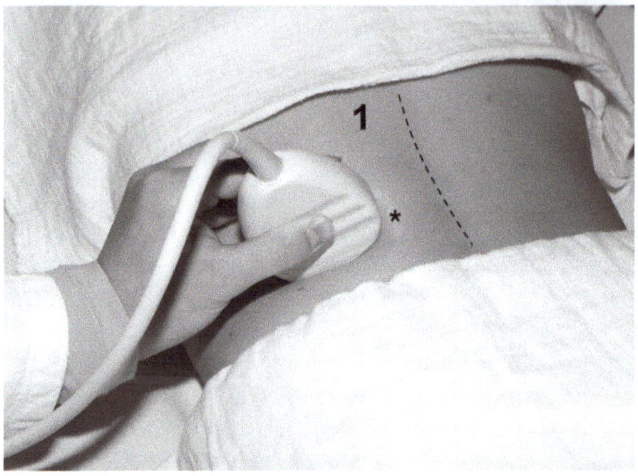

c

Fig. 7.7a–c. Sonographic guided psoas compartment block (L2–L3). **a** Sonogram. **b** Corresponding line drawing and recommended position of needle (*arrow*). **c** Position of the transducer in transverse plane with site of needle insertion medial to the transducer (*asterisk*) and dotted line through spinous processes. Through the erector spinae muscle (*1*) the posterior part of the psoas major muscle (*2*) is reached lateral to the third lumbar vertebra (*3*). Note the close relationship to the kidney (*4*). Quadratus lumborum muscle (*5*)

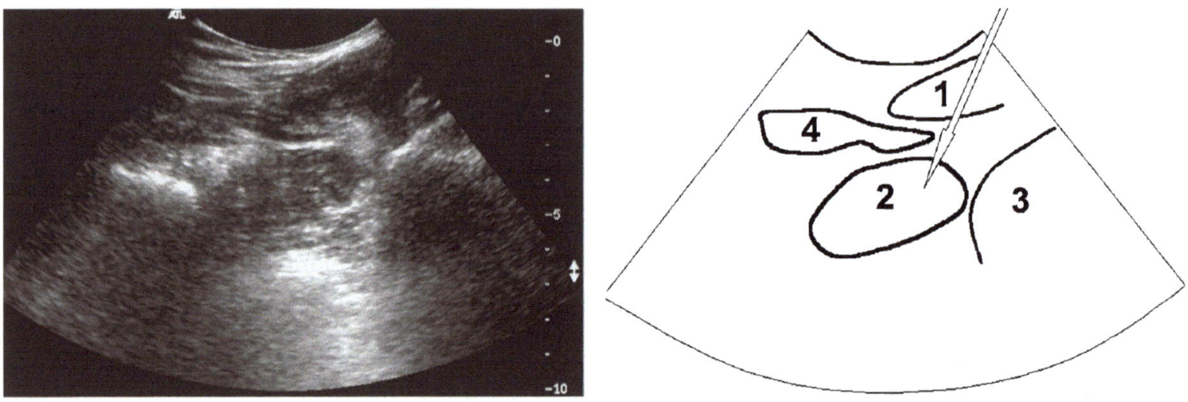

a b

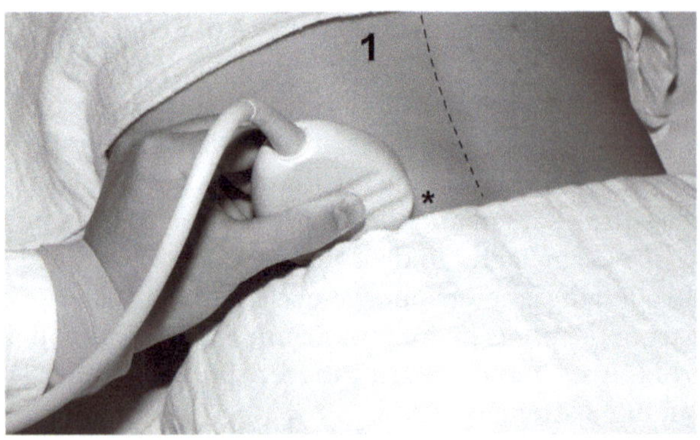

c

Fig. 7.8a–c. Sonographic guided psoas compartment block (L4–L5). **a** Sonogram. **b** Corresponding line drawing and recommended position of needle (*arrow*). **c** Position of the transducer in transverse plane with site of needle insertion medial to the transducer (*asterisk*) and dotted line through spinous processes. Erector spinae muscle (*1*), psoas major muscle (*2*), fifth lumbar vertebra (*3*), quadratus lumborum muscle (*5*) ily and a direct visualization of the spread of local anesthetic ensured additionally (Marhofer et al. 1997). Nevertheless, only the femoral nerve is infiltrated directly, whereas the lateral femoral cutaneous nerve is reached indirectly by lateral spread, and the anterior branch of the obturator nerve by medial spread of the local anesthetics. However, the posterior branch of the obturator nerve is reached neither by guided nor non guided blocks (Marhofer et al. 2000). In children ultrasound guided femoral (and sciatic) nerve blocks are also approved to be a safe technique leading to longer duration of sensory blockade although smaller amounts of anesthetic are administered (Oberndorfer et al. 2007).

7.2.2.3 Sciatic Nerve Block

The non-guided block of the large sized sciatic nerve is successful in 87%–97%, but subtotal anesthesia is reported, which may be due to anatomic variations in separation of the tibial and the common fibular nerve. The nerves may separate in the distal thigh, the proximal thigh or even inside the pelvis. These variations are visible sonographically leading to a modified needle position during administration of anesthetic.

The sciatic nerve and its branches may be reached in the subgluteal region (Karmakar et al. 2007), the midfemoral region (Domingo-Triado et al. 2007), or the popliteal fossa (McCartney et al. 2004; Gray et al. 2004). In the subgluteal region the patient is positioned laterally and a low frequency transducer is used. In the mid-femoral and popliteal region the high frequency linear transducer is placed on the posterior thigh, whereas the needle is advanced from the lateral thigh anterior to the tendon of biceps femoris muscle to administer anesthetic around the nerve (Fig. 7.10). In a prospective, randomized study Domingo-Triado et al. found complete sensory block in 96.7% of ultrasound guided and in 71% of non-guided procedures.

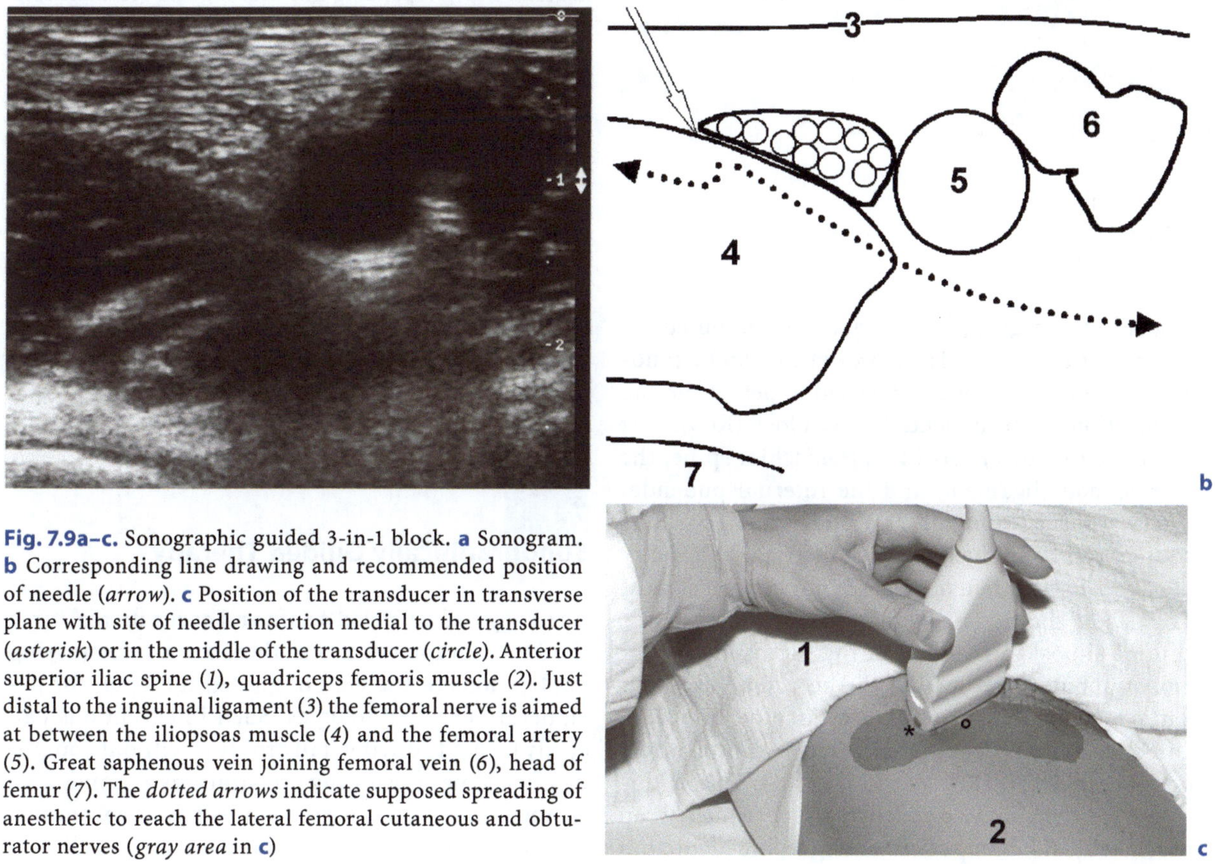

Fig. 7.9a–c. Sonographic guided 3-in-1 block. **a** Sonogram. **b** Corresponding line drawing and recommended position of needle (*arrow*). **c** Position of the transducer in transverse plane with site of needle insertion medial to the transducer (*asterisk*) or in the middle of the transducer (*circle*). Anterior superior iliac spine (*1*), quadriceps femoris muscle (*2*). Just distal to the inguinal ligament (*3*) the femoral nerve is aimed at between the iliopsoas muscle (*4*) and the femoral artery (*5*). Great saphenous vein joining femoral vein (*6*), head of femur (*7*). The *dotted arrows* indicate supposed spreading of anesthetic to reach the lateral femoral cutaneous and obturator nerves (*gray area* in **c**)

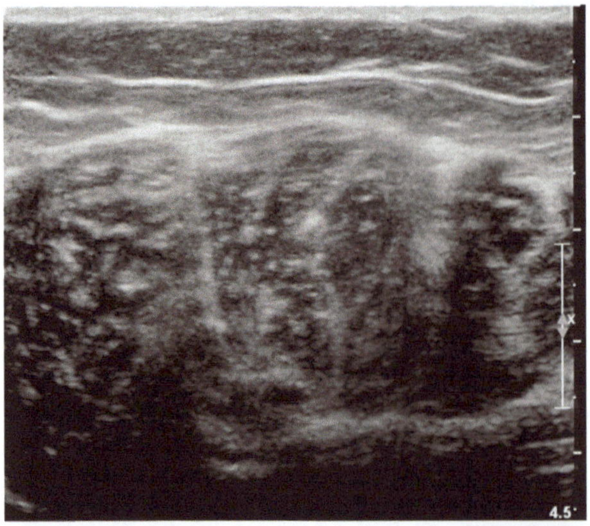

a

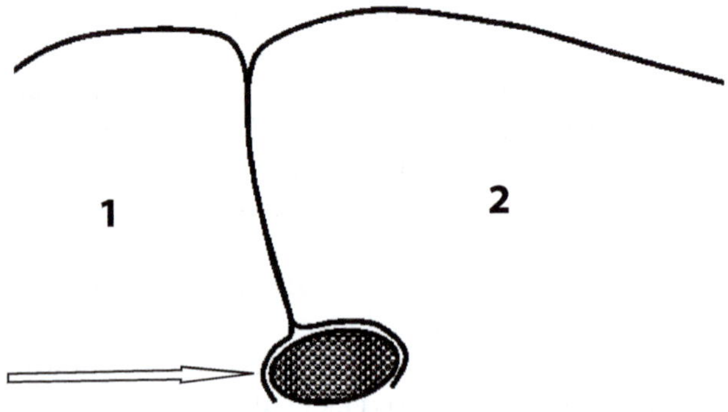

b

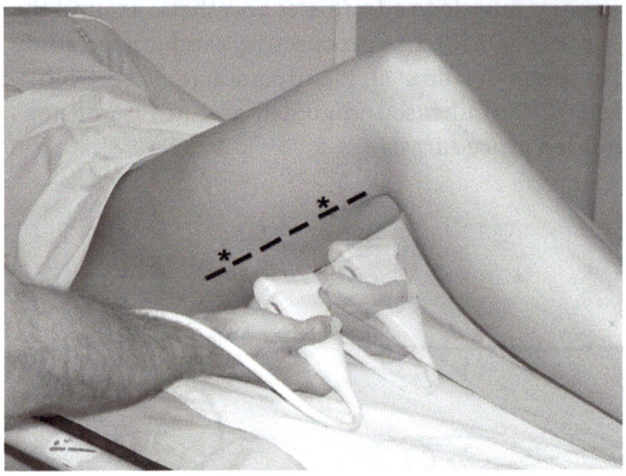

c

Fig. 7.10a–c. Sonographic guided sciatic nerve block. **a** Sonogram. **b** Corresponding line drawing and recommended position of needle (*arrow*). **c** Position of the transducer in transverse plane with sites of needle insertions (*asterisks*) lateral just dorsal to the tendon or through the belly of femoral biceps muscle (broken line, *1* in **b**). Semitendinosus and semimembranosus muscle (*2*)

7.2.2.4 Pudendal Nerve Block

Instead of non-guided techniques or computed tomography guidance (Thoumas et al. 1999), sonographic guidance can also be used to depict the site of injection for the pudendal nerve block (Kovacs et al. 2001). In a prone position, the ischial spine, the sacrospinous ligament, and the internal pudendal artery, which accompanies the pudendal nerve at its course, can be delineated by sonography although the nerve itself can in most cases not be seen clearly. The needle should be advanced under sonographic control almost to the level of the sacrospinous ligament about 5 mm medial to the artery or about 8 mm medial to the tip of the sciatic spine (Fig. 7.11). Direct depiction of the pudendal nerve is only rarely possible in 47.2% (Kovacs et al. 2001). This is due to the adipose and connective tissue which wrap the nerve and hamper its sonographic depiction (Gruber et al. 2001). However, a clear sonographic depiction of the region mentioned above suffices as the anesthetics spread if administered in the correct fascial space also around the nerve and provoking a highly effective block.

7.3 Sonographically Guided Therapy

As sonography proved a safe and accurate real-time modality for interventions, there are also increasing applications in the field of guided therapies for peripheral nerve pathologies. Such interventions can easily be made during daily routine without complicated or time consuming preparations and may also be repeated. As these procedures have evolved just over the last few years, evaluations on the clinical

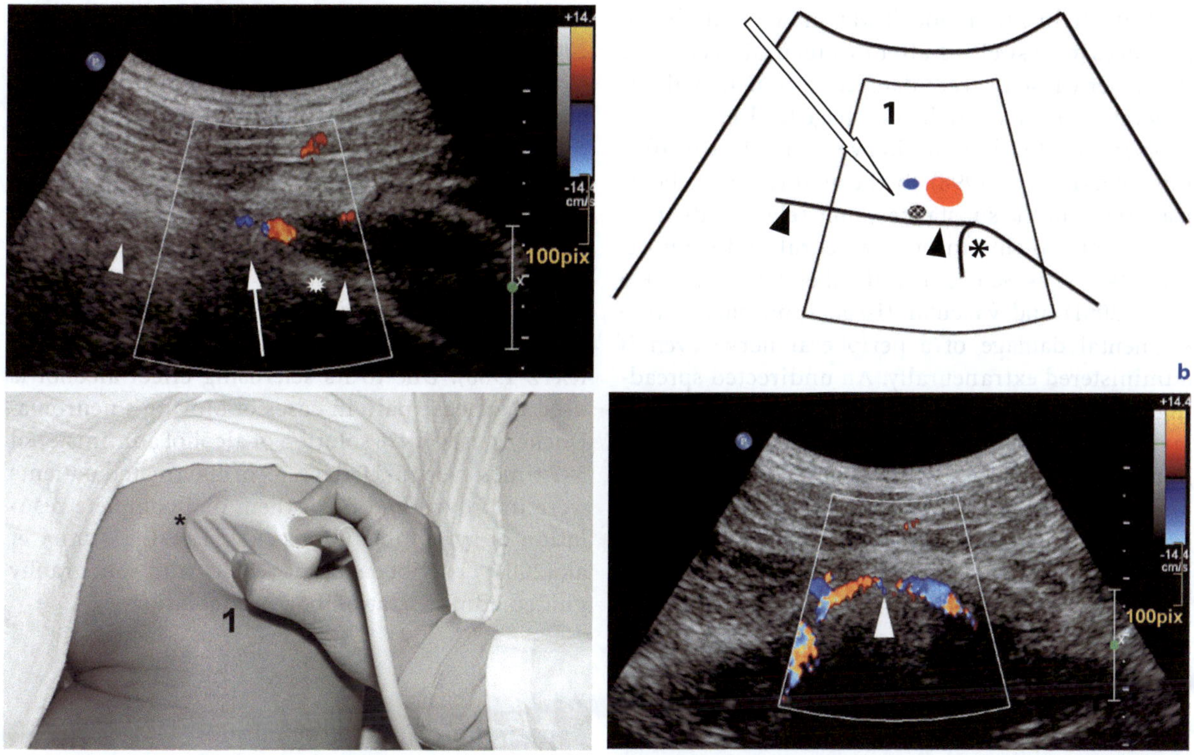

Fig. 7.11a–d. Sonographic guided pudendal nerve block. **a** Sonogram. **b** Corresponding line drawing and recommended position of needle (*open arrow*). **c** Position of the transducer in almost transverse plane with site of needle insertion medial to the transducer (*asterisk*). The needle should be advanced through the gluteus maximus muscle (*1*) close to the ischial spine (*star*) and the sacrospinous ligament (*arrowheads*). Using color coded Doppler sonography the internal pudendal artery (*red*) and vein (*blue*) can be identified as guidance to the pudendal nerve (*arrow*). **d** Almost longitudinal sonogram of the internal pudendal artery (changing from red to blue due to flow to and from the transducer) crossing the sacrospinous ligament (*arrowhead*)

evidence for these therapies are often still work-in-progress and only case series and pilot studies are published, which are often promising indeed. In the following we try to figure out the "what" and "how" and give hints on clinical and therapeutic problems emerging with concerned patients.

7.3.1 Therapeutic Agents

7.3.1.1 Steroids

Steroids decrease inflammatory reactions and reduce edema at the site of, e.g., neuroma formations and help to loosen the connective tissue surrounding the nerve, thereby reducing compression of the nerve by encasing connective tissue. Depending on the galenic preparation they are more or less long acting drugs. However, applications should never be performed intraneurally (Al-Nasser 2007). Steroid injections may be used both to treat painful lesions in large nerves, such as the sciatic nerve (Hanania and Kitain 1998) and for painful neuromas of small nerves, such as in treatment of Morton's neuroma of interdigital nerves (Rasmusen et al. 1996). However, localized applications of rather high steroid-doses at the site of, e.g., a neuroma formation is not known to cause critical systemic reactions, whereas local problems, such as local atrophy of fat tissue may develop (Fredberg 1997).

7.3.1.2 Phenol

Besides type A botulinum toxin, phenol has been used for decades to treat muscle spasticity with blind intramuscular injections (Maher 1964) and pain with perineural and intraneural injections (Mooney et al. 1969). In a rat model it was shown that phenol produces focal swelling after intraneural injections. It further caused severe demyelination, axonal degeneration, edema and hemorrhage leading to complete architectural disruption verifiable 1 week after injection (Lu et al. 1998). By the mainly direct chemical effects of the substance a non-selective disintegration of proteins in proper neural and supporting tissue – as Schwann cell tubes (Westerlund et al. 2001) and vascular tissue – produce severe segmental damage of a peripheral nerve even if administered extraneurally. An undirected spreading of phenol is promoted additionally by its apolar chemical benzol-structure. In summary, phenol damages the peripheral nerves in a combined toxic and ischemic way, but more severely after intraneural than extraneural administration (Westerlund et al. 2001). Despite this profound and actually irreversible reactions to phenol instillation, signs of nerve regeneration are detected about 2 weeks after, when axonal sprouts become visible (Westerlund et al. 2001). In a similar setting Tsukazaki et al. (1993) reported on a significant increase of neuronal recovery at 4 weeks after phenol injection followed by total recovery at 8 weeks. This fast and complete recovery may be the reason for the reports on only transient effects of imprecise neurolytic blocks with phenol (Mooney et al. 1969).

In contrast to surgical neuroma resection, the development of secondary neuromas is avoided when axons sprout through the toxic nerve lesion (Myers and Katz 1988). After treatment with phenol Westerlund et al. (2001) report broken basal laminae. Axonal sprouts seem to be guided by the fragments of basal laminae and the lesion recovers without significant misrouting of the sprouts.

In the precisely sonographically guided treatment of painful stump neuromas the damage to conduction on the peripheral nerve following phenol injection plays the most important role. Although the tendency of nerve recovery has to be determined in follow-up studies (Westerlund et al. 2001), whereas our experiences so far also show at least promising long time results over 6 months in more than 80 treated persons.

7.3.1.3 Glycerol

Compared with phenol, glycerol causes similar effects on the nerve fibers, but never produces ischemia with hemorrhagic necrosis and is less effective in breaking the basal laminae (Westerlund et al. 2001). Due to its viscosity it is difficult to be injected with fine needles and, therefore, more difficult to handle.

7.3.1.4 Alcohol

In comparison with phenol, alcohol has a slower action, is more irritating to adjacent tissues and more likely to cause painful neuritis (Myers and Katz 1988). Due to its sclerosing effect alcohol is used to release pain in cases of Morton´s neuroma. Dockery used a 4% solution of alcohol administered 3–7 times every 5–10 days. 89 of 100 treated patients were improved and 82 of them had complete resolution of symptoms (Dockerey 1999). Masala et al. (2001) described similar results with sonography guided administration of a 30% solution.

7.3.2 Sonographic Guided Techniques

Thomas et al. (1999) administered local anesthetic around neuromas under sonographic control to confirm the neuroma being the reason for stump pain. Afterwards they marked the neuroma with breast localization wires to allow for minimally invasive surgical resection of the lesion.

The great advantage of sonographic guided instillations is the accuracy with which it can be performed: on the one hand due to the resolution power of sonography, and on the other hand due to the realtime depiction by which these procedures are realized. At present several applicators with (attachable) needle-steering devices are available which should help to find the correct path to intended structure. This works well for, e.g., amniocentesis where the structures of interest are in a respectable depth to the body surface. Peripheral neural structures are usually found in the immediate near-field on the one hand, and due to changing topographic situations very standardized entryways are usually counterproductive on the other. Thus free-hand puncture techniques are considered to be more comfortable, more easily to perform and more accurate although persistent exercising is essential.

Overall, sonographic guided techniques show a very low complication rate and are also relatively comfortable for the patient (Holm and Skjoldbye 1996).

7.3.3
Indications for Guided Therapy

7.3.3.1
Instillations at the Spine

Severe pain in the spine – often known as diffuse back pain – is the most frequent reason for (at least temporary) disablement in the western world (Pelz and Haddad 1989; Diamond and Borenstein 2006). To control the life quality reducing pain symptoms in the lumbar and cervical spine several strategies have been defined so far, based on surgical, physiotherapeutic procedures and on anti-inflammatory procedures and applications (Albert and Murrell 1999; Indahl 2004; Diamond and Borenstein 2006). To propose and discuss all these possibilities would clearly be beyond the scope of this book, but we want to identify where sonography can be helpful doing simple interventions.

Most importantly, in the cervical and lumbar spine – which are usually compromised by radiculopathies or facet joint pain at several levels – it has been shown that local instillations of anti-inflammatory agents such as corticoid suspensions are often more effective than systemic medications or surgery (Riew et al. 2000; Manchikanti et al. 2006).

Galiano et al. (2005a,b, 2006) showed that the sonographic approach to the lumbar and cervical spine is possible. Using 22G needles (always of a sufficient length) it was shown that sonography is more than sufficient for the guidance to the according landmarks at the facet joints or the spinal nerve roots to administer therapeutic agents at according doses (Fig. 7.12). It has also been shown that, as well as saving time, these procedures need no ionizing radiation – as in guidance by fluoroscopy and computed tomography – and show less complications. This is due to the fact that sonographic interventions are always real-time procedures, where the sonographer watches the needle at all times during advancement.

7.3.3.2
Corticoid Instillations in Compression Syndromes

Peripheral nerve compression due to so called "tunnel syndromes" are often not only a challenge in the diagnostic (see Chap. 3) but also in the therapeutic field (Spinner 2006). So far it has been proven that decompression surgery is the gold-standard therapy, whereas there still seems to be discussion on when is the correct time for surgery and how it should be performed (Heckler and Jabaley 1986; Tennent and Goddard 1997; McNally and Hales 2003). However, surgery of decompression syndromes – particularly of the median and the ulnar nerve – is far from being without controversy: often even the initial outcome is insufficient and compression syndromes frequently recur secondarily, often presumably due to unintended scar formations (Mackinnon 1991). Actually, in contrast to the aforementioned, it was also shown by Agarwal et al. (2005) that, e.g., in compressions of the median nerve in the carpal tunnel local instillations of corticoid suspensions also are highly effective. They could show that after 3 months over 90% and after 16 months about 80% of the treated patients reported a marked improvement, which could be significantly fortified by the appropriate conduction parameters. Based on our own experiences we can approve these data. Using sonography in this context assures non-intended injuries and painful punctures of the nerve. Peri-neural instillations of the corticoid suspensions is thereby very comfortable and easy to perform (Fig. 7.13).

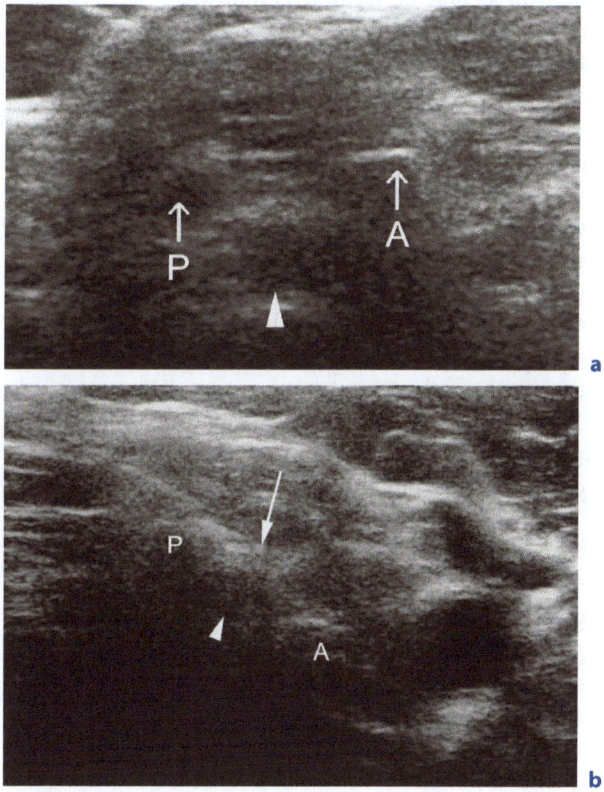

Fig. 7.12a,b. Sonographic guided cervical instillation. **a** Transverse sonogram depicting the anterior (*A*) and posterior (*P*) tubercle of the 6th cervical vertebra and the emerging nerve root of C6 (*arrowhead*). **b** The needle is advanced from lateral until the tip (*arrow*) reaches the nerve root (*arrowhead*)

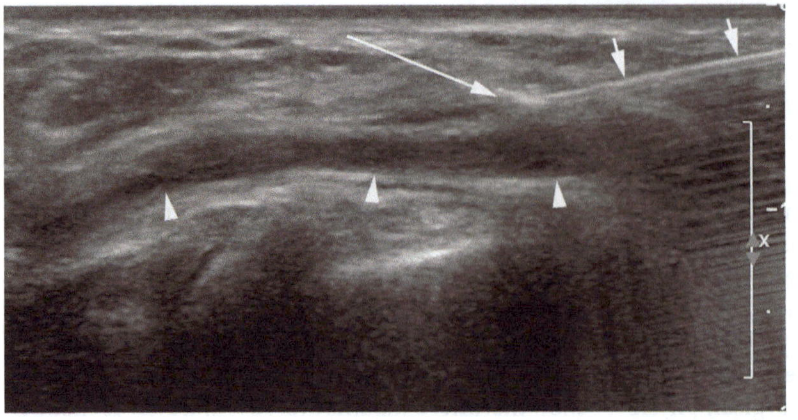

Fig. 7.13. Sonographic guided corticoid instillation. Longitudinal sonogram of the ulnaris nerve (*arrowheads*) in the "sulcus nervi ulnaris" showing the advanced needle (*arrows*) and fluid with air bubbles around the nerve (*long arrow*)

7.3.3.3 Agent Induced Pain Therapy

The formation of neuromas is part of the normal regeneration process after nerve injury. After amputations stump neuromas may lead to pain, such as stump pain or phantom limb pain. These painful neuromas may be treated as follows:

- With surgical interventions
- With instillation of therapeutic agents

There is a wide range of possible surgical techniques for treatment of neuroma including nerve-to-nerve repair after nerve dissection or transection. After amputations the stump neuroma may be surgically exposed and capped with some inert material, but according to the literature implantation of the resected nerve stump into the adjacent muscle or even between muscle and bone is considered to be the most efficient treatment option (Dellon et al. 1984; Dellon and Mackinnon 1986).

The therapeutic agents used for instillations include steroids, phenol, alcohol and glycerol.

In this context we performed a study in which we accurately administered phenol directly into the neck of painful stump neuromas under sonographic guidance (Gruber et al. 2004). According to the reported procedure, local anesthetics are used first to release pain, by the infiltration of the soft tissues surrounding the neuroma and the neuroma itself. If this procedure releases pain sufficiently a subsequent setting is performed. In this following session – after a sufficient local anesthesia – the needle is advanced into the nerve proximal to the neuroma and 0.3–0.5 ml of phenol are injected under direct sonographic control. During injection swelling of the nerve fascicles or injected air within the nerve can be delineated and visually confirm a successful application (Fig. 7.14). After injection the syringe must be flushed with saline to avoid spreading of phenol into the adjacent tissue when pulling back the needle. If necessary, the procedure can be repeated after several days. Six months after a standardized protocol of treatment there was either still significant cessation or at least a remarkable decrease of pain in these patients.

References

Agarwal V, Singh R, Sachdev A, Wiclaff, Shekhar S, Goel D (2005) A prospective study of the long-term efficacy of local methyl prednisolone acetate injection in the management of mild carpal tunnel syndrome. Rheumatology 44(5):647–650

Aida S, Takahashi H, Shimoji K (1996) Renal subcapsular hematoma after lumbar plexus block. Anesthesiology 84:452–455

Albert TJ, Murrell SE (1999) Surgical management of cervical radiculopathy. J Am Acad Orthop Surg 7(6):368–376

Al-Nasser B (2007) Intraneural injection of local anesthetics during ultrasound-guided peripheral nerve block may lead to nerve injury. Anesthesiology 106(6):1245–1246; author reply 1247

Bedder MD, Kozody R, Cronig DB (1988) Comparison of bupivacaine and alkalinised bupivacaine in brachial plexus anesthesia. Anesth Analg 67:48–52

Bridenbaugh LD (1988) The upper extremity: somatic blockade. In: Cousins MJ, Bridenbaugh PO (eds) Neural blockade in clinical anesthesia and management of pain. Lippincott, Philadelphia, pp 387–416

Buckenmaier CC III, Bleckner LL (2005) Anaesthetic agents for advanced regional anaesthesia: a North American perspective. Drugs 65(6):745–759

Chan VW, Perlas A, Rawson R, Odukoya O (2003) Ultrasound-guided supraclavicular brachial plexus block. Anesth Analg 97:1514–1517

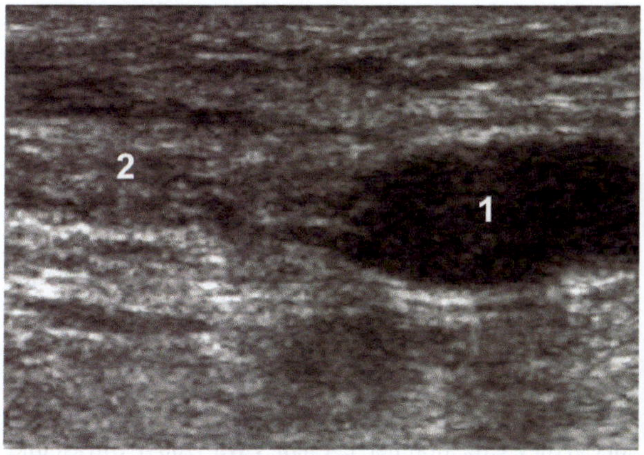

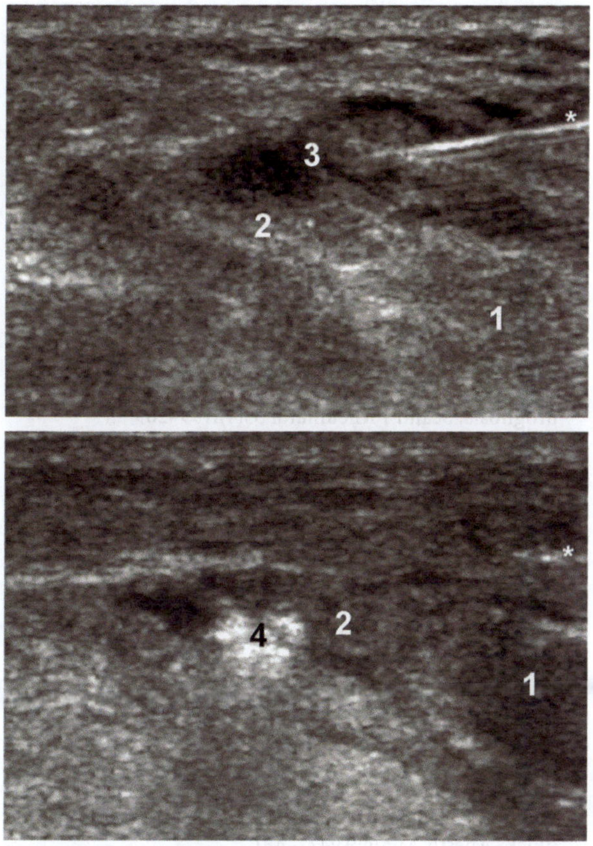

Fig. 7.14a–c. Intraneural injection of phenol for treatment of painful neuroma. **a** Depiction of a stump neuroma (*1*) at the end of the sciatic nerve (*2*) in a 56-year-old male patient. **b** A needle (*asterisk*) is advanced to the nerve proximal to the neuroma and 5 ml of local anesthetic (*3*) is administered. **c** The needle is advanced further into the nerve and 0.5 ml of phenol (with air bubbles (*4*)) are injected directly into the nerve

Dellon AL, Mackinnon SE (1986) Treatment of the painful neuroma by neuroma resection and muscle implantation. Plast Reconstr Surg 77:427–436

Dellon AL, Mackinnon SE, Pestronk A (1984) Implantation of sensory nerve into muscle: preliminary clinical and experimental observations on neuroma formation. Ann Plast Surg 12:30–40

Diamond S, Borenstein D (2006) Chronic low back pain in a working-age adult. Best Pract Res Clin Rheumatol 20(4):707–720

Dockery GL (1999) The treatment of intermetatarsal neuromas with 4% alcohol sclerosing injections. J Foot Ankle Surg 38:403–408

Domingo-Triado V, Selfa S, Martinez F, Sanchez-Contreras D, Reche M, Tecles J, Crespo MT, Palanca JM, Moro B (2007) Ultrasound guidance for lateral midfemoral sciatic nerve block: a prospective, comparative, randomized study. Anesth Analg 104:1270–1274

Dupuy DE, Rosenberg AE, Punyaratabandhu T, Tan MH, Mankin HJ (1998) Accuracy of CT-guided needle biopsy of musculoskeletal neoplasms. AJR Am J Roentgenol 171(3):759–762

Fredberg U (1997) Local corticosteroid injection in sport: review of literature and guidelines for treatment. Scand J Med Sci Sports 7(3):131–139

Galiano K, Obwegeser AA, Bodner G, Freund M, Maurer H, Kamelger FS, Schatzer R, Ploner F (2005a) Ultrasound guidance for facet joint injections in the lumbar spine: a computed tomography-controlled feasibility study. Anesth Analg 101(2):579–583

Galiano K, Obwegeser AA, Bodner G, Freund MC, Gruber H, Maurer H, Schatzer R, Ploner F (2005b) Ultrasound-guided periradicular injections in the middle to lower cervical spine: an imaging study of a new approach. Reg Anesth Pain Med 30(4):391–396

Galiano K, Obwegeser AA, Bodner G, Freund MC, Gruber H, Maurer H, Schatzer R, Fiegele T, Ploner F (2006) Ultrasound-guided facet joint injections in the middle to lower cervical spine: a CT-controlled sonoanatomic study. Clin J Pain 22(6):538–543

Goldberg ME, Gregg C, Larijani GE, Norris MC, Marr AT, Seltzer JL (1987) Comparison of three methods of axillary approach to brachial plexus blockade for upper extremity surgery. Anesthesiology 66:814–816

Graf BM, Martin E (2001) Peripheral neuronal blockade. A review of new developments of an old technique [German]. Anaesthesist 50:312–322

Gray AT, Huczko EL, Schafhalter-Zoppoth I (2004) Lateral popliteal nerve block with ultrasound guidance. Reg Anesth Pain Med 29:507–509

Gruber H, Kovacs P, Piegger J, Brenner E (2001) New, simple, ultrasound-guided infiltration of the pudendal nerve: topographic basics. Dis Colon Rectum 44:1376–1380

Gruber H, Kovacs P, Peer S, Frischhut B, Bodner G (2004) Sonographically guided phenol injection in painful stump neuroma. AJR Am J Roentgenol 182(4):952–954

Hanania M, Kitain E (1998) Perisciatic injection of steroid for the treatment of sciatica due to piriformis syndrome. Reg Anesth Pain Med 23:223–228

Hansen E, Wolff N, Knuechel R, Ruschoff J, Hofstaedter F, Taeger K (1995) Tumor cells in blood shed from the surgical field. Arch Surg 130(4):387–393

Heckler FR, Jabaley ME (1986) Evolving concepts of median nerve decompression in the carpal tunnel. Hand Clin 2(4):723–736

Holm HH, Skjoldbye B (1996) Interventional ultrasound. Ultrasound Med Biol 22(7):773–789

Indahl A (2004) Low back pain: diagnosis, treatment, and prognosis. Scand J Rheumatol 33(4):199–209

Jandrasits O, Likar R, Marhofer P, Weinstabl C, Kapral S (1998) The use of ultrasonography for regional anesthetic techniques: upper extremity blockades. Acta Anaesthesiol Scand 42:48–51

Kapral S, Krafft P, Eibenberger K, Fitzgerald R, Gosch M, Weinstabl C (1994) Ultrasound-guided supraclavicular approach for regional anesthesia of the brachial plexus. Anesth Analg 78:507–513

Karmakar MK, Kwok WH, Ho AM, Tsang K, Chui PT, Gin T (2007) Ultrasound-guided sciatic nerve block: description of a new approach at the subgluteal space. Br J Anaesth 98:390–395

Kirchmair L, Entner T, Wissel J, Moriggl B, Kapral S, Mitterschiffthaler G (2001) A study of the paravertebral anatomy for ultrasound-guided posterior lumbar plexus block. Anesth Analg 93:477–481

Kirchmair L, Entner T, Kapral S, Mitterschiffthaler G (2002) Ultrasound guidance for the psoas compartment block: an imaging study. Anesth Analg 94:706–710

Kovacs P, Gruber H, Piegger J, Bodner G (2001) New, simple, ultrasound-guided infiltration of the pudendal nerve: ultrasonographic technique. Dis Colon Rectum 44:1381–1385

Kransdorf MJ (1995a) Benign soft-tissue tumors in a large referral population: distribution of specific diagnoses by age, sex, and location. AJR Am J Roentgenol 164(2):395–402

Kransdorf MJ (1995b) Malignant soft-tissue tumors in a large referral population: distribution of diagnoses by age, sex, and location. AJR Am J Roentgenol 164(1):129–134

Lu L, Atchabahian A, Mackinnon SE, Hunter DA (1998) Nerve injection injury with botulinum toxin. Plast Reconstr Surg 101:1875–1880

Mackinnon SE (1991) Secondary carpal tunnel surgery. Neurosurg Clin N Am 2(1):75–91

Maher RM (1964) The medical treatment of spasticity. Proc R Soc Med 57:720–723

Manchikanti L, Damron K, Cash K, Manchukonda R, Pampati V (2006) Therapeutic cervical medial branch blocks in managing chronic neck pain: a preliminary report of a randomized, double-blind, controlled trial: clinical trial NCT0033272. Pain Physician 9(4):333–346

Marhofer P, Chan VW (2007) Ultrasound-guided regional anesthesia: current concepts and future trends. Anesth Analg 104:1265–1269

Marhofer P, Schrögendorfer K, Koinig H, Kapral S, Weinstabl C, Mayer N (1997) Ultrasonographic guidance improves sensory block and onset time of three-in-one blocks. Anesth Analg 85:854–857

Marhofer P, Schrögendorfer K, Wallner T, Koinig H, Mayer N, Kapral S (1998) Ultrasonographic guidance reduces the amount of local anesthetic for 3-in-1 blocks. Reg Anesth 23:584–588

Marhofer P, Nasel C, Sitzwohl C, Kapral S (2000) Magnetic resonance imaging of the distribution of local anesthetic during the three-in-one block. Anesth Analg 90:119–124

Marhofer P, Greher M, Kapral S (2005) Ultrasound guidance in regional anaesthesia. Br J Anaesth 94:7–17

Masala S, Fanucci E, Ranconi P, Sodani G, Taormina P, Romagnoli A, Simonetti G (2001) Treatment of intermetatarsal neuromas with alcohol injection under US guidance [Italian]. Radiol Med (Torino) 102:370–373

McCartney CJL, Brauner I, Chan VWS (2004) Ultrasound guidance for a lateral approach to the sciatic nerve in the popliteal fossa. Anaesthesia 59:1023–1025

McNally SA, Hales PF (2003) Results of 1245 endoscopic carpal tunnel decompressions. Hand Surg 8:111–116

Mooney V, Frykman G, McLamb J (1969) Current status of intraneural phenol injections. Clin Orthop 63:122–129

Moore D (1954) Regional block. Thomas, Springfield, IL, p 60

Moorthy SS, Schmidt SI, Dierdorf SF, Rosenfeld SH, Anagnostou JM (1991) A supraclavicular lateral approach for brachial plexus regional anesthesia. Anesth Analg 72:241–244

Myers RR, Katz J (1988) Neuropathy of neurolytic and semidestructive agents. In: Cousins MJ, Bridenbaugh PO (eds) Neural blockade in clinical anesthesia and management of pain. Lippincott, Philadelphia, pp 1031–1051

Oberndorfer U, Marhofer P, Bösenberg A, Willschke H, Felfernig M, Weintraud M, Kapral S, Kettner SC (2007) Ultrasonographic guidance for sciatic and femoral nerve blocks in children. Br J Anaesth 98:797–801

Ogilvie CM, Torbert JT, Finstein JL, Fox EJ, Lackman RD (2006) Clinical utility of percutaneous biopsies of musculoskeletal tumors. Clin Orthop Relat Res 450:95–100

Ootaki C, Hayashi H, Amano M (2000) Ultrasound-guided infraclavicular brachial plexus block: an alternative technique to landmark-guided approaches. Reg Anesth Pain Med 25:600–604

Pelz DM, Haddad RG (1989) Radiologic investigation of low back pain. Can Med Assoc J 140(3):289–295

Rasmussen MR, Kitaoka HB, Patzer GL (1996) Nonoperative treatment of plantar interdigital neuroma with a single corticosteroid injection. Clin Orthop 326:188–193

Retzl G, Kapral S, Greher M, Mauritz W (2001) Ultrasonographic findings of the axillary part of the brachial plexus. Anesth Analg 92:1271–1275

Riew KD, Yin Y, Gilula L, Bridwell KH, Lenke LG, Lauryssen C, Goette K (2000) The effect of nerve-root injections on the need for operative treatment of lumbar radicular pain. A prospective, randomized, controlled, double-blind study. J Bone Joint Surg Am 82-A(11):1589–1593

Sandhu NS, Maharlouei B, Patel B, Erkulwater E, Medabalmi P (2006a) Simultaneous bilateral infraclavicular brachial plexus blocks with low-dose lidocaine using ultrasound guidance. Anesthesiology 104:199–201

Sandhu NS, Manne JS, Medabalmi PK, Capan LM (2006b) Sonographically guided infraclavicular brachial plexus block in adults: a retrospective analysis of 1146 cases. J Ultrasound Med 25:1555–1561

Shives TC (1993) Biopsy of soft-tissue tumors. Clin Orthop Relat Res 289:32–35
Singh HK, Kilpatrick SE, Silverman JF (2004) Fine needle aspiration biopsy of soft tissue sarcomas: utility and diagnostic challenges. Adv Anat Pathol 11(1):24–37
Spinner RJ (2006) Outcomes for peripheral nerve entrapment syndromes. Clin Neurosurg 53:285–294
Tennent TD, Goddard NJ (1997) Carpal tunnel decompression: open vs endoscopic. Br J Hosp Med 58(11):551–554
Thomas AJ, Bull MJ, Howard AC, Saleh M (1999) Peri operative ultrasound guided needle localization of amputation stump neuroma. Injury 30:689–691
Thoumas D, Leroi AM, Mauillon J, Muller JM, Benozio M, Denis P, Freger IP (1999) Pudendal neuralgia: CT-guided pudendal nerve block technique. Abdom Imaging 24:309–312
Ting PL, Sivagnanaratnam V (1989) Ultrasonographic study of the spread of local anesthetic during axillary brachial plexus block. Br J Anaesth 63:326–329
Torriani M, Etchebehere M, Amstalden E (2002) Sonographically guided core needle biopsy of bone and soft tissue tumors. J Ultrasound Med 21(3):275–281
Tsukazaki T, Ito N, Maeda H, Iwasaki K (1993) Effect of phenol block on peripheral nerve: morphometric and histochemical study in rats [Japanese, abstract]. Nippon Seikeigeka Gakkai Zasshi 67:473–479
Tuominen M, Haasio J, Hekali R, Rosenberg PH (1989) Continuous interscalene brachial plexus block: clinical efficacy, technical problems and bupivacaine plasma concentrations. Acta Anaesthesiol Scand 33:84–88
Westerlund T, Vuorinen V, Röyttä M (2001) Same axonal regeneration rate after different endoneurial response to intraneural glycerol and phenol injection. Acta Neuropathol 102:41:54
Winnie AP (1993) Axillary perivascular technique of brachial plexus block. In: Winnie AP, Håkansson L (eds) Plexus anesthesia, vol 1, edn 3. WB Saunders, Philadelphia, pp 121–143
Winnie AP, Ramamurthy S, Durrani Z (1973) The inguinal perivascular technique of lumbar plexus anesthesia: the 3-in-1 block. Anesth Analg 52:989–996
Winnie AP, Radonjic R, Akkineni SR, Durrani Z (1979) Factors influencing distribution of local anesthetic injected into the brachial plexus sheath. Anesth Analg 58:225–234
Yang WT, Chui PT, Metreweli C (1998) Anatomy of the normal brachial plexus revealed by sonography and the role of sonographic guidance in anesthesia of the brachial plexus. AJR Am J Roentgenol 171:1631–1636

The Surgeon's Perspective

8

Hildegunde Piza-Katzer

CONTENTS

8.1 Anatomy of the Peripheral Nerve

Operative repair and reconstruction of damaged nerves presupposes a very clear knowledge of the gross anatomy of the peripheral nerve. Use of clearly defined terms is a prerequisite for understanding and precisely describing the pathophysiological sequelae and the morphological consequences of nerve injury.

8.1.1 Nerve Fiber

The basic structural unit of the peripheral nerve at the microscopic level is the nerve fiber which is responsible for conducting impulses to and from the peripheral organs. The nerve fiber has a complex structure. The central core is the axon which is enveloped in a complex covering of a single layer of linked Schwann cells – with and without a myelin component.

8.1.2 Fascicle

Nerve fibers are bundled together to form a fascicle which is a macroscopic unit of the peripheral nervous system. Endoneurial space refers to tissue spaces within the nerve fascicle. Each fascicle is surrounded by the perineurium. It has important barrier functions, protecting the fascicle from interfascicular tissue fluids and from infection.

H. Piza-Katzer, MD
Professor and Head, Department of Plastic and Reconstructive Surgery, Ludwig Boltzmann Institute for Quality Control in Plastic and Reconstructive Surgery, Innsbruck Medical University, Anichstrasse 35, 6020 Innsbruck, Austria

8.1.3
Nerve Trunk

Many fascicles are bundled together by the epineurium to form a nerve. There are monofascicular nerves composed of a single fascicle, and polyfascicular nerves composed of a few large fascicles or entirely of small fascicles of the same size or a combination of large and small fascicles. These anatomical details play a role in determining the severity of injury and in the choice of the appropriate method of surgical repair of nerve lesions.

There are three different types of nerve fibers – motor, sensory and sympathetic. Sensory and motor nerves contain both myelinated and unmyelinated nerve fibers. The postganglionic sympathetic nerves containing unmyelinated fibers innervate the skin, blood vessels and hair follicles.

8.1.4
Vascular Supply

Extensively interconnected microvascular systems ensure that the peripheral nerves are adequately vascularized. Intraneural microvessels extend longitudinally within the epineurium, with this system being reinforced by extrinsic segmental regional blood vessels. There are vascular plexi within the perineurium and within the fascicles. Intimate knowledge of the intraneural microvascular system is a precondition for microsurgical procedures on nerves.

8.2
Nerve Injury, Degeneration and Regeneration

Traumatic injury to a nerve might consist only of focal demyelination demonstrated by local conduction block. Regeneration in this case represents local myelin repair, resulting in restoration of excitability and conduction of nerve fibers.

Trauma that results in transection of the nerve fibers sets in motion several pathophysiological processes. There is focal demyelination at the site of injury, Wallerian degeneration distally and proximally (Waller 1850), and depending on the site of injury, cell body death (Kristensson 1981). The more proximal the injury, the greater is the danger of cell body death. When axons undergo damage, their transport functions – anterograde and retrograde – fail, causing structural and functional changes also in the nerve cell body (Gelbermann 1991), and, under certain conditions, death of the neuron. The process of regeneration consists in the surviving axons sprouting regenerating units proximally under the influence of neurotrophic factors (Varon and Adler 1989), and their establishing contact with the corresponding part of the distal nerve. This results in functional recovery (sensory, motor, sympathetic) to a greater or less extent. If the gap between the transected ends is large, the axon sprouts may fail to reach the distal stump, or they may be misdirected. In the former case, painful neuromas may develop and the peripheral target structures may suffer irreversible damage (Mumenthaler et al. 1998). In the latter case, incorrect reinnervation of targets will occur.

8.3
Classification of Nerve Injuries

8.3.1
Classification of Nerve Injuries According to Functional Loss and Severity

Sunderland (1951) classified nerve injuries into five types, according to the extent of damage that has occurred.

Neuropraxia is first degree injury; axonometsis consists of axon damage alone (second degree injury); axon severance with damage to endoneurial sheaths, but with intact perineurium and maintenance of fascicular continuity represents third degree injury; fourth degree injury comprises axonal severance with damage to the endoneurium and the perineurium; neurotmesis, the most severe form of injury with transected nerve trunk and complete loss of nerve continuity represents fifth degree injury.

Spontaneous and complete regeneration can occur after first and second degree injuries. Spontaneous recovery after third degree injury may also occur, but is mostly incomplete. The more proximal the injury, the poorer the prognosis since proximally, fascicles are mixed, and distally they comprise either motor or sensory fibers alone. Mismatch of regenerating fibers is possible in the former case and is not likely in the latter case. Spontaneous recovery cannot be expected in fourth degree injury where the perineurium is damaged. Fifth degree injuries involving complete severance of a nerve can only be managed surgically.

In sixth degree injury (Mackinnon and Dellon 1988), also called neuroma-in-continuity, all five or varying combinations of the five types of injuries mentioned above are present within one and the same nerve.

Nerve injuries are followed by temporary or long-lasting loss of sensory and motor function and in some cases by pain. The type of nerve injury will determine both the method of repair to be employed and the prognosis of recovery of motor and sensory functions and alleviation of pain symptoms after surgical repair.

8.3.2 Classification of Nerve Injuries According to Their Etiology

A nerve injury is defined as any damage caused to a nerve by a physical force applied externally or generated by a disturbed internal anatomical situation. Neuropathy refers to nerve lesions caused not by physical injury but by underlying systemic diseases, metabolic and toxic disturbances, and primary vascular disease. Causes of nerve injuries include:

- Compression – Compression trauma can occur with closed or open wounds.
- Acute compression can be caused by exogenous or endogenous forces (blow from a blunt object, tight bandages, tourniquet, splints and plaster casts, dislocated bone, etc. The severity of the injury can vary. Recovery should occur spontaneously and completely by six months after injury at the latest.
- Chronic compression develops slowly and can be progressive or intermittent. There are irregular remissions and exacerbations in the signs and symptoms associated with these lesions. The severity of the injury can progress from first degree to even fourth degree damage unless the nerve is decompressed.

Regardless of the cause of the pathology, the injured nerve fibers suffer progressive segmental demyelination, axon thinning and destruction of the axon with Wallerian degeneration.

8.3.2.1 Nerve Entrapment Lesions

Nerve entrapment lesions are mechanically caused nerve injuries. They develop in anatomical regions where a nerve runs through a confined space, and is fixed in some confined position because of adhesions. In compartment compression, the nerve is not fixed to any tissue, but suffers injury because of compression. The key pathogenetic factor in entrapment nerve lesions is local inflammatory reactions to repeated mechanical irritations.

Some classical examples of nerve compression injuries and entrapment in the upper extremity include: median and ulnar nerve at the wrist – carpal tunnel, Guyon's canal – ulnar and median nerve compression, and radial sensory nerve entrapment in the forearm, and ulnar nerve compression and radial nerve entrapment at the elbow.

8.3.2.1.1 Traction

Traction injury can be acute or chronic. In the former, an abruptly applied force causes destructive structural changes in a nerve and results in immediate loss of function. In the latter, a nerve is stretched gradually and symptoms of appear only after considerable deformation has taken place.

When a nerve has a short free-running course and is fixed at one or both ends, such as, for instance, the suprascapular nerve, the elastic limit of the nerve is rapidly exceeded when it is stretched. The axillary nerve, the median and ulnar nerves at the elbow joint and the common peroneal nerve at the knee joint are particularly vulnerable to traction injuries after joint dislocation.

8.3.2.2 Ischemic Lesions

These may result from compression, stretch or damage to the arteries supplying the nerve. The severity of the consequences of ischemia – disturbances in motor and sensory functions – will depend on the duration of ischemia and whether collateral circulation is available.

8.3.2.2.1 Complete Transection

Injuries resulting in loss of continuity of the nerve trunk can present in basically three different forms:

(1) clean severance; (2) severance with lacerated, crushed and contused nerve ends; (3) trauma causing destruction of a nerve segment, so that there is nerve defect that will have to be bridged. In each of these situations, the methods of nerve repair employed are distinctly different.

8.4 Surgical Nerve Repair and Reconstruction: Techniques

8.4.1 Nerve-0in-Continuity

8.4.1.1 Neurolysis

Scar tissue can cause compression, adhesion and thus loss of longitudinal mobility. When the expected spontaneous regeneration does not take place within the normal period of time (8–12 weeks) and the patient complains of pain, exploration is necessary.

In external neurolysis, a nerve is freed segment by segment by removing adhesions and by resection of constrictive scar tissue from around the nerve, taking care not to injure regional blood vessels. In epineuriotomy, the fibrotic superficial epineurium is opened under microscope to decompress the fascicles contained within it.

In epifascicular epineuriectomy, the thickened fibrotic tissue surrounding the nerve is totally or partially resected to free the nerve from compression.

Interfascicular epineuriectomy is performed in cases where deep layers and larger areas of the interfascicular epineurium are fibrotic.

However, internal neurolysis is rarely performed except where there is no alternative (Fig. 8.1a–h).

Removal of epineural scar tissue will damage the blood vessels that run on the surface of the superficial and in the deeper interfascicular epineurium and compromise blood supply to the nerve; additional scar tissue that develops during the healing process will again lead to nerve compression (Rydevik et al. 1976; Frykman et al. 1981; Lundborg 1988). The problem of ischemia can be avoided if at least a part of the longitudinal blood supply is maintained (Millesi 1992).

8.4.1.2 Mobilization

Nerves may need to be extensively mobilized so that they can be transposed to a new bed or for joining nerve ends with a wide gap between them in tensionless coaptation. Mobilization carries several risks such as destruction of the complex fascicular plexus and unintentional severance of nutrient vessels. All mobilization requires stripping of branches and sacrifice of some nutrient blood vessels. How much sacrifice is needed for mobilization and how much is permissible without causing additional lesions are issues that an experienced surgeon will have to decide case by case (Sunderland 1991).

8.4.1.3 Transposition

This is performed in cases where an injured nerve needs a new bed for regeneration after extensive injury to the original bed, to shorten the course of a nerve to enable joining the ends of a transected nerve or to protect a repaired nerve from undue tension.

8.4.2 Nerve Injury with Loss of Continuity

8.4.2.1 Coaptation

8.4.2.1.1 Epineural Repair

Depending on the type of nerve continuity loss, different methods of repair will have to be employed. If there is clean severance, and the nerve ends can be brought together without tension, primary repair with end-to-end coaptation can be performed using epineural suture. With this method, nerve trunk continuity is restored and if correct axial alignment of the nerve ends is established, fascicular continuity can be achieved.

8.4.2.1.2 Group Fascicular Repair

Epineural repair that unavoidably results in opposing fascicular tissue at one end of the nerve to interfascicular tissue at the other end may result in major loss of regenerating axons that get lost in

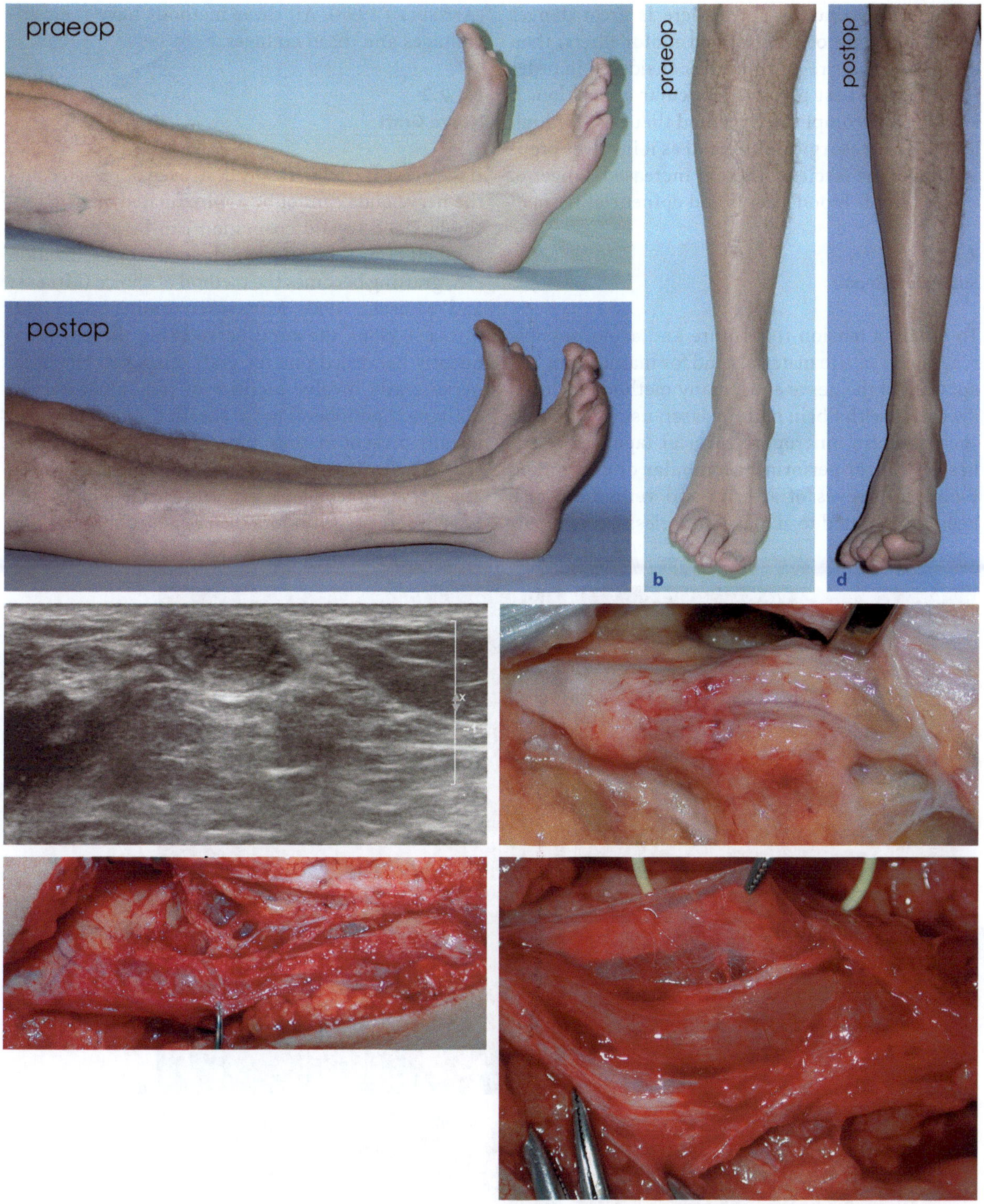

a c b d e f g h

Fig. 8.1a–h. A 43-year-old male patient after surgery performed elsewhere for removal of peroneal nerve cyst. **a,b** Condition before revision surgery – foot and toe extensor muscle weakness. **c,d** Condition 4 years after revision surgery – marked improvement in foot and toe extensor muscle weakness. **e** Longitudinal sonogram: suspicion of endoneural neuroma. **f** Intraoperative view of exploration of the peroneal nerve at the popliteal cavity and proximal lower leg – nerve enveloped by scar tissue. **g** Marked compression of the peroneal nerve, neurolysis, intraneural cysts. **h** After epineurotomy and partial epineurectomy and intraneural preparation of single fascicle groups, in the cranial part, expelled fascicle caused by cystic alterations remains the interfascicular tissue. If there is great danger of mismatching of sensory and motor fibers, then group fascicular repair must be considered in order to obtain the best possible fascicular apposition. It is a long and complicated method that calls for high levels of microsurgical skills and as it involves preparation of the fascicles, there is increased danger of trauma to the blood vessels and epineurial tissue.

8.4.2.1.3 Sutureless Repair

To obtain a tension-free suture and avoid possible reaction to suture materials and for maintaining coaptation of the nerve ends, many methods are used – welding with fibrin glue, by laser, using adhesives such as fibrin, micropore surgical tape, tissue adhesives etc., or performing a tubular or cuff union. Biological sleeves of arteries and veins have also been investigated to achieve sutureless nerve repair (Ansselin 1998). All these methods have their advantages and disadvantages.

8.4.2.2 Nerve Graft

If the nerve is traumatically destroyed or resected and the nerve ends cannot be approximated and no tensionless end-to-end coaptation can be achieved despite all efforts to gain length such as mobilization etc., grafting becomes the method of choice (Millesi and Meissel 1981; Miyamoto and Tsuge 1981; Millesi 1986), the sural nerve being the most frequently harvested one for graft purposes. However, nerve grafts involve sacrifice of functional nerves. Malignant peripheral nerve sheath tumors (MPNST) usually present in close proximity of a nerve trunk (Fig. 8.2a–j). The most common sites include the sciatic nerve, brachial plexus, and sacral plexus – or benign soft tissue tumors such as neurofibromas and

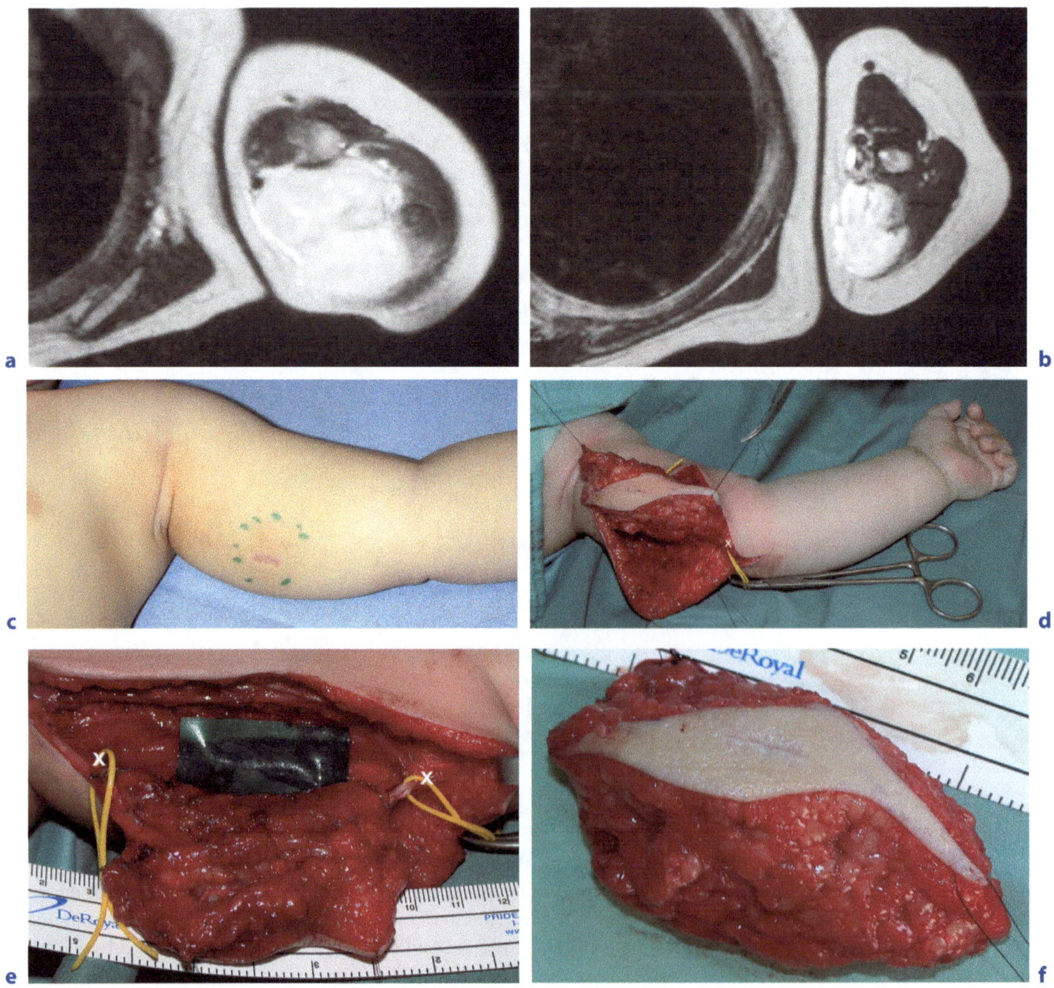

▷▷

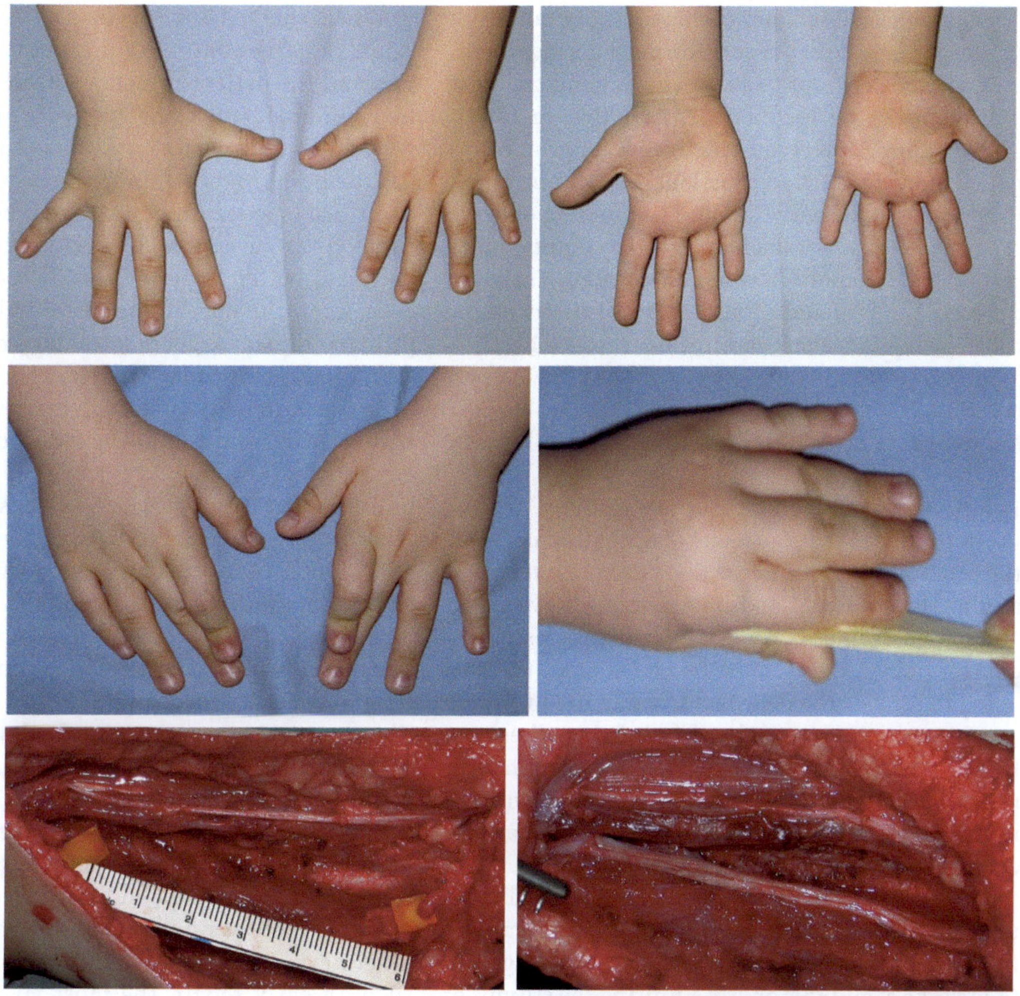

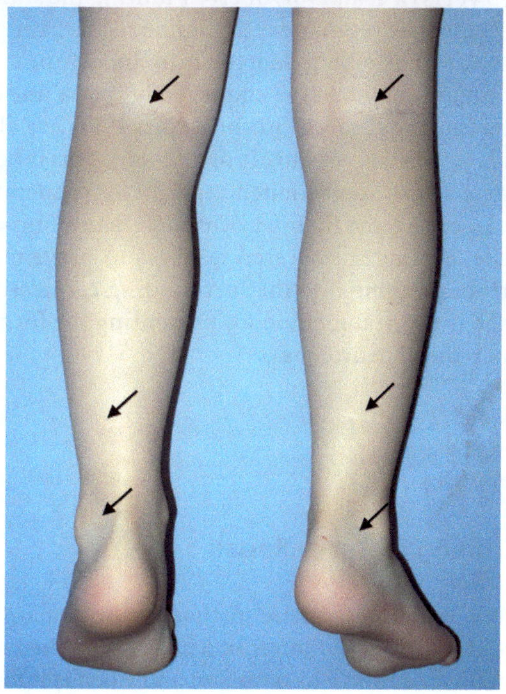

Fig. 8.2a–j. A 9-month-old male patient. **a** Infantile fibrosarcoma, left upper arm – CT. **b** After preoperative therapy consisting of four cycles according to protocol CWS 96, marked volume reduction in tumor mass – control CT. **c** After biopsy and chemotherapy. **d** Operation including removal of a skin spindle – radical tumor resection. **e** The ulnar nerve runs through the tumor and has to be resected along with the tumor. **f** Resection specimen. **g** Intraoperative – 7-cm long defect of the ulnar nerve (nerve ends beneath a sheath). **h** Reconstruction with 4×7-cm long sural nerve transplant. **i** Scars on both lower legs after harvest of the sural nerves. **j** At 3 years post surgery – no limitations in mobility of the left hand, the child uses his hand during play normally

schwannomas. Resections of these tumors can result in a large nerve defect. A surgeon must decide whether a nerve defect represents a serious handicap or is a disability with which a patient can live; re-educational training and reconstructive surgery can help a patient adjust to certain functional loss, for instance, irreparable radial nerve lesion. The function of nerve repair is not just to establish nerve continuity but to restore lost functions (Sunderland 1991). There are different kinds of nerve grafts such as full thickness, cable, group fascicular and free neurovascular.

8.4.2.2.1 Neuromas

Painful neuromas can develop on an injured nerve in continuity, at the suture site of a repaired nerve, at the proximal end of a nerve that cannot be repaired and at the proximal end of a severed nerve in an amputated stump. If conservative measures fail to control pain, surgery must be considered, the aim being to remove the neuroma from an area where it is subject to pressure and to free it from adhesions. However, timing of resection is crucial. Premature resection might result in further suture site neuromas that may be even more troublesome than the original one.

One way to deal with neuromas would be to disregulate or prevent such regeneration. However, all the methods currently available such as fascicle ligation (Battista et al. 1981) or cross-uniting the stumps of severed nerves in order to confine regenerating axon to the anastomotic loop (Wood and Mudge 1987), implanting the nerve end directly into a muscle after cutting it short (Sunderland 1991) are all only about 80% successful (Tupper 1986). This is because axons have an unlimited capacity to regenerate and can even force their way through dense fibrous tissue. Sealing the severed fascicles to prevent axons from escaping into the surrounding connective tissue is the best method for preventing the formation of painful neuromas.

8.5 Timing of Nerve Repair

When are conservative methods to be employed and when is surgical intervention indicated? When is it too soon for surgical intervention and when is it too late?

When a nerve has been cleanly severed, and there is loss of nerve continuity without loss of nerve tissue, and the patient presents within a few hours of injury, immediate primary repair is advisable for reestablishing continuity. Although primary repair has the best prognosis under the wound conditions described above, unless skilled and experienced surgeons are available for performing primary repair, it is better to perform early secondary repair even when the conditions of wound would justify primary repair. A good secondary repair is better than inefficient primary repair.

In blunt injuries involving massive tissue damage, bleeding and contaminated wounds with danger of infection, primary nerve repair should not be attempted. It may take 3–4 weeks before the extent of nerve damage can be ascertained (Zachary et al. 1987). In most trauma surgery units, often a skilled surgeon specialized in the microsurgical techniques of nerve repair may not be available and, quite simply, the necessary operative conditions for optimal nerve surgery are often fulfilled. The negative consequences of delay can probably be reduced by a so-called delayed primary repair for establishing nerve continuity (Millesi 1992) – this means wound closure on the day of injury and then a few days later, under optimal institutional and personnel conditions, reopening of the wound which has not yet healed, in order to perform nerve repair. If the wound does not permit such an early repair, the most favorable time for repair is 3–5 weeks after injury.

Closed injuries require different timing of repair. The patient is monitored over a period of 3 months. If at the end of this period, there are some clinical signs of recovery or some electrical evidence of regeneration, then it would be worth waiting for complete recovery to take place, while monitoring the patient carefully. If, however, after a 3-month waiting period, no signs of recovery are present, the nerve needs to be surgically explored.

The maximum tolerated interval between injury and recovery of function depends on whether the loss involved is motor or sensory. This can vary depending on the muscles involved. The smaller intrinsic muscles in the hand must be innervated even sooner than that in order to reinstate motor function. But the time interval between injury and repair should never exceed 4–5 months. The time limits on sensory return are different from those of motor; return of sensation can be achieved many years after repair of injury to the nerve.

The situation is different when the closed nerve injury is in an area which has a known predilection for compression of nerves. In such cases, it is recommended that surgery be performed immediately in order to decompress the nerve. For instance, in a patient presenting with traumatic injury to the hand or forearm associated with deficits in sensory and motor functions, one should suspect an acute carpal tunnel syndrome and immediate decompression of the nerve involved should be performed.

8.6 Prognosis

The success of nerve repair depends on a large number of factors that have to do with the kind of nerve injured (monofascicular, polyfascicular), the level of injury, the kind and severity of injury, factors operating at and below the site of repair, the time between injury and repair, the skill of the surgeon carrying out the microsurgical procedures and the techniques employed, to name just a few (Lundborg 2000). One extremely critical factor is that of timing. The longer a nerve injury is left untreated, the greater are the chances of endoneurial tube atrophy, fascicular shrinkage and intrafascicular fibrosis, end organ atrophy because of denervation and consequently the poorer is the chance of recovery of function.

Generally speaking, the more proximal the lesion, the poorer is the prognosis. Age is also a relevant factor. Better recovery can be achieved in younger than in older patients, and the very young have a decided advantage.

Post-operative procedures also contribute significantly to recovery. Training and practice do contribute to improvement of motor performance and the sharpening of sensory perceptions. Even if nerve repair is followed by residual sensory and motor deficits, it should be kept in mind that with training (for instance, with sensory reeducation consisting of desensitization, early phase discrimination and localization and late phase discrimination and tactile gnosis), a patient can be helped to learn to deal with new and altered patterns of innervation (Lundborg and Rosen 2001). The role of cortical plasticity in regaining function after nerve injury should not be underestimated (Lundborg 2000, 2003).

Furthermore, the condition of the patient is important – whether he is a smoker, an alcoholic or has underlying systemic diseases etc. are factors that will affect the final results of nerve repair.

8.7 Iatrogenic Nerve Injuries

Iatrogenic nerve injuries are lesions caused to the central or peripheral nervous system during simple or complex surgical procedures performed for diagnostic or therapeutic purposes.

It is estimated that nearly 10% of all peripheral nerve lesions are iatrogenic in character. One can distinguish between direct and indirect injuries.

Direct injuries are, for example, severance of a nerve, injury caused by fixing screws, nails, traction caused during coaptation of nerves, puncture of a nerve during an injection etc. (Piza-Katzer et al 1994, 1995).

Some examples of indirect injuries are those caused by postoperative hematomas, scar tissue resulting in nerve compression (Fig. 8.3a–h), or ischemic injuries to the nerve caused by blood vessel damage or compression caused by malpositioning of a patient during surgery.

The clinical symptoms of injuries depend on the kind of nerve fibers affected.

Loss of sensation (for example, of position, vibration, temperature, surface sensibility) after injury occurs to sensory fibers, muscle weakness and loss of motor function after injury to motor fibers. Reflex sympathetic dystrophy and pain can also occur. Clinical assessment of peripheral nerve lesions consists in determining the severity and cause of lesions, interval between injury and diagnosis and also functional significance of the affected nerves.

As a result of an information campaign addressed to our professional colleagues who are responsible for referring patients to us regarding possibilities of surgical revision after nerve lesions, we have seen and treated an increasing number of iatrogenic nerve lesions. Patients were referred to us by surgeons (33%), by GPs (30%), by neurologists (13%) and by other specialists (13%). We have no information on 9% of cases, and 2% were referred to us by the pain clinic. Over a period of 3 years, we repaired seven lesions in the face and neck region (three facial nerves and four cases of the accessory nerve lesion).

In the upper extremity, 44 lesions were repaired: one brachial plexus injury, one musculocutaneous

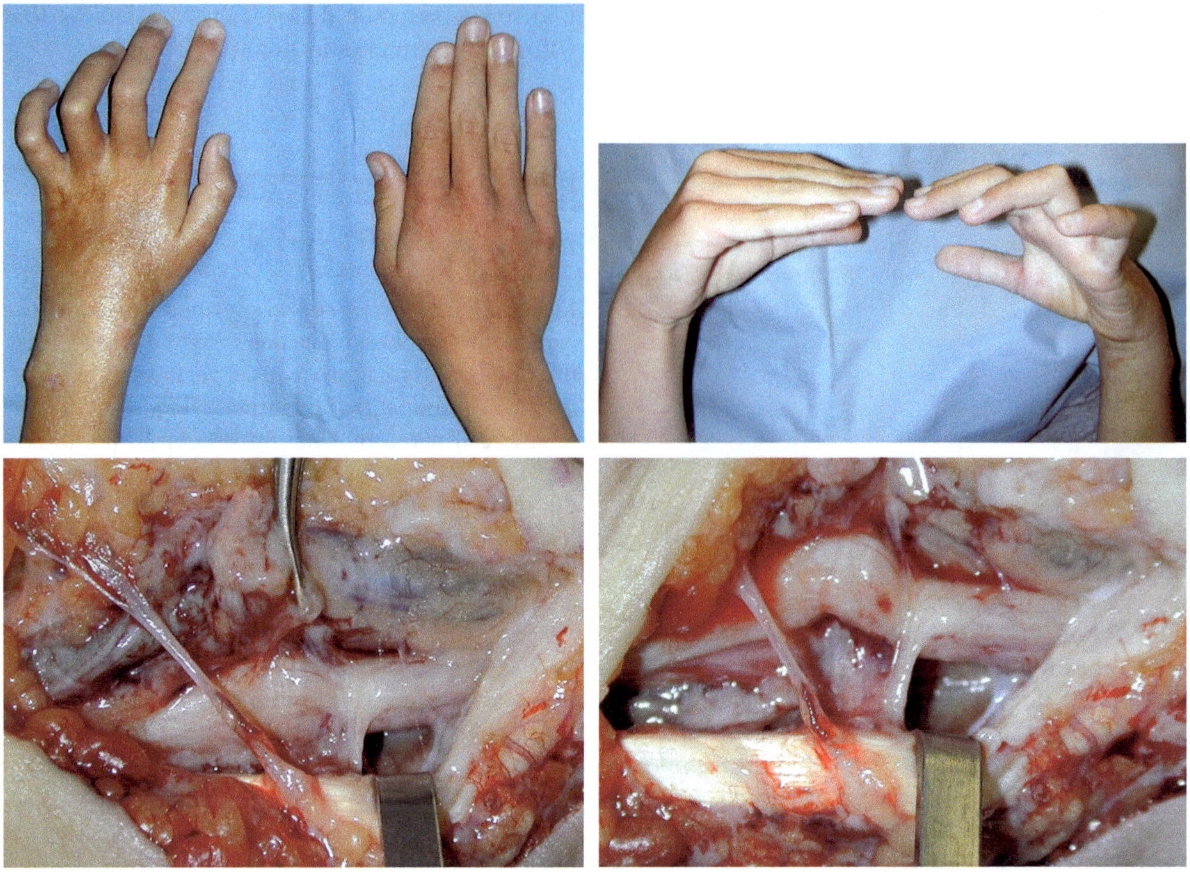

a b c d

Fig. 8.3a–h. A 12-year-old male patient. Fall during excursion – distal forearm fracture left – closed repositioning and plaster cast; 3 days after the accident, K-wire fixation of the distal radius and ulna. **a,b** At 4 weeks after the accident, massive ulnar paresis with atrophy of intrinsic muscles of the entire hand, loss of sensibility in digits IV, V; EMG shows complete conduction block with acute denervation. No evidence of reinnervation. **c** At 12 weeks after the accident – surgical release of the ulnar nerve at the distal forearm –debridement of scar tissue compressing the ulnar nerve (the adhesive band had developed along the path of the K wire). **d** Compression of the ulnar nerve by the scar. **e** After removal of the adhesive band and external neurolysis and epineurotomy of the ulnar nerve. **f–h** Control 1 year after neurolysis of the ulnar nerve; very good regeneration of sensibility and motor function. Gross grip right 29 – left 23 kg, key grip right 6.5 – left 5.6 kg, pinch grip I/II right 3.6 – left 3.5 kg, 90° flexion in the MP joints, powerful finger abduction and adduction

nerve lesion, four radial, 18 ulnar, 17 median and three finger nerve injuries.

In the lower extremity, 45 nerve lesions were repaired: two cutaneous femoral, 13 femoral, six sciatic, nine tibial, 13 peroneal, and two sural nerve lesions.

We used the following treatment methods: in 50 cases, neurolysis was performed, in six cases epineurotomy, in two cases epineurectomy, in two cases intraneural neurolysis, in three cases direct nerve coaptation, in 23 cases nerve transplantation and neurotisation in three cases. Neuromas were resected in nine cases and five cases were treated conservatively.

Surgeons must keep in mind the possibility of iatrogenic nerve injuries in their patients. Although avoiding them is the best policy, the next best is to recognise them by adequate follow-up care and take prompt steps to get them treated by colleagues with special training in nerve repair procedures. Failure to do so may result in irreversible damage to patients.

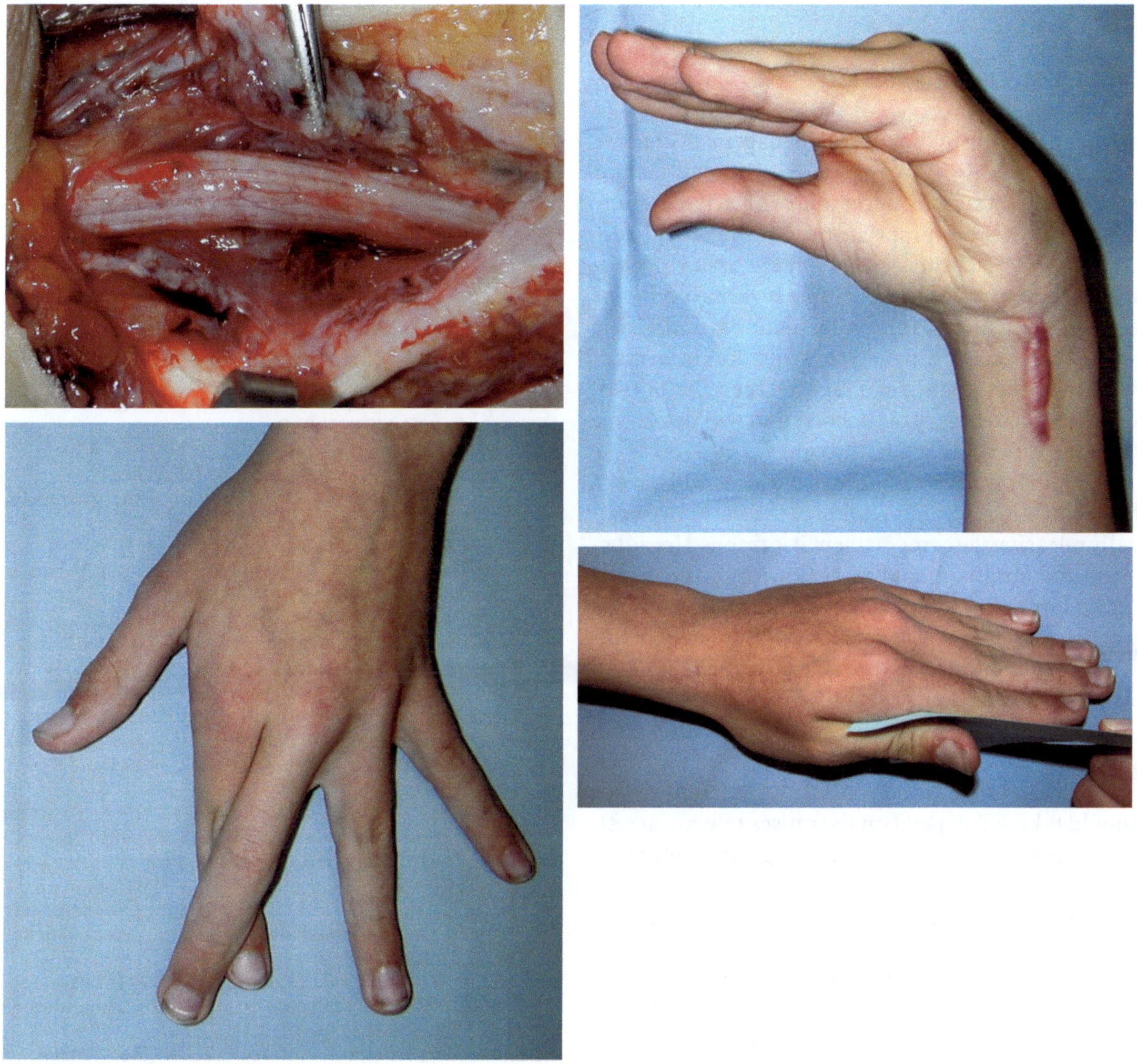

e f g h

8.8 Future Directions in Peripheral Nerve Surgery

Successful nerve repair is based on how issues of proper axial alignment and fascicular approximation are resolved. Atraumatic surgical techniques currently offer the only method to keep scarring to the minimum. Several in vitro experiments have shown that survival of nerve cells and axon growth depend on biomolecules such as nerve growth factor, fibroblast growth factor (Morrison et al. 1986) etc., which are produced by peripheral target cells and transmitted via the retrograde axonal transport along the axon to the nerve cell body and exert a trophic influence on them (Hansson et al. 1986). Promotion and acceleration of nerve regeneration and selective reinnervation after injury might be achieved by altering the microenvironment with the help of various neurotrophic factors administered in the region between the nerve stumps. Gene therapy holds out the promise of delivering a gene together with its necessary regulatory elements to the cell surface, using a vector to mediate the transfer across cell membrane and in some cases into the nuclei. This might prove to be useful in stimulating the growth of adult nerve cells. Thus, despite the remarkable advances in peripheral nerve repair made in the past five decades, several problems remain to be addressed in the future.

8.9 Summary and Conclusion

Decision making in the clinical management of nerve injury and repair is a complex and difficult task. A patient presenting with nerve injury must be carefully investigated with appropriate methods in order to determine the exact site, accompanying tissue involvement, the nerve affected, cause, severity and time elapsed since injury, prior interventions, underlying systemic diseases if any, and consequences in terms of functional disturbance of injury. All these factors will play a role in recovery of function and will determine the surgeon's approach to the case.

A compartment entrapment syndrome will have to be dealt with by decompression of the nerve by surgically releasing the compartment it is trapped in, adhesions and fibrosis should be dealt with by the appropriate form of neurolysis etc. Complex nerve lesions where different fascicles have suffered injuries of different grades of severity present a great challenge to even the most experienced and skilled surgeon.

Where there is no evidence of recovery after a period of 3 months following injury, the need for surgical intervention must be considered. What form this should take will depend on the causes that are arresting or preventing recovery and regeneration. Since every such intervention represents additional trauma and causes scar tissue, surgery should be an option only when no spontaneous regeneration can be expected. Furthermore, the longer the period of denervation of end organs and distal receptors, the less complete will be the recovery. Surgical nerve repair is an extremely demanding and skillful task – it should be undertaken only by a surgeon with deep knowledge of the complex and often variable anatomy of the peripheral nervous system, special training in microsurgical techniques and extensive experience.

References

Ansselin AD, Fink T, Davey DF (1998) An alternative to nerve grafts in peripheral nerve repair: nerve guides seeded with adult Schwann cells. ACA 30 [Suppl 147]:19–124

Battista AF, Cravioto HM, Budzilovich GN (1981) Painful neuroma: changes produced in peripheral nerve after fascicle ligation. Neurosurgery 9:589

Frykman GK, Adams J, Bowen WW (1981) Neurolysis. Orthop Clin North Am 12:325

Gelbermann RH (1991) Operative nerve repair and reconstruction, vol. 1. J.B. Lippincott Company, Philedelphia

Hansson HA, Dahlin LB, Danielsen N et al. (1986) Evidence indicating trophic importance of IGF-1 in regenerating peripheral nerves. Acta Physiol Scand 126:609–614

Kristensson K (1981) Retrograde signalling of nerve cell body response to trauma. In: Gorio A, Millesi H, Mingrino S (eds)Posttraumatic peripheral nerve regeneration. Raven Press, New York, pp 27–34

Lundborg G (1988) Nerve injury and repair. Churchill Livingstone, Edinburg, p 105

Lundborg G (2000) A 25-year perspective of peripheral nerve surgery: evolving neuroscientific concepts and clinical significance. J Hand Surg 25A:391–414

Lundborg G (2000) Brain plasticity and hand surgery: an overview. J Hand Surg 25B:2422–2252

Lundborg G, Rosen B (2001) Sensory relearning after nerve repair. Lancet 358:809–810

Lundborg G (2003) Nerve injury and repair – a challenge to the plastic brain. J Periph Nerv Sys 8:209–226

Mackinnon SE, Dellon AL (1988) Surgery of the peripheral nerve. Thieme Medical Publishers, New York

Millesi H (1986) The nerve gap. Hand Clin 2:651–663

Millesi H (1992) Chirurgie der peripheren Nerven. Urban & Schwarzenberg, München

Millesi H, Meissel G (1981) Consequences of tension at the suture line. In: Gorio A, Millesi H, Mingrino S (eds) Posttraumatic peripheral nerve regeneration. Raven Press, New York, p 277

Miyamoto Y, Tsuge K (1981) Grafting vs end-to-end coaptation of nerves. In: Gorio A, Millesi H, Mingrino S (eds) Posttraumatic peripheral nerve regeneration. Raven Press, New York, p 351

Morrison RS, Sharma A, de Vellis J et al. (1986) Basic fibroblast growth factor supports the survival of cerebral cortical neurons in primary culture. Proc Natl Acad Sci USA 83:7537–7541

Mumenthaler M, Schliack H, Stöhr M (1998) Läsionen peripherer Nerven und radikuläre Syndrome. Georg Thieme Verlag, Stuttgart

Piza-Katzer H, Herczeg E, Balogh B et al. (1994) Intra- und postoperative Nervenläsionen und ihre Behandlung. Nervenarzt 65:375–380

Piza-Katzer H, Balogh B, Herczeg E et al. (1995) Iatrogene Nervenläsionen und ihre mikrochirurgische Behandlung. Chirurg 66:1146–1153

Rydevik B, Lundborg G, Nordborg C (1976) Intraneural tissue reactions induced by internal neurolysis. Scan J Plast Reconstr Surg 10:3

Sunderland S (1951) A classification of peripheral nerve injuries producing loss of function. Brain 74:491

Sunderland S (1991) Nerve injuries and their repair: a critical appraisal. Churchill Livingstone, New York

Tupper JW (1986) Discussion of paper by Dellon AL and Mackinnon SE, 1986. J Plas Reconstr Surg 77:437

Varon S, Adler R (1989) Nerve growth factors and control of nerve growth. Curr Top Dev Biol 16: 207–252

Waller AV (1850) Experiments on the glossopharyngeal and hypoglossal nerves of the frog and observations produced thereby in the structure of their primitive fibers. Phil Trans R Soc Lond 140:423

Wood VE, Mudge MK (1987) Treatment of neuromas about a major amputation stump. J Hand Surg 12A:302

Zachary LS, Dellon AL, Seiler WA (1987) Relationship of intraneural damage in the rat sciatic nerve to the method of injury. Microsurgery 8:182–185

Subject Index

A

B

C

E

F

G

R

S

T

U

W

X

List of Contributors

GERD BODNER, MD
Professor, Department of Radiology
St. Bernards Hospital
Europort 1–4
Gibraltar

Email: Gerd.Bodner@gha.gi

HANNES GRUBER, MD
Associate Professor, Department of Radiology
Innsbruck Medical University
Anichstrasse 35
6020 Innsbruck
Austria

Email: hannes.gruber@uibk.ac.at

STEFAN KIECHL, MD
Professor, Department of Neurology
Section for Electrodiagnosis (EMG/NLG)
Innsbruck Medical University
Anichstrasse 35
6020 Innsbruck
Austria

Email: Stefan.Kiechl@uibk.ac.at

PETER KOVACS, MD
Department of Radiology
Innsbruck Medical University
Anichstrasse 35
6020 Innsbruck
Austria

Email: peter.kovacs@uibk.ac.at

SIEGRIED PEER, MD
Professor, Department of Radiology
Section for Diagnostic and
Interventional Sonography
Innsbruck Medical University
Anichstrasse 35
6020 Innsbruck
Austria

Email: siegfried.peer@i-med.ac.at

HILDEGUNDE PIZA-KATZER, MD
Professor, Department of Plastic and
Reconstructive Surgery
Ludwig Boltzmann Institute for Quality Control
in Plastic
and
Reconstructive Surgery
Innsbruck Medical University
Anichstrasse 35
6020 Innsbruck
Austria

Email: hildegunde.piza@uibk.ac.at

Medical Radiology Diagnostic Imaging and Radiation Oncology

Titles in the series already published

Diagnostic Imaging

Innovations in Diagnostic Imaging
Edited by J. H. Anderson

Radiology of the Upper Urinary Tract
Edited by Erich K. Lang

The Thymus - Diagnostic Imaging, Functions, and Pathologic Anatomy
Edited by E. Walter, E. Willich, and W. R. Webb

Interventional Neuroradiology
Edited by A. Valavanis

Radiology of the Pancreas
Edited by A. L. Baert. Co-edited by G. Delorme

Radiology of the Lower Urinary Tract
Edited by Erich K. Lang

Magnetic Resonance Angiography
Edited by I. P. Arlart, G. M. Bongartz, and G. Marchal

Contrast-Enhanced MRI of the Breast
S. Heywang-Köbrunner and R. Beck

Spiral CT of the Chest
Edited by M. Rémy-Jardin and J. Rémy

Radiological Diagnosis of Breast Diseases
Edited by M. Friedrich and E. A. Sickles

Radiology of Trauma
Edited by M. Heller and A. Fink

Biliary Tract Radiology
Edited by P. Rossi. Co-edited by M. Brezi

Radiological Imaging of Sports Injuries
Edited by C. Masciocchi

Modern Imaging of the Alimentary Tube
Edited by A. R. Margulis

Diagnosis and Therapy of Spinal Tumors
Edited by P. R. Algra, J. Valk, and J. J. Heimans

Interventional Magnetic Resonance Imaging
Edited by J. F. Debatin and G. Adam

Abdominal and Pelvic MRI
Edited by A. Heuck and M. Reiser

Orthopedic Imaging
Techniques and Applications
Edited by A. M. Davies and H. Pettersson

Radiology of the Female Pelvic Organs
Edited by E. K. Lang

Magnetic Resonance of the Heart and Great Vessels
Clinical Applications
Edited by J. Bogaert, A. J. Duerinckx, and F. E. Rademakers

Modern Head and Neck Imaging
Edited by S. K. Mukherji and J. A. Castelijns

Radiological Imaging of Endocrine Diseases
Edited by J. N. Bruneton in collaboration with B. Padovani and M.-Y. Mourou

Radiology of the Pancreas
2nd Revised Edition
Edited by A. L. Baert. Co-edited by G. Delorme and L. Van Hoe

Trends in Contrast Media
Edited by H. S. Thomsen, R. N. Muller, and R. F. Mattrey

Functional MRI
Edited by C. T. W. Moonen and P. A. Bandettini

Emergency Pediatric Radiology
Edited by H. Carty

Liver Malignancies
Diagnostic and Interventional Radiology
Edited by C. Bartolozzi and R. Lencioni

Spiral CT of the Abdomen
Edited by F. Terrier, M. Grossholz, and C. D. Becker

Medical Imaging of the Spleen
Edited by A. M. De Schepper and F. Vanhoenacker

Radiology of Peripheral Vascular Diseases
Edited by E. Zeitler

Diagnostic Nuclear Medicine
Edited by C. Schiepers

Radiology of Blunt Trauma of the Chest
P. Schnyder and M. Wintermark

Portal Hypertension
Diagnostic Imaging and Imaging-Guided Therapy
Edited by P. Rossi. Co-edited by P. Ricci and L. Broglia

Virtual Endoscopy and Related 3D Techniques
Edited by P. Rogalla, J. Terwisscha van Scheltinga, and B. Hamm

Recent Advances in Diagnostic Neuroradiology
Edited by Ph. Demaerel

Multislice CT
Edited by M. F. Reiser, M. Takahashi, M. Modic, and R. Bruening

Pediatric Uroradiology
Edited by R. Fotter

Transfontanellar Doppler Imaging in Neonates
A. Couture and C. Veyrac

Radiology of AIDS
A Practical Approach
Edited by J. W. A. J. Reeders and P. C. Goodman

CT of the Peritoneum
Armando Rossi and Giorgio Rossi

Magnetic Resonance Angiography
2nd Revised Edition
Edited by I. P. Arlart, G. M. Bongartz, and G. Marchal

Pediatric Chest Imaging
Chest imaging in Infants and Children
Edited by Javier Lucaya and Janet L. Strife

Applications of Sonography in Head and Neck Pathology
Edited by J. N. Bruneton in collaboration with C. Raffaelli and O. Dassonville

3D Image Processing
Techniques and Clinical Applications
Edited by D. Caramella and C. Bartolozzi

Imaging of the Larynx
Edited by R. Hermans

Pediatric ENT Radiology
Edited by S. J. King and A. E. Boothroyd

Imaging of Orbital and Visual Pathway Pathology
Edited by W. S. Müller-Forell

Radiological Imaging of the Small Intestine
Edited by N. C. Gourtsoyiannis

Imaging of the Knee
Techniques and Applications
Edited by A. M. Davies and V. N. Cassar-Pullicino

Perinatal Imaging
From Ultrasound to MR Imaging
Edited by Fred E. Avni

Radiological Imaging of the Neonatal Chest
Edited by V. Donoghue

Diagnostic and Interventional Radiology in Liver Transplantation
Edited by E. Bücheler, V. Nicolas, C. E. Broelsch, X. Rogiers, and G. Krupski

Radiology of Osteoporosis
Edited by S. Grampp

Imaging Pelvic Floor Disorders
Edited by C. I. Bartram and J. O. L. DeLancey
Associate Editors: S. Halligan, F. M. Kelvin, and J. Stoker

High-Resolution Sonography of the Peripheral Nervous System
Edited by S. Peer and G. Bodner

Imaging of the Pancreas
Cystic and Rare Tumors
Edited by C. Procacci and A. J. Megibow

Imaging of the Foot & Ankle
Techniques and Applications
Edited by A. M. Davies, R. W. Whitehouse, and J. P. R. Jenkins

Radiological Imaging of the Ureter
Edited by F. Joffre, Ph. Otal, and M. Soulie

Radiology of the Petrous Bone
Edited by M. Lemmerling and S. S. Kollias

Imaging of the Shoulder
Techniques and Applications
Edited by A. M. Davies and J. Hodler

Interventional Radiology in Cancer
Edited by A. Adam, R. F. Dondelinger, and P. R. Mueller

Imaging and Intervention in Abdominal Trauma
Edited by R. F. Dondelinger

Radiology of the Pharynx and the Esophagus
Edited by O. Ekberg

Radiological Imaging in Hematological Malignancies
Edited by A. Guermazi

Functional Imaging of the Chest
Edited by H.-U. Kauczor

Duplex and Color Doppler Imaging of the Venous System
Edited by G. H. Mostbeck

Multidetector-Row CT of the Thorax
Edited by U. J. Schoepf

Multislice CT
2nd Revised Edition
Edited by M. F. Reiser, M. Takahashi, M. Modic, and C. R. Becker

Radiology and Imaging of the Colon
Edited by A. H. Chapman

Intracranial Vascular Malformations and Aneurysms
From Diagnostic Work-Up to Endovascular Therapy
Edited by M. Forsting

Coronary Radiology
Edited by Matthijs Oudkerk

Multidetector-Row CT Angiography
Edited by C. Catalano and R. Passariello

Focal Liver Lesions
Detection, Characterization, Ablation
Edited by R. Lencioni, D. Cioni, and C. Bartolozzi

Imaging in Treatment Planning for Sinonasal Diseases
Edited by R. Maroldi and P. Nicolai

Clinical Cardiac MRI
With Interactive CD-ROM
Edited by J. Bogaert, S. Dymarkowski, and A. M. Taylor

Dynamic Contrast-Enhanced Magnetic Resonance Imaging in Oncology
Edited by A. Jackson, D. L. Buckley, and G. J. M. Parker

Contrast Media in Ultrasonography
Basic Principles and Clinical Applications
Edited by Emilio Quaia

Paediatric Musculoskeletal Disease
With an Emphasis on Ultrasound
Edited by D. Wilson

MR Imaging in White Matter Diseases of the Brain and Spinal Cord
Edited by M. Filippi, N. De Stefano, V. Dousset, and J. C. McGowan

Imaging of the Hip & Bony Pelvis
Techniques and Applications
Edited by A. M. Davies, K. Johnson, and R. W. Whitehouse

Imaging of Kidney Cancer
Edited by Ali Guermazi

Magnetic Resonance Imaging in Ischemic Stroke
Edited by R. von Kummer and T. Back

Diagnostic Nuclear Medicine
2nd Revised Edition
Edited by Christiaan Schiepers

Imaging of Occupational and Environmental Disorders of the Chest
Edited by P. A. Gevenois and P. De Vuyst

Virtual Colonoscopy
A Practical Guide
Edited by P. Lefere and S. Gryspeerdt

Contrast Media
Safety Issues and ESUR Guidelines
Edited by H. S. Thomsen

Head and Neck Cancer Imaging
Edited by R. Hermans

Vascular Embolotherapy
A Comprehensive Approach
Volume 1: *General Principles, Chest, Abdomen, and Great Vessels*
Edited by J. Golzarian. Co-edited by S. Sun and M. J. Sharafuddin

Vascular Embolotherapy
A Comprehensive Approach
Volume 2: *Oncology, Trauma, Gene Therapy, Vascular Malformations, and Neck*
Edited by J. Golzarian. Co-edited by S. Sun and M. J. Sharafuddin

Vascular Interventional Radiology
Current Evidence in Endovascular Surgery
Edited by M. G. Cowling

Ultrasound of the Gastrointestinal Tract
Edited by G. Maconi and G. Bianchi Porro

Parallel Imaging in Clinical MR Applications
Edited by S. O. Schoenberg, O. Dietrich, and M. F. Reiser

MRI and CT of the Female Pelvis
Edited by B. Hamm and R. Forstner

Imaging of Orthopedic Sports Injuries
Edited by F. M. Vanhoenacker, M. Maas, J. L. Gielen

Ultrasound of the Musculoskeletal System
S. Bianchi and C. Martinoli

Clinical Functional MRI
Presurgical Functional Neuroimaging
Edited bei C. Stippich

Radiation Dose from Adult and Pediatric Multidetector Computed Tomography
Edited by D. Tack and P. A. Gevenois

Spinal Imaging
Diagnostic Imaging of the Spine and Spinal Cord
Edited by J. Van Goethem, L. van den Hauwe, and P. M. Parizel

Computed Tomography of the Lung
A Pattern Approach
J. A. Verschakelen and W. De Wever

Imaging in Transplantation
Edited by A. Bankier

Radiological Imaging of the Neonatal Chest
2nd Revised Edition
Edited by V. Donoghue

Radiological Imaging of the Digestive Tract in Infants and Children
Edited by A. S. Devos and J. G. Blickman

Pediatric Chest Imaging
Chest Imaging in Infants and Children
2nd Revised Edition
Edited by J. Lucaya and J. L. Strife

Color Doppler US of the Penis
Edited by M. Bertolotto

Radiology of the Stomach and Duodenum
Edited by A. H. Freeman and E. Sala

Imaging in Pediatric Skeletal Trauma
Techniques and Applications
Edited by K. J. Johnson and E. Bache

Image Processing in Radiology
Current Applications
Edited by E. Neri, D. Caramella, and C. Bartolozzi

Screening and Preventive Diagnosis with Radiological Imaging
Edited by M. F. Reiser, G. van Kaick, C. Fink, and S. O. Schoenberg

Percutaneous Tumor Ablation in Medical Radiology
Edited by T. J. Vogl, T. K. Helmberger, M. G. Mack, and M. F. Reiser

Liver Radioembolization with ^{90}Y Microspheres
Edited by J. I. Bilbao and M. F. Reiser

Pediatric Uroradiology
2nd Revised Edition
Edited by R. Fotter

Radiology of Osteoporosis
2nd Revised Edition
Edited by S. Grampp

Gastrointestinal Tract Sonography in Fetuses and Children
A. Couture, C. Baud, J. L. Ferran, M. Saguintaah, and C. Veyrac

Intracranial Vascular Malformations and Aneurysms
Edited by M. Forsting and I. Wanke

High-Resolution Sonography of the Peripheral Nervous System
Edited by S. Peer and G. Bodner

Springer